MUDRAS

FOR HEALING AND TRANSFORMATION

Joseph and Lilian Le Page

Integrative Yoga Therapy

Le Page, Joseph and Lilian
Illustrations by Sergio Rezek and Carlos Eduardo Barbosa
Graphic Design by Alan Pedro
Mudras for healing / Joseph and Lilian Le Page

ISBN 978-0-9744303-4-0

Integrative Yoga Therapy website: www.iytyogatherapy.com

Integrative Yoga Therapy
e-mail: info@iytyogatherapy.com

We wish to thank the Sanskrit scholars and health professionals who reviewed this material including:
Carlos Eduardo Barbosa, Professor of Sanskrit
Jessica Byron, MD
Cheryl Van Demark, PT

We wish to thank all those who assisted in typing and editing the manuscript including:
Brynn Byrne
Jean Farkas
Daniel Gamito
Beth Gibbs
Victoria Gigante
Julia Hough
Cynthia Lawrence
Nancy Levenson
Julie Lusk
Natalie Nardi
Marielle Poss
Cathy Prescott
Jennifer Reis
Tina Romenesko
Miriam Seidel
Adriana Saldana

We would especially like to thank Kelly Birch for her valuable editorial input as well as all of our Integrative Yoga Therapy students who practiced the mudras and commented on the text.

MUDRAS FOR HEALING AND TRANSFORMATION

By Joseph & Lilian Le Page

This book is dedicated to Richard Miller, PhD, who opened the door to mudras for us.

With deep gratitude for the unconditional love of Cecília and Luiz de Aboim Costa and family

"What more should I tell Thee?
In short, there is nothing in this world like mudras
for giving quick success (along the spiritual path)."
Gheranda Samhita, verse 100

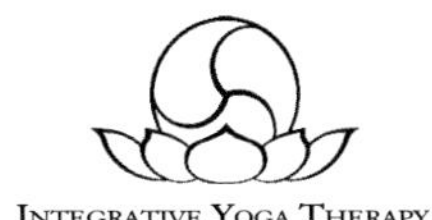

Integrative Yoga Therapy

Index

IV - MANOMAYA KOSHA - The Emotional Dimension

V - VIJNANAMAYA KOSHA - The Wisdom Dimension

VI - ANANDAMAYA KOSHA - The Bliss Dimension

VII - APPENDICES

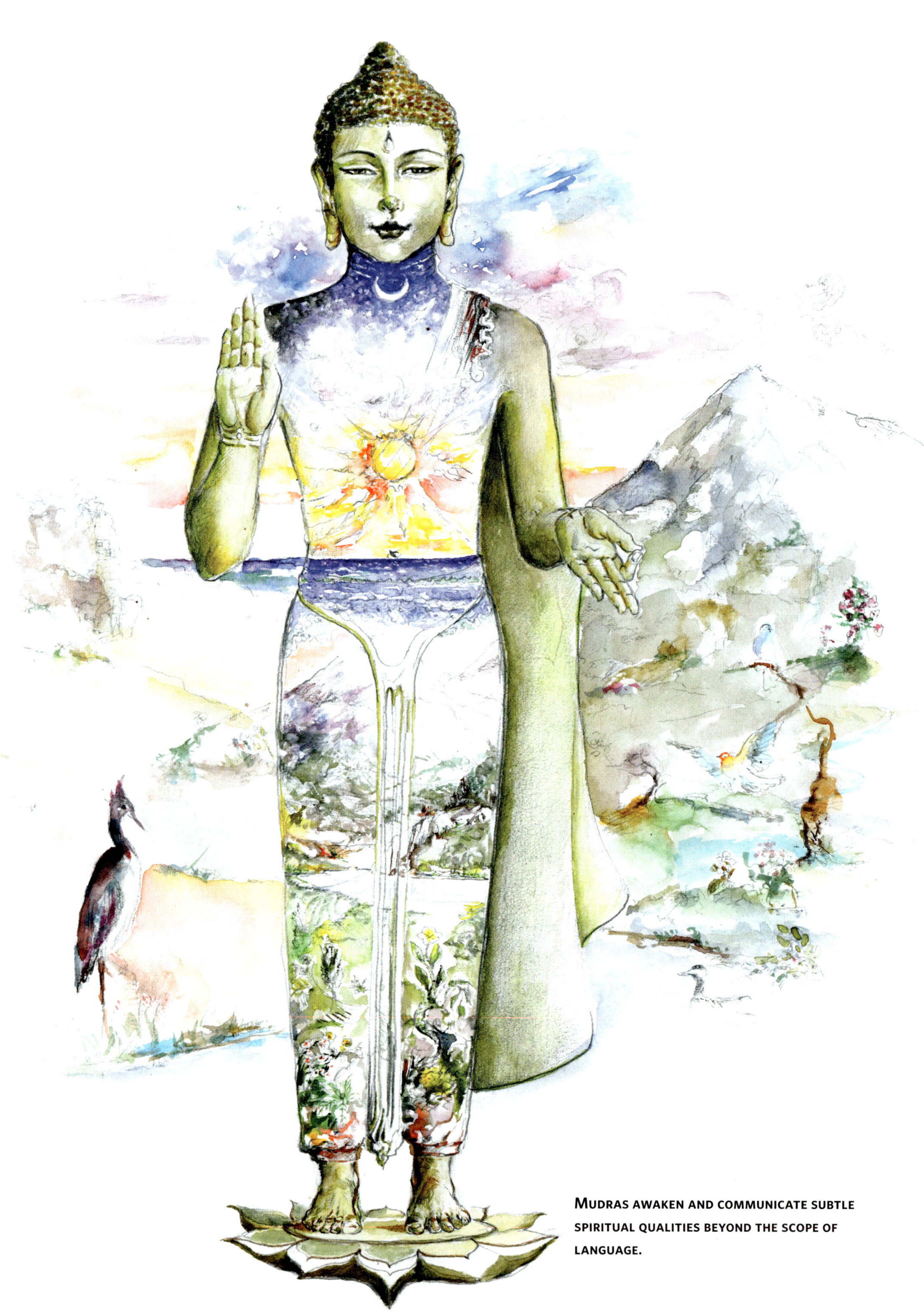

Mudras awaken and communicate subtle spiritual qualities beyond the scope of language.

Chapter One

Introduction

THE UNIVERSE OF MUDRAS

Mudras are gestures of the hands, face and body that promote physical health, psychological balance and spiritual awakening. The Sanskrit word mudra, with the emphasis on the final "a," can be translated as "gesture," "seal," "attitude" or "signature." Mudras are gestures that evoke psychological and spiritual attitudes, each with its own specific quality or "signature." The word mudra is derived from two root words: *mud,* which means "delight," "pleasure" or "enchantment," and *rati*, which means "to bring forth." Mudras bring forth our own inherent delight and enchantment, which are always present and waiting to be awakened.

The use of mudras is most strongly identified with Indian spiritual traditions in which they have been used for more than two thousand years. However, mudras are also found in various religious traditions around the world, including Christianity, where Christ is often depicted using hand gestures. Some mudras are almost universal, and one of the most easily recognized is the prayer position in which the hands are placed together in front of the heart as a symbol of reverence and devotion. Within the Indian spiritual tradition, this gesture is called Anjali mudra.

Origin and Evolution of Mudras

Gestures of the hands, face and body are part of our everyday body language. When the arms are crossed in front of the chest, it sends a message of defensiveness. When the head hangs forward, it may send a message of sadness. Clenched fists are often a sign of anger. Touching the tips of the fingers together suggests a pensive mood and raised eyebrows can show surprise or disbelief. These gestures are a non-verbal language that, often unconsciously, communicates moods, intentions and attitudes.

When gestures of the hands, face or body are consciously used to evoke psychological or spiritual attitudes, they are called mudras. Subtle qualities, such as unity and limitlessness, which cannot easily be expressed within the confines of language, find full expression through the use of mudras. In Shamanism, one of the earliest forms of spirituality, sound, movement, and gestures of the hands, face and body are used to invoke the deeper sacred energies of the universe. The shaman transmits these energies through rituals that include the use of gestures to support health, healing and spiritual connection. Various forms of Shamanism are found around the globe, but in India, the impulse to unite with the sacred source of creation evolved into an in-depth science, with mudra as one of its facets.

The *Rishis*, the great sages of ancient India, explored states of deep spiritual union through meditation. Mudras arose naturally as an expression of these meditative states; they were then employed to call forth these same experiences and share them with their initiated disciples. The ultimate wisdom revealed within the meditative experiences of the ancient seers is one of unity beyond all dualities. The journey toward unity encompasses a wide range of spiritual qualities, such as discernment, limitlessness, wholeness and compassion. Mudras are vehicles to awaken these individual qualities, naturally leading us toward a global vision of unity.

Each of the deities within Indian art and sculpture embodies a specific spiritual quality. Many of these deities are depicted holding mudras that reflect and communicate these qualities. The large number of statues and images showing the deities holding mudras highlights their important role within the development of spirituality on the Indian subcontinent. Among the oldest of these images are statues and paintings of the Buddha in the *Ellora* and *Ajanta* caves in India from approximately 2,000 years ago.

During the period of *Tantra* in India, ranging from the fifth to the fifteenth centuries, the use of mudra evolved into the fully developed form we know today. In Tantra, the body is seen as a sacred sanctuary of spirit, a microcosm of the Divine. The transformation of the physical body into a temple of spirit occurs through the performance of elaborate rituals that make use of sacred sounds, called *mantras*, sacred geometrical forms, called *yantras*, and the extensive use of mudras.

Beginning in the eleventh century, the body-positive approach of Tantra gave birth to the science of *Hatha Yoga*. This approach to Yoga uses the physical body as a primary vehicle for spiritual development, leading to liberation. The texts of the Hatha Yoga tradition outline the practices of Yoga within a framework of stages or limbs, which include mudra. The importance given to mudras within these texts is highlighted in numerous sutras, including the following from the seventeenth century Hatha Yoga text, the *Gheranda Samhita* (sutra 100):

"What more shall I tell thee? There is nothing in this world like mudras for giving quick success (along the spiritual path)."[1]

The importance given to mudras in iconography, Tantric ritual, and the texts of Hatha Yoga demonstrates the key role they have played within the overall evolution of Indian spirituality.

The Special Role of Hand Mudras

There are several categories of mudras. Facial gestures, such as Shambhavi mudra (turning the eyes upward toward the third eye point), serve to awaken subtle spiritual energies. There are also full body mudras that resemble Hatha Yoga postures, such as Viparita Karani mudra (similar to the Half Shoulder Stand), which enhance and maintain the flow of subtle energy for extended periods. Mudras are also used extensively in Indian classical dance to evoke the essence and feeling of each part of the dance sequence.

The type of mudra that is most widely used, both in the context of dance and as a vehicle for healing and awakening, is the hand gesture. These gestures, which are the subject of this book, are held in high esteem for several reasons:

- Our fingers contain a large number of sensory and motor nerve endings, making them a powerful vehicle for communicating directly with the brain and the rest of the body.
- The hands and fingers are extremely dexterous, creating a wide range of possibilities for awakening psychological and spiritual qualities.
- Each finger is traditionally related to one of the five elements, and specific finger combinations offer a wide range of possibilities for balancing the elements, and thereby optimizing health.
- The hand gestures support the health of the hands themselves and can aid in the prevention and treatment of arthritis when practiced moderately and regularly.

The Mudra Core Qualities

"Core Qualities" are the inherent positive qualities that mudras evoke within us. These qualities are reflections of our deeper spiritual essence, which is already present as a potential, waiting to be awakened. Mudras function as energetic keys that unlock these qualities. The Sanskrit names of the mudras usually reveal, or at least give clues to, their related Core Qualities. For example, *rupa* means "form," and Rupa mudra instills a sense of stability and embodiment. *Dirgha svara* means "lengthened breath," and Dirgha Svara mudra supports the full expansion of the rib cage and lungs, enhancing breath capacity.

Many of the mudras bear the names of Indian deities, and these mudras awaken the Core Qualities that these gods and goddesses embody. For example, *Kubera* is the god of wealth, and Kubera mudra instills a sense of intrinsic self-worth. *Ganesha* is the deity of protection and remover of obstacles, and Ganesha mudra instills a deep sense of trust and protection.

By highlighting the Core Qualities awakened by each mudra, we emphasize that the gestures are not ends in themselves, nor are they "magic bullets" for curing health conditions, but vehicles for unfolding the inherent positive qualities of our true being, thereby supporting our journey of health, healing and awakening.

Guided Meditations to Awaken the Core Qualities

Each of the 108 gestures in this book is accompanied by a Guided Meditation that supports the unfolding of each gesture's Core Quality. These meditations allow us to sense and integrate the Core Qualities more easily as a lived experience within our bodies, thereby enhancing the benefits of mudra practice. These Guided Meditations can be read aloud to a group, or individually by a teacher or a spiritual guide. You can read to yourself silently or aloud as you practice each gesture, or listen to the audio recordings of the Guided Meditations, read by Joseph and Lilian Le Page. One of the best ways to use the Guided Meditations is to work in pairs, taking turns reading and then sharing the experience.

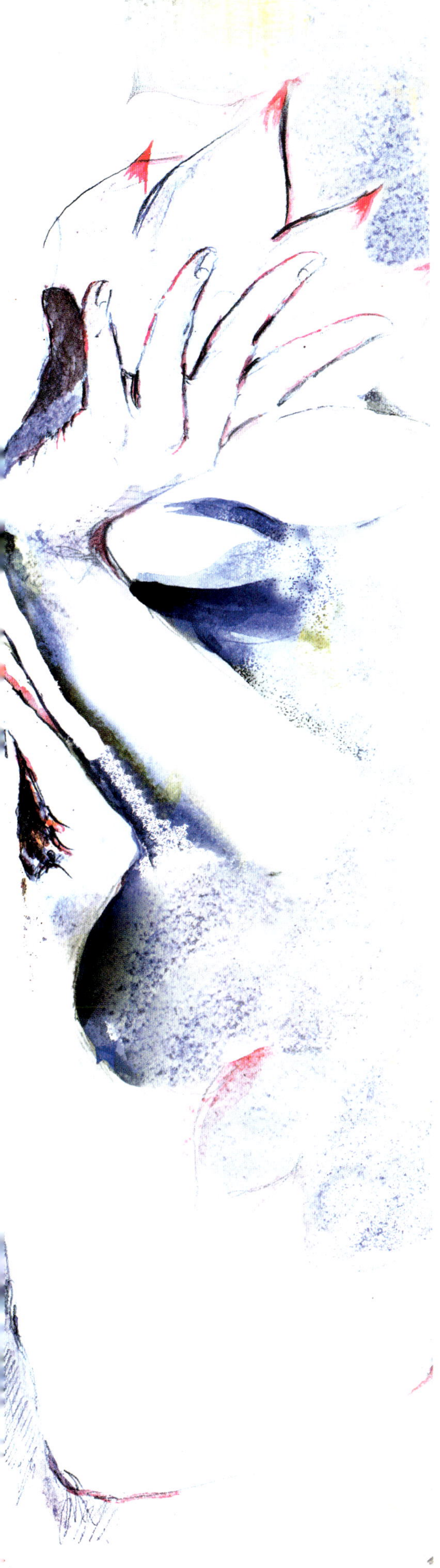

Mudras as Vehicles for Experiencing the Yoga Tradition Directly

Mudras for Healing and Transformation uses hand gestures as vehicles for exploring the most important facets of Yoga philosophy and psychology, including the five *koshas*, the five elements, the seven *chakras* and the eight limbs of Yoga. When these facets of Yoga are explored with the support of the mudras, our understanding of Yoga becomes direct and immediate, and its benefits for health, healing and awakening are enhanced greatly. Using the mudras as energetic keys, the profound insights of Yoga are naturally awakened and integrated within all dimensions of our being.

Mudras as Vehicles for Health and Healing

The power of mudras to support health and healing rests in their ability to cultivate balance and harmony within all dimensions of our being. At the physical level, mudras direct breath and awareness to particular areas of the body, enhancing our awareness and deepening our ability to recognize and respond to the body's messages more easily. Mudras also support optimal breathing. In mudra practice, the gesture itself guides the breath and has the ability to change the speed, focus, quality and location of our breathing almost instantly. As mudras bring awareness and breath into specific areas, a massaging effect is created that increases circulation to the areas where the breath is directed.

As mudras expand and channel the breath, they also promote balance within our subtle anatomy. The breath is a primary vehicle for *prana*, the "life force energy." By channeling the breath into specific areas of the body, mudras enhance our sensitivity to the flow of subtle energy, removing energy blockages and thereby reestablishing the free flow of prana. Specific gestures cultivate balance within each facet of our subtle anatomy, including the energy centers, the *chakras*; the energy currents, the *prana vayus*; and the energy channels, the *nadis*.

At the psychological level, mudras evoke moods and feelings that range from calming to energizing. There are specific gestures for instilling relaxation and serenity while others enhance enthusiasm, optimism and vitality. Mudras support the cultivation of a wide range of psycho-emotional qualities, including self-confidence, courage and self-esteem. Mudras also support us in perceiving and releasing the limiting beliefs that sustain challenging thoughts and feelings. As limiting beliefs are released, space is created for the unfolding of our innate positive qualities. The integration of all of these Core Qualities naturally reveals our true being, experienced as freedom and unity.

Our Approach to the Universe of Mudras

Mudras are a vast science that includes ritual, dance and iconography. Within this universe of mudras, our particular focus is the use of the gestures as energetic keys for awakening Core Qualities, leading to a vision of unity. Our journey within the mudra tradition began in the early 1990s through studies with Richard Miller, PhD. Richard organized the mudras into families and we have expanded his concept to include the whole of Yoga philosophy and psychology. Numerous other teachers have inspired our spiritual path, including Kali Ray, Vayuananda, Eneida de Oliveira, Glória Arieira and all the faculty at Kripalu Center. Over the years, we have developed a unique experiential framework for mudra practice within the model of the five *koshas* - the five dimensions of our being. We have shared this model with thousands of students in our *Integrative Yoga Therapy* training programs (www.iytyogatherapy.com). We have also used the gestures extensively in therapeutic settings at the *Enchanted Mountain Center* in Brazil (www.enchanted-mountain.org). Most importantly, mudras have been an essential vehicle within our own journey of health, healing and awakening. It is this personal experience that forms the foundation and essence of this book. Welcome to the Journey!

How To Use This Book

The mudras in this book are organized within the model of the *Koshas* (see chapter five), the five dimensions of our being, beginning at the physical level and culminating at the spiritual level.

• Chapters one through five offer an introduction to mudras, enhancing sensitivity and providing a foundation for experiencing the effects of the gestures.
• Chapters six through eight explore the use of mudras within our physical dimension, the *Annamaya kosha*, including gestures for specific health conditions as well as mudras for activating each of the five elements and balancing the ayurvedic *doshas*.
• Chapters nine through eleven explore the use of mudras within our subtle anatomy, the *Pranamaya kosha*, including gestures for the *prana vayus*, *chakras* and *nadis*.
• Chapters twelve and thirteen explore the use of mudras for cultivating balance in the mind and emotions, the *Manomaya kosha*.
• Chapters fourteen and fifteen present mudras for supporting the journey of spiritual purification, leading to the awakening of our wisdom dimension, the *Vijnanamaya kosha*.
• Chapters sixteen and seventeen explore the use of mudras for awakening our spiritual essence, the *Anandamaya kosha*, and integrating our inherent spiritual qualities into daily living.

Mudra practice allows us to explore and integrate all the dimensions of our being, supporting our journey toward health, healing and awakening.

How to Begin Mudra Practice

We recommend that you begin your mudra journey with the Hasta mudras. Once comfortable with the gestures of this family, you may work through the book chapter by chapter, exploring the various dimensions of your being, or choose an area of special interest or a particular health challenge that you are working with. You may also choose Core Qualities that you would like to cultivate, such as self-esteem, from the list of Core Qualities (see appendix F). As you practice, your sensitivity will deepen, and the mudras themselves will begin to speak to you, allowing you to sense intuitively which gestures are especially appropriate for a particular moment in your journey.

An excellent way to get to know each mudra is to hold it silently, deepening your sensitivity, exploring its effects at each level of your being: physical, energetic, psycho-emotional and spiritual. We recommend that you stay with each mudra long enough to begin to sense the awakening of its Core Quality. You can begin holding each mudra for five to ten breaths, gradually working up to holding each gesture for up to five minutes, three times a day. The duration of the Guided Meditations that accompany each mudra also serves as an appropriate guide to a gesture's holding time. You can assess a gesture's effects by noting the changes in all dimensions of your being, including improved vitality and energy, greater calm and clarity, and a growing ability to meet life's challenges more openly.

General Guidelines for Mudra Practice

• If you are in treatment for any health challenge, be sure to monitor any significant changes, such as in your blood pressure, with medical supervision. Mudras should never be used as a substitute for medical treatment.
• Each mudra in this book is accompanied by a description of cautions and contraindications in the left-hand column. These should be reviewed before practicing any of the gestures.
• Throughout this book, detailed benefits for each mudra are presented. Since little research has been done on the effects of mudras, these should be considered as possible benefits only.
• A short body relaxation, part by part, together with hand warm-ups, is helpful for releasing tension before mudra practice.
• The effects of a particular mudra may not appear immediately. Allow the process to unfold gradually, understanding that feeling the full effects of each gesture is a journey in itself.
• Many of the mudras open us to subtle energies that may be unfamiliar or uncomfortable. You should never force the practice of any gesture, but rather, always stay within your level of comfort.
• Some gestures may not be right for you at a particular time. For this reason, each gesture lists "Mudras with similar effects." An individual may find that one of the similar mudras is especially helpful for them. The Guided Meditation for the principal mudra can usually be used with the "Mudras with similar effects" as well.
• The recommended pressure for holding a mudra is similar to that of tuning a stringed instrument, neither too loose nor too tight. The contact in mudra practice is always skin to skin, which may involve cutting the nails or adjusting your fingers until you find the point of optimal contact.
• Mudras can be practiced while lying down, sitting or standing. The seated meditation position with the spine naturally aligned is ideal while the restorative position, lying on the back supported by bolsters or firm blankets, is especially helpful when using mudras for healing.
• The speed of the breath and length of the inhale and exhale are naturally controlled by the mudra itself. Simply allow the gesture to guide your breath.
• An empty stomach is optimal for mudra practice. If practicing after meals, wait thirty to forty-five minutes.
• Mudras can be practiced anywhere, any time and in any state of mind. Dawn and dusk are optimal times.
• Only relaxing, calming and soothing mudras should be practiced before bedtime. Many mudras are formed with the palms facing upward; turning the palms downward will produce a more calming effect, which is especially recommended for the evening.
• Discomfort in the hands and fingers can occur if complex mudras are held for long periods of time. It is fine to begin holding a mudra, release it as needed while visualizing it, and then return to it when you are comfortable.
• The support and guidance of an experienced Yoga teacher, Yoga therapist or spiritual guide is recommended, especially when working with health conditions or with mudras that explore the more subtle realms of being.

The format of *Mudras for Healing and Transformation* allows you to access all of the essential information about each mudra quickly and easily. This page outlines how the information for each mudra is organized.

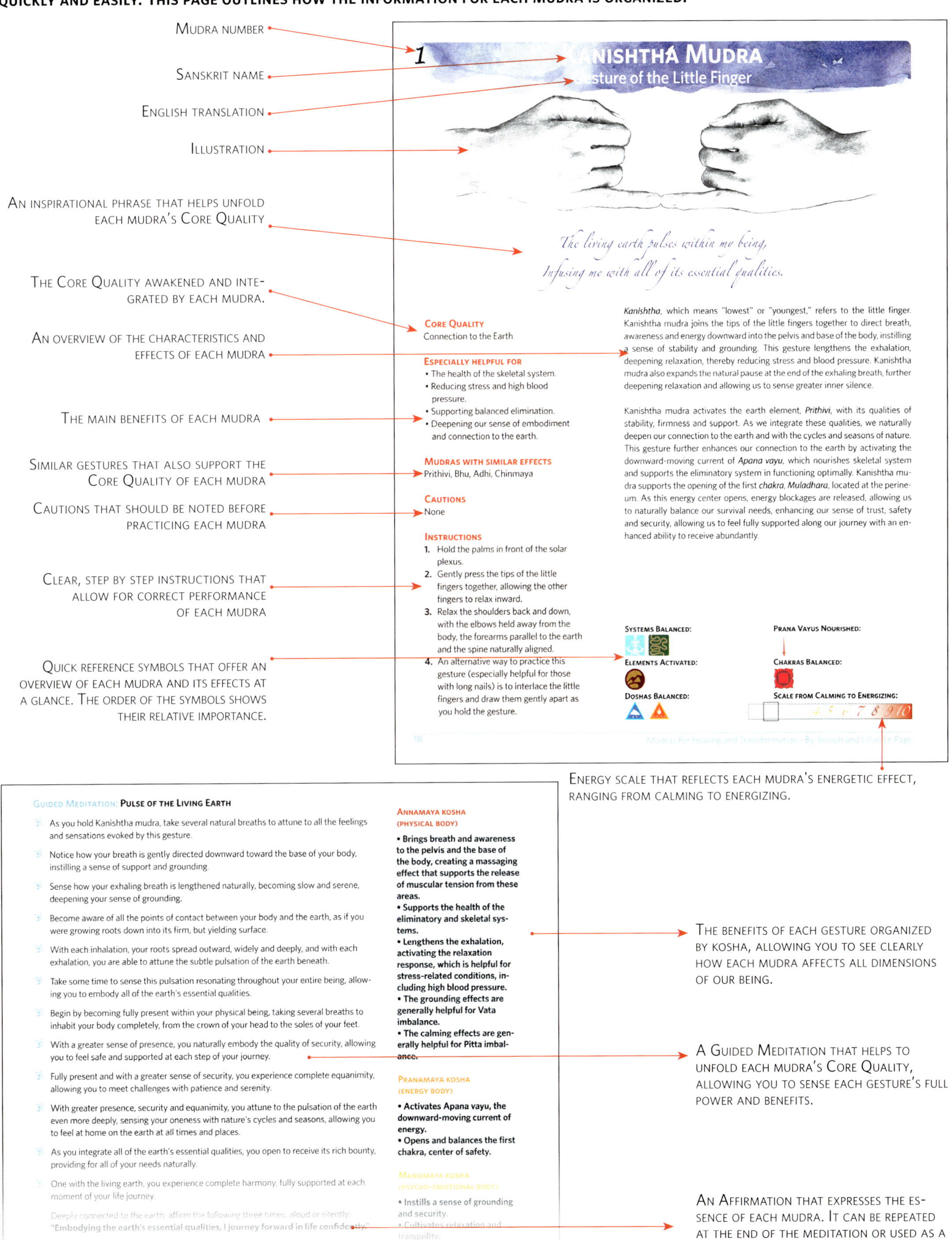

Guide to the Symbols Found in this Book

A quick reference to the main focus and effects of each mudra are presented at the bottom of the first page of each mudra's two-page spread. Symbols are used to represent the primary physical and subtle systems that each mudra activates or balances. These systems include the twelve physiological systems, the five elements, the five prana vayus, the seven chakras and the three ayurvedic doshas. Within each mudra, these symbols are organized by the intensity of the effects produced by a particular gesture.

Symbols that represent the Physiological Systems of the Body (for more information, see chapter six)

Skeletal	Muscular	Respiratory	Digestive	Eliminatory	Urinary
Consists of bones. Related to the Earth element & the qualities of solidity & density.	Consists of muscles, ligaments & tendons. Related to the Water element & the qualities of fluidity & flexibility.	Consists of the nose, sinuses, trachea, bronchial tree, alveoli & other lung tissues. Related to the Air element & the quality of exchange.	Consists of the mouth, esophagus, stomach, small intestine & auxiliary organs. Related to the Fire element & the quality of transformation.	Consists of the large intestine & anus. Primarily related to the Earth element & the quality of elimination.	Consists of the kidneys, bladder, ureters & urethra. Related to the Water element & the quality of filtration.

Reproductive	Cardiovascular	Endocrine	Lymphatic	Immune	Nervous
Consists of the reproductive organs & glands. Related to the Water element & the qualities of procreation & pleasure.	Consists of the heart, arteries, veins & blood. Related to the Air element & the qualities of vitality and circulation.	Consists of the endocrine glands & their respective hormones. Related to the Space element & the quality of communication.	Consists of the lymph nodes, ducts, & lymphatic fluid. Related to the Water element & the quality of purification.	Consists of immune cells, antibodies, thymus gland & spleen. Related to the Air element & the quality of integrity.	Consists of the brain, spinal cord, & all neural tissues. Related to the Space element & the quality of orchestration.

Symbols that represent the Five Elements (for more information, see chapter seven)

Earth	Water	Fire	Air	Space
Embodies the qualities of solidity, stability, immobility & density. Related to the sense of smell.	Embodies the qualities of fluidity, flexibility, refreshment, hydration & adaptability. Related to the sense of taste.	Embodies the qualities of heat, light, transformation & purification. Related to the sense of sight.	Embodies the qualities of movement, lightness, sensitivity & exchange. Related to the sense of touch.	Embodies the qualities of expansiveness, limitlessness, vastness & subtlety. Related to the sense of hearing.

Symbols that represent the Five Prana Vayus (for more information, see chapter nine)

Apana Vayu	Prana Vayu	Samana Vayu	Udana Vayu	Vyana Vayu
The downward current of energy. Related to the exhalation; nourishes the pelvis, reproductive & eliminatory systems.	The upward current of energy. Related to the inhalation; nourishes the chest, cardio-respiratory & immune systems.	The horizontal current of energy. Expands on inhalation & softens on exhalation; nourishes the solar plexus & the digestive system.	The uppermost current of energy. Rises on inhalation & circulates on exhalation; nourishes the neck, head, nervous & endocrine systems.	The all-pervading current of energy. Expands on exhalation & concentrates on inhalation; supports circulation to the extremities.

Symbols that represent the Seven Chakras (for more information, see chapter ten)

Muladhara	Svadhisthana	Manipura	Anahata	Vishuddha	Ajna	Sahasrara
Located at the perineum, with four red petals. Related to the Earth element & the qualities of stability & safety.	Located below the navel, with six orange petals. Related to the Water element & the qualities of fluidity & self-nourishment.	Located at the solar plexus, with ten golden petals. Related to the Fire element & the qualities of energy & self-confidence.	Located at the heart, with twelve emerald green petals. Related to the Air element & the qualities of love & compassion.	Located at the throat, with sixteen sky blue petals. Related to the Space element & the quality of spiritual purification.	Located at the third eye, with two violet petals. Integrates all of the elements & awakens the qualities of wisdom & clarity.	Located at the crown, with one thousand crystal light petals. Source of the elements; awakens the qualities of freedom & unity.

Symbols for the Ayurvedic Doshas (see chapter eight)

Vata	Pitta	Kapha
Comprised of Air & Space. Tends toward creativity & versatility. Imbalanced qualities include fear, confusion & hyperactivity.	Comprised of Fire & Water. Tends toward organization & leadership. Imbalanced qualities include perfectionism & criticism.	Comprised of Earth & Water. Tends toward consistency, loyalty & good humor. Imbalanced qualities include lethargy & excessive attachment.

Special Symbol

All Systems
Supports the health of all the systems of the body.

Scale from Calming to Energizing: rated from zero to ten with zero being the most relaxing and ten being the most energizing (see chapter four)

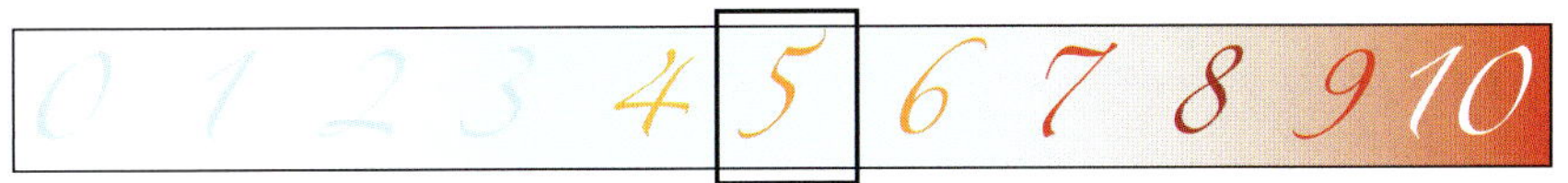

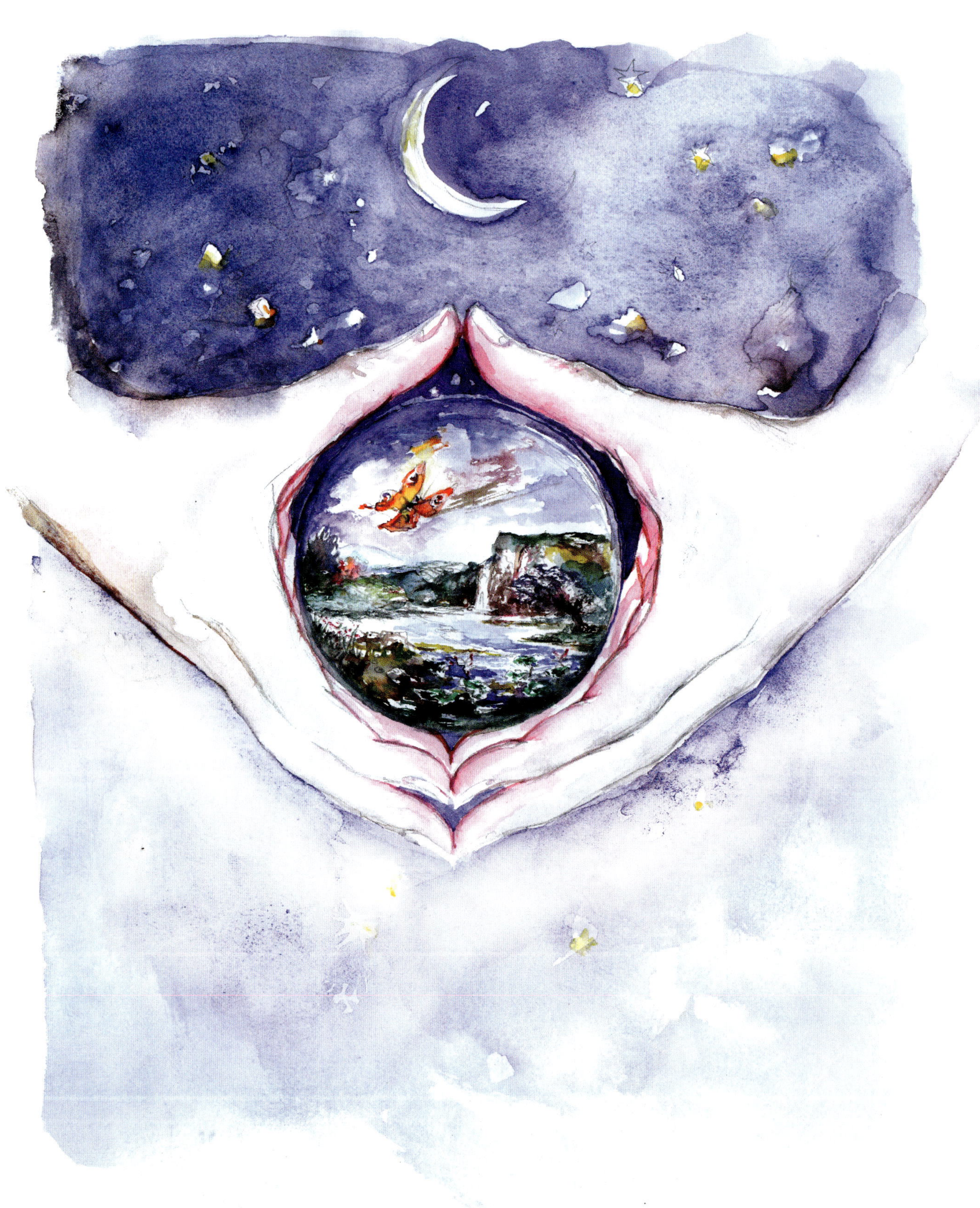

As we deepen our sensitivity,
mudras open a doorway to a subtle realm of magic and beauty.

Chapter Two

Expanding Awareness

THE HASTA MUDRAS

Hasta means "hand," and the *Hasta Mudras* serve as an introduction to the practice of the hand gestures. In this first family of mudras, one of the fingertips touches the same fingertip of the opposite hand, directing breath, awareness and energy to a specific area of the body. For example, touching the tips of the little fingers directs breath, awareness and energy into the pelvic floor. As we change finger positions, our focus rises upward, culminating at the throat as the thumbs are brought together in Angushtha mudra. The final gesture in this family, Hakini mudra, brings all of the fingertips and the thumbs together to support the integration of the whole body. The following table shows the relationship between each mudra and the specific area of the body awakened. Each of these gestures is also associated with a particular element, chakra, prana vayu and Core Quality.

Mudra	Breathing Area	Element	Chakra	Prana Vayu	Core Quality
Kanishtha	Pelvic floor	Earth - Prithivi	Muladhara	Apana	Connection to the Earth
Anamika	Pelvis	Water - Jala	Svadhisthana	Apana	Self-healing
Madhyama	Solar plexus	Fire - Tejas	Manipura	Samana	Balanced Energy
Tarjani	Chest	Air - Vayu	Anahata	Prana	Opening the Heart
Angushtha	Neck	Space - Akasha	Vishuddha	Udana	Inner Listening
Hakini	Integration of the whole body	All elements	First through sixth	All prana vayus, with a focus on Vyana	Integration

1

Kanishtha Mudra

Gesture of the Little Finger

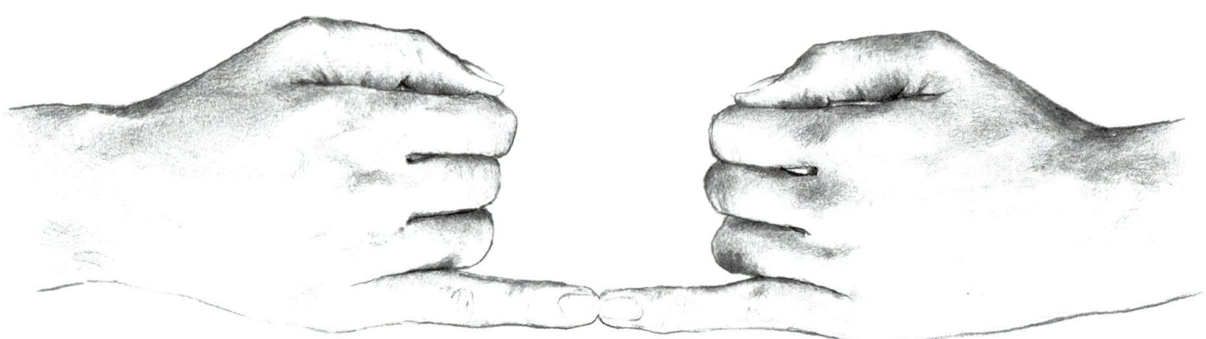

The living earth pulses within my being,
Infusing me with all of its essential qualities.

Core Quality

Connection to the Earth

Especially helpful for

- Deepening our sense of embodiment and connection to the earth.
- The health of the skeletal system.
- Reducing stress and high blood pressure.
- Supporting balanced elimination.

Mudras with similar effects

Prithivi, Bhu, Adhi, Chinmaya

Cautions

None

Instructions

1. Hold the palms in front of the solar plexus.
2. Gently press the tips of the little fingers together, allowing the other fingers to relax inward.
3. Relax the shoulders back and down, with the elbows held away from the body, the forearms parallel to the earth and the spine naturally aligned.
4. An alternative way to practice this gesture (especially helpful for those with long nails) is to interlace the little fingers and draw them gently apart as you hold the gesture.

Kanishtha, which means "lowest" or "youngest," refers to the little finger. Kanishtha mudra joins the tips of the little fingers together to direct breath, awareness and energy downward into the base of the body, instilling a sense of stability and grounding. This gesture lengthens the exhalation, deepening relaxation, thereby reducing stress and blood pressure. Kanishtha mudra also expands the natural pause at the end of the exhaling breath, further deepening relaxation and allowing us to sense greater serenity.

Kanishtha mudra activates the earth element, *Prithivi*, with its qualities of stability, firmness and support. As we integrate these qualities, we naturally deepen our connection to the natural world and its cycles and seasons. This gesture further enhances our connection to the earth by activating the downward moving current of *Apana vayu*, which nourishes the skeletal system and supports the eliminatory system in functioning optimally. Kanishtha mudra supports the opening of *Muladhara chakra*, located at the perineum. As this energy center opens, subtle blockages related to survival needs are released, enhancing our sense of trust, safety and security. With a greater sense of security, we move forward along our journey, more able to receive the earth's rich bounty.

Systems Balanced:

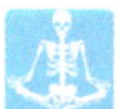
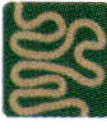

Elements Activated:

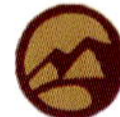

Doshas Balanced:

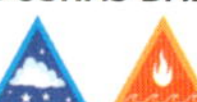

Prana Vayus Nourished:

Chakras Balanced:

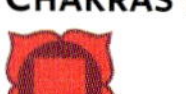

Scale from Calming to Energizing:

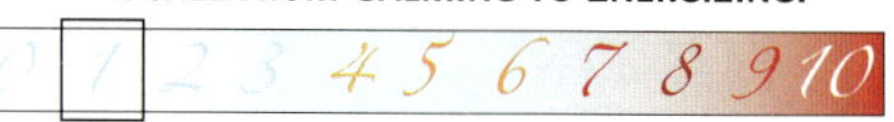

Guided Meditation: **Pulse of the Living Earth**

- As you hold Kanishtha mudra, take several natural breaths to attune to all the feelings and sensations evoked by this gesture.
- Notice how your breath is gently directed downward toward the base of your body, instilling a sense of support and grounding.
- Sense how your exhaling breath is lengthened naturally, becoming slow and serene, deepening your sense of grounding.
- Become aware of all the points of contact between your body and the earth, as if you were growing roots down into its firm, but yielding, surface.
- With each inhalation, your roots spread outward, widely and deeply, and with each exhalation, you are able to attune to the subtle pulsation of the earth beneath.
- Take some time to sense this pulsation resonating throughout your entire being, allowing you to embody all of the earth's essential qualities.
- Begin by becoming fully present within your physical being, taking several breaths to inhabit your body completely, from the crown of your head to the soles of your feet.
- With a greater sense of presence, you naturally embody the quality of security, allowing you to feel safe and supported at each step of your journey.
- Fully present and with a greater sense of security, you experience complete equanimity, allowing you to meet challenges with patience and serenity.
- With greater presence, security and equanimity, you attune to the pulsation of the earth even more deeply, sensing your oneness with nature's cycles and seasons, allowing you to feel at home on the earth at all times and places.
- As you integrate all of the earth's essential qualities, you open to receive its rich bounty, providing for all of your needs naturally.
- One with the living earth, you experience complete harmony, fully supported at each moment of your life journey.
- Deeply connected to the earth, affirm the following three times, aloud or silently: **"Embodying the earth's essential qualities, I journey forward in life confidently."**
- Now, slowly release the gesture, taking several breaths to sense your oneness with the living earth.
- When you are ready, open your eyes, returning slowly and gently, continuing your journey with a deeper sense of support and grounding.

Annamaya kosha (physical body)

- **Directs breath and awareness to the pelvis and the base of the body, creating a massaging effect that supports the release of muscular tension from these areas.**
- **Supports the health of the eliminatory and skeletal systems.**
- **Lengthens the exhalation, activating the relaxation response, which is helpful for stress-related conditions, including high blood pressure.**
- **The grounding effects of this gesture are generally helpful for Vata imbalance.**
- **The calming effects are generally helpful for Pitta imbalance.**

Pranamaya kosha (energy body)

- **Activates Apana vayu, the downward moving current of energy.**
- **Opens and balances the first chakra, center of safety.**

Manomaya kosha (psycho-emotional body)

- **Instills a sense of grounding and security.**
- **Cultivates relaxation and tranquility.**

Vijnanamaya kosha (wisdom body)

- **As our sense of grounding increases, we attune more easily to our true inner being, whose essential nature is safety.**

Anandamaya kosha (bliss body)

- **As we become more embodied and connected to the earth, a deep sense of comfort and well-being naturally arise from within the base of the body.**

2 Anamika Mudra
Gesture of the Ring Finger

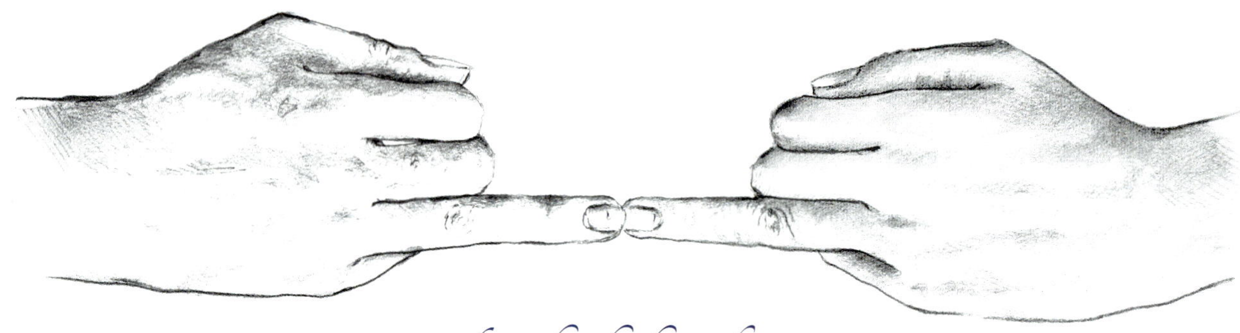

Attuned to the rhythms of my inner sea,
I am nourished by waves of healing energy.

Core Quality
Self-healing

Especially helpful for
- Cultivating self-healing.
- Supporting the health of the reproductive and urinary systems.
- Developing healthy intimate relationships.
- Overcoming addictions and codependency.

Mudras with similar effects
Svadhisthana, Shankha, Yoni, Trimurti

Cautions
None

Instructions
1. Hold the palms in front of the solar plexus.
2. Gently press the tips of the ring fingers together, allowing the other fingers to relax inward.
3. Relax the shoulders back and down, with the elbows slightly away from the body, the forearms parallel to the earth and the spine naturally aligned.
4. An alternative way to practice this gesture is to interlace the ring fingers and draw them gently apart as you hold the gesture.

Anamika is the "ring finger," and Anamika mudra joins the tips of the ring fingers together to direct breath, awareness and energy into the pelvis, cultivating a sense of inner nourishment and self-healing. As we practice this gesture, we sense a subtle internal massage within the pelvis, experienced as waves of healing energy flowing out from the center of our pelvis to nourish our entire being. The nourishing massage cultivated by this gesture instills a sense of coming home to ourselves, allowing us to experience complete comfort and ease. As our sense of inner comfort deepens, we connect to our inherent wholeness, deepening our ability to remain centered within our own being no matter what is happening in our surroundings. This enhanced self-nourishment and centering supports the development of relationships that are genuinely healing.

The pelvic area is the seat of the water element, *Jala*, and Anamika mudra cultivates the qualities of water, including fluidity, flexibility and adaptability. This enhanced sense of fluidity is supported by the activation of *Apana vayu*, the downward moving current of energy. The soothing qualities of water combined with the downward flow of Apana vayu support the health of the urinary and reproductive systems. Anamika mudra opens and balances *Svadhisthana chakra*, releasing energy blockages from the pelvis while cultivating a sense of self-nourishment and self-healing that support the release of second chakra issues, including feelings of abandonment, addictions and codependency.

Systems Balanced:

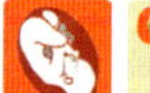 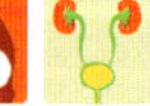

Elements Activated:

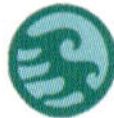

Doshas Balanced:

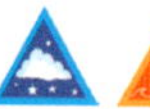

Prana Vayus Nourished:

Chakras Balanced:

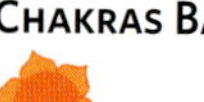

Scale from Calming to Energizing:

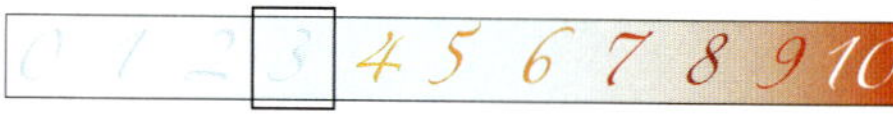

Guided Meditation: **Sea of Nourishment and Healing**

- As you hold Anamika mudra, take several natural breaths to attune to all the feelings and sensations evoked by this gesture.
- Notice how your breath is gently directed down into your pelvis, massaging you internally with soft waves of nourishing energy.
- As your pelvis is immersed in gentle waves of comfort and ease, experience this area of your being as an inner sea of healing.
- Take several breaths to sense soft waves of nourishing energy bathing your pelvic area completely, supporting all of its glands and organs in functioning optimally.
- Now, as you inhale, attune to your inner sea, and as you exhale, allow soft waves to flow downward into your legs and feet, taking several breaths to experience your lower extremities bathed in healing energy.
- Now, with your next inhalation, return to your sea of healing, and as you exhale, sense waves of nourishment flowing into your abdomen, solar plexus, low and mid back, allowing these areas to soften and completely relax.
- With your next inhalation, attune to the soft sea at the center of your being, and as you exhale, allow your heart, lungs, chest and upper back to be infused with healing energy.
- Waves of self-healing now flow upward from your inner sea to gently bathe your shoulders, cascading down into your arms and hands, all the way to your fingertips, filling these areas with healing and nourishment.
- With your next inhalation, return to the center of your being, and as you exhale, sense your spinal column bathed in soft waves of healing. Take several breaths to allow healing energy to lubricate each disc and vertebra.
- With your spinal column nourished completely, waves of healing energy naturally flow up into your neck and head, soothing your senses and allowing them to deeply rest.
- As your entire being is bathed in soft waves of nourishment and healing, you naturally experience absolute calm and serenity.
- Affirm your source of self-healing, repeating the following three times, aloud or silently: **" As waves of nourishment bathe my being, I experience complete inner healing."**
- Slowly release the gesture, taking several breaths to sense complete inner nourishment.
- When you are ready, open your eyes, returning slowly and gently, with a greater sense of self-healing.

Annamaya kosha (physical body)

• Directs breath and awareness to the pelvis, creating a massaging effect that helps release muscular tension from this area.
• Improves circulation to the pelvis, which supports the health of the reproductive and urinary systems.
• Cultivates a feeling of fluidity in all the joints of the body, especially the hips.
• The nourishing effects cultivated by this gesture are generally helpful for Vata imbalance.
• The calming effects are generally helpful for Pitta imbalance.

Pranamaya kosha (energy body)

• Activates Apana vayu, the downward moving current of energy.
• Opens and balances the second chakra, center of self-nourishment.

Manomaya kosha (psycho-emotional body)

• Cultivates comfort and ease with our own sexuality.
• Supports the process of overcoming addictions and codependency.

Vijnanamaya kosha (wisdom body)

• Awakens a sense of inner contentment that frees us from the need to seek nourishment compulsively in the outside world.

Anandamaya kosha (bliss body)

• As we sense greater inner nourishment and self-healing, feelings of wholeness and well-being arise from within the pelvis.

3

Madhyama Mudra

Gesture of the Middle Finger

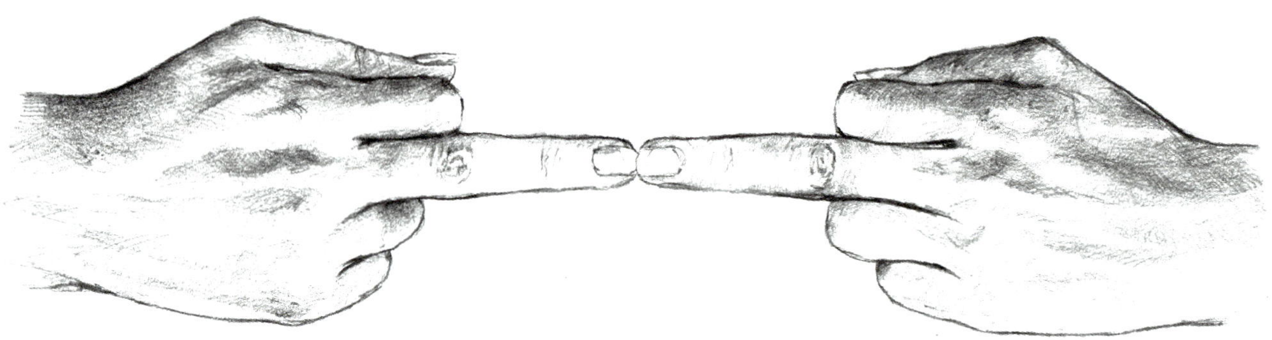

Cultivating balance in all of my activities,
I experience greater energy and vitality.

Core Quality

Balanced Energy

Especially helpful for

- Stabilizing our level of energy.
- Supporting optimal digestion.
- Releasing tension from the mid back.
- Balancing giving and receiving.
- Unfolding all of our potential.

Mudras with similar effects

Pushan, Kubera, Surya

Cautions

None

Instructions

1. Hold the palms in front of the solar plexus.
2. Gently press the tips of the middle fingers together, allowing the other fingers to relax inward.
3. Release the shoulders back and down, with the elbows held slightly away from the body, the forearms parallel to the earth and the spine naturally aligned.
4. An alternative way to practice this gesture (especially helpful for those with long nails) is to interlace the middle fingers and draw them gently apart as you hold the gesture.

Madhyama means "middle," and refers to the middle finger. Madhyama mudra joins the tips of the middle fingers together to direct breath, awareness and energy into the solar plexus, the body's storehouse of personal power. As we attune to this area more deeply, we naturally recognize the importance of balancing our level of energy. This gesture supports us in evaluating both balance and imbalance in our level of energy. With greater awareness, we are able to conserve energy consciously, thereby cultivating abundant vitality for all of our activities. This gesture activates *Samana vayu*, the horizontal current of energy, supporting optimal digestion at the physical and subtle levels, thereby enhancing our ability to balance our level of energy.

Madhyama mudra gently activates the fire element, *Tejas*, with its qualities of warmth, brilliance, light and transformation, enhancing our ability to balance our level of energy. Madhyama mudra opens and balances *Manipura chakra*, located at the solar plexus. As this chakra opens, energetic blockages in the solar plexus are released, naturally cultivating self-esteem, personal power and vitality. By bringing awareness to our storehouse of energy and enhancing our ability to maintain balance, we are able to channel this energy consciously to unfold all of our talents and possibilities.

Systems Balanced:

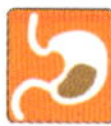

Elements Activated:

Doshas Balanced:

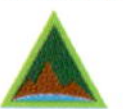
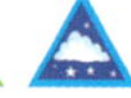

Prana Vayus Nourished:

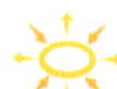

Chakras Balanced:

Scale from Calming to Energizing:

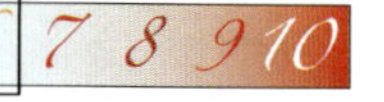

Guided Meditation: Cultivating Balanced Energy

- As you hold Madhyama mudra, take several natural breaths to attune to all the feelings and sensations awakened by this gesture.
- Notice how your breath is gently directed into your solar plexus, instilling a sense of energy and vitality that radiates outward from the center of your being.
- Take several breaths to attune to your solar plexus as a storehouse of energy, providing radiant vitality for all of your activities.
- As you attune to your center of vital energy more deeply, you are able to sense the importance of cultivating energetic balance at all levels of your being.
- Begin by sensing energetic balance within your physical body. Visualize all of your cells working in harmony, taking in exactly what they need, while supporting each other in a spirit of cooperation and unity.
- Take several breaths to reflect on your ability to cultivate this same harmony within your own body by taking in nutritious foods, fresh air, and living in healthy, natural surroundings.
- Envision the changes in your diet and environment that would support your ability to maintain a balanced level of energy within your physical body.
- Next, assess energetic balance within your daily routine. To what extent do you consciously harmonize periods of rest with periods of activity?
- Take several breaths to envision changes in your daily routine that would support balanced use of energy within all of your activities.
- Now, sense your energetic balance within your relationships, family, friends and community. Take several breaths to reflect on your ability to care for your own needs while contributing to the benefit of other beings.
- Envision the changes you could make in your relationships that would allow you to balance your own energy while participating more fully in your community.
- Now, take several breaths to envision yourself living with balanced energy in your body, daily routine, relationships and surroundings, allowing you to appreciate life more deeply while unfolding all of your talents and possibilities.
- Affirm your balanced energy as you repeat the following three times, aloud or silently: **"With balanced energy at all levels of my being, I live fully and vibrantly."**
- Slowly release the gesture, taking several breaths to sense energetic balance.
- When you are ready, open your eyes, returning slowly and gently, with a greater sense of balance in all of your activities.

Annamaya kosha (physical body)

• Directs breath and awareness to the solar plexus, creating a massaging effect that supports the release of muscular tension from this area.
• The enhanced breathing in the abdomen creates a massaging effect that supports the health of the digestive system.
• Massages the mid back, which may be helpful for back pain.
• The massage of the middle back improves circulation to the area of the kidneys and adrenal glands.
• The mildly energizing effects of this gesture are generally helpful for Kapha imbalance.
• The warming and balancing effects are generally helpful for Vata imbalance.

Pranamaya kosha (energy body)

• Activates Samana vayu, the horizontal current of energy.
• Opens and balances the third chakra, center of personal power.

Manomaya kosha (psycho-emotional body)

• Instills self-esteem and confidence.

Vijnanamaya kosha (wisdom body)

• Cultivates awareness of our actions, supporting us in using our energy wisely.

Anandamaya kosha (bliss body)

• As we become balanced energetically, radiance and clarity arise naturally.

4

Tarjani Mudra

Gesture of the Index Finger

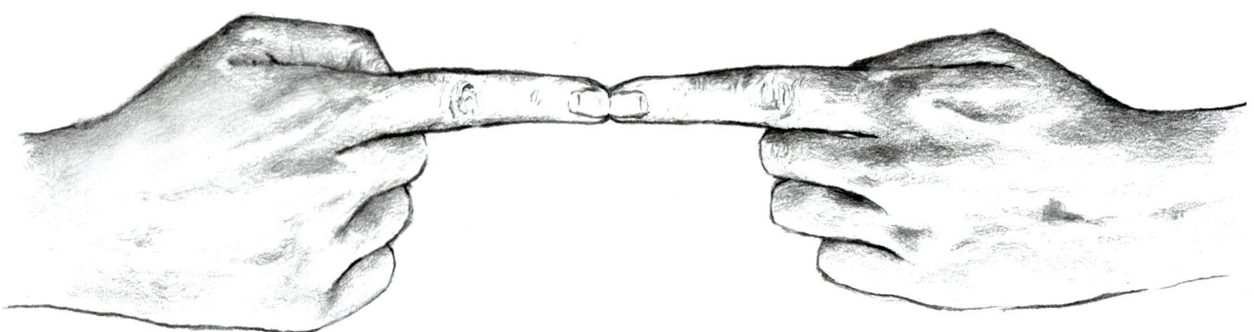

Attuned to my heart's inner symphony,
I live with joy and vitality.

Core Quality

Opening the Heart

Especially helpful for

- Opening the subtle heart.
- Releasing constriction from the chest.
- Expanding breath capacity.
- Enhancing enthusiasm, which may be helpful for depression.

Mudras with similar effects

Padma, Purna Hridaya, Vajrapradama

Cautions

None

Instructions

1. Hold the palms in front of the solar plexus.
2. Gently press the tips of the index fingers together, allowing the other fingers to relax inward.
3. Release the shoulders back and down, with the elbows held slightly away from the body, the forearms parallel to the earth and the spine naturally aligned.
4. An alternative way to practice this gesture (especially helpful for those with long nails) is to interlace the index fingers and draw them gently apart as you hold the gesture.

Tarjani is the "index finger," and Tarjani mudra brings the tips of the index fingers together to direct breath, awareness and energy to the chest, heart and lungs, instilling a sense of expansion and openness. This gesture expands the rib cage on all four sides, optimizing breath capacity and releasing muscular tension from the thoracic area. The opening of the chest facilitated by this gesture supports the optimal functioning of the cardio-respiratory system. This mudra also creates a massaging effect in the area of the thymus gland, supporting the health of the immune system.

Tarjani mudra activates the air element, *Vayu*, cultivating the qualities of lightness, gracefulness, ease and sensitivity. This gesture also activates the upward moving current of *Prana vayu*, instilling a sense of enthusiasm and uplifting energy. Tarjani mudra supports the awakening of *Anahata chakra*, releasing energetic blockages from the chest, side ribs and upper back. This release enhances our ability to welcome feelings more easily, creating an open space in which our heart's essential qualities unfold naturally. These qualities include self-acceptance, gratitude, compassion and communion with all beings. As these qualities unfold, they naturally lead to the awakening of unconditional love, which unites all of them into a harmonious symphony.

Systems Balanced:

 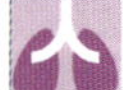

Elements Activated:

Doshas Balanced:

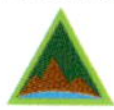 

Prana Vayus Nourished:

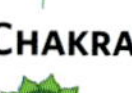

Chakras Balanced:

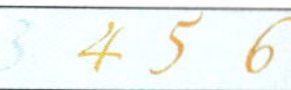

Scale from Calming to Energizing:

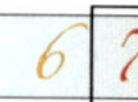 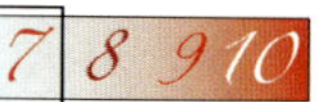

Guided Meditation: Symphony of the Heart

- ॐ As you hold Tarjani mudra, take several natural breaths to attune to all the feelings and sensations awakened by this gesture.
- ॐ Notice how your breath is gently directed into your chest, side ribs and upper back, instilling a sense of openness.
- ॐ Sense how each inhalation expands your rib cage in all directions simultaneously, while each exhaling breath allows this area to soften and relax completely.
- ॐ Allow this natural rhythm of expansion and release to create a space in which you deepen your sensitivity to all of your heart's essential qualities.
- ॐ These qualities are like musical instruments that, when played in harmony, allow all of your life's activities to be integrated into a melodious symphony.
- ॐ Begin by opening to receive the quality of self-acceptance, taking several breaths to embrace all that you have done and been, realizing that there are no mistakes in life, only lessons that teach you to play with greater harmony.
- ॐ As you embrace self-acceptance, the quality of gratitude unfolds, allowing you to welcome each moment of life as a precious gift to be unwrapped carefully and savored completely.
- ॐ As gratitude unfolds within your being, take several breaths to allow the quality of compassion to join your symphony, opening the eyes of your heart to see that all beings seek the same happiness and harmony.
- ॐ As compassion awakens, your heart opens naturally, allowing you to sense your communion with all beings, serving others with sincerity and caring as one extended family.
- ॐ Now, all of these qualities merge harmoniously, revealing universal love as the conductor of your symphony, your heart's essence, which radiates out to touch all beings.
- ॐ Affirm your heart's opening, repeating the following three times, aloud or silently: **"Attuned to my heart's essential qualities, unconditional love unfolds naturally."**
- ॐ Slowly release the gesture, taking several breaths to rest within your heart's true essence.
- ॐ When you are ready, open your eyes, returning slowly and gently, more attuned to your heart's essential harmony.

Annamaya kosha (physical body)

• Directs breath and awareness to the chest, enhancing breath capacity and supporting the release of muscular tension from this area.
• Enhances circulation to the area of the thymus gland.
• The mildly energizing effects of this gesture along with the opening of the chest are generally helpful for Kapha imbalance.
• The heart-opening qualities are generally helpful for Pitta imbalance.

Pranamaya kosha (energy body)

• Activates Prana vayu, the upward moving current of energy.
• Opens and balances the fourth chakra, center of unconditional love.

Manomaya kosha (psycho-emotional body)

• Cultivates enthusiasm and uplifting energy.
• Opens the heart and deepens our sensitivity to its subtle qualities.

Vijnanamaya kosha (wisdom body)

• Cultivates a sense of spaciousness in the heart where emotions can be welcomed, integrated and released, thereby revealing our essential positive qualities.

Anandamaya kosha (bliss body)

• Awakens the qualities of the subtle heart, including compassion and unconditional love.

5

Angushtha Mudra

Gesture of the Thumb

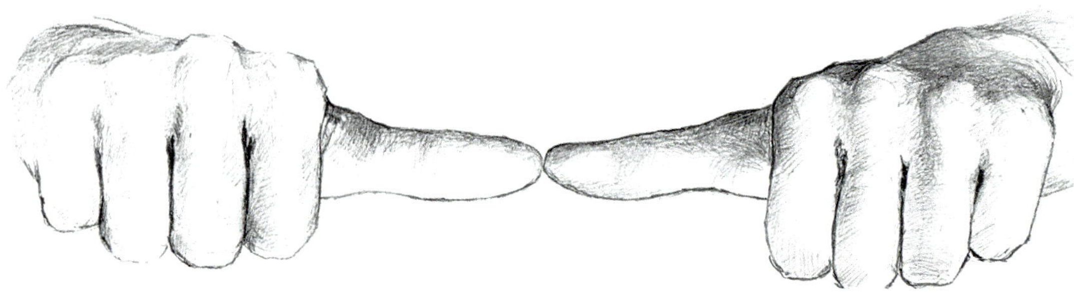

Through deeper listening and enhanced sensitivity,
I receive the guidance of my inner being.

Core Quality

Inner Listening

Especially helpful for

- Receiving inner guidance and expressing it clearly in the world.
- Releasing tension from the shoulders, throat and neck.
- Aligning the cervical spine.
- Supporting the health of the thyroid.
- Enhancing speaking and singing.

Mudras with similar effects

Garuda, Vishuddha, Akasha, Shunya

Cautions

None

Instructions

1. Hold the palms in front of the solar plexus.
2. Gently press the tips of the thumbs together, allowing the other fingers to relax inward.
3. Release the shoulders back and down, with the elbows held slightly away from the body, the forearms parallel to the earth and the spine naturally aligned.
4. Alternatively, you may practice this gesture by interlacing the thumbs and drawing them gently apart.

Angushtha is the "thumb," and Angushtha mudra joins the tips of the thumbs together to direct breath, awareness and energy into the uppermost parts of the chest, collarbones, throat and neck. The enhanced breathing and awareness in these areas helps release tension from the shoulders, throat and neck. As tension is released, this gesture supports correct alignment of the cervical spine, alleviating one of the possible causes of neck pain. Angushtha mudra activates the uppermost current of *Udana vayu*, nourishing the nervous and endocrine systems, as well as the senses. As this gesture enhances the flow of breath and energy to the neck, circulation is increased to the area of the thyroid gland, supporting balanced metabolism.

Angushtha mudra activates the space element, *Akasha*, whose qualities include expansion, limitlessness and an opening to the subtle energies of our being. Opening to our subtle dimension supports us in cultivating the qualities of non-attachment, spiritual purification and clear communication. As this gesture releases tension from the throat and neck, energetic blockages are released, allowing *Vishuddha chakra*, our center of spiritual purification, to open naturally. This opening enhances our power of inner listening, allowing us to receive the messages that guide our life journey. Angushtha mudra also supports the awakening of our inner voice, allowing us to express the guidance we receive more clearly.

Systems Balanced:

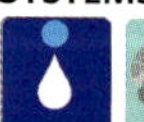 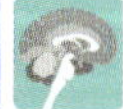

Elements Activated:

Doshas Balanced:

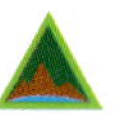

Prana Vayus Nourished:

Chakras Balanced:

Scale from Calming to Energizing:

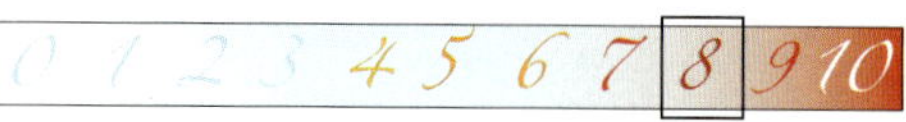

Guided Meditation: Space of Inner Listening

- As you hold Angushtha mudra, take several natural breaths to attune to all the feelings and sensations awakened by this gesture.
- Notice how your breath is gently directed into your throat and neck, instilling a sense of spaciousness.
- As spaciousness expands throughout this area of your being, you are able to hear your inner voice more clearly, allowing its messages to guide your life journey.
- These messages may be received as words, images, symbols, intuition or subtle feelings.
- In order to cultivate inner listening, take several breaths to bring to mind an issue calling for guidance in your life at this time.
- Take some time to attune to your inner voice, listening to the messages you receive, inviting clarity for the issue you are exploring.
- As this guidance is received, envision how it might be integrated into all dimensions of your life journey.
- See yourself making the changes you need to honor the guidance you have received, allowing it to be manifest as a lived reality.
- Affirm your deeper listening, repeating the following three times, aloud or silently: **"Listening to the voice of my inner being, I receive clear guidance for my life journey."**
- Now, slowly release the gesture, taking several breaths to integrate the wisdom you have received.
- When you are ready, open your eyes, returning slowly and gently, more sensitive to the inner voice that guides your journey.

Annamaya kosha (Physical Body)

• Directs breath and awareness to the throat and neck, helping to release tension from this area.
• Enhances circulation to the area of the thyroid gland.
• Supports the lengthening of the cervical spine and aligns the head over the torso.
• Supports the health of the vocal cords.
• The energizing effects of this gesture are generally helpful for Kapha imbalance.

Pranamaya kosha (Energy Body)

• Activates Udana vayu, the uppermost current of energy.
• Opens and balances the fifth chakra, the center of spiritual purification.

Manomaya kosha (Psycho-Emotional Body)

• Enhances clear communication.
• Deepens sensitivity and inner listening.

Vijnanamaya kosha (Wisdom Body)

• As we learn to listen to our own inner voice, we receive guidance for our life journey, free of the habitual, conditioned responses of the personality.

Anandamaya kosha (Bliss Body)

• As tension is released from the neck and throat, we naturally experience greater clarity.

6

Hakini Mudra

Gesture of the Goddess Hakini

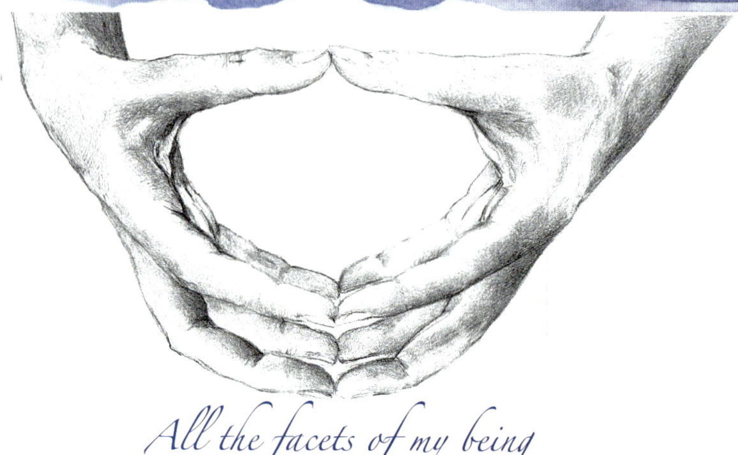

All the facets of my being
Are integrated as a seamless unity.

Core Quality

Integration

Especially helpful for

- Instilling a sense of wholeness and integration.
- Facilitating Full Yogic Breathing.
- Supporting overall health and healing.
- Enhancing body awareness.

Mudras with similar effects

Dharma Chakra, Dharma Pravartana, Mandala

Cautions

None

Instructions

1. Hold the hands facing each other in front of the solar plexus.
2. Gently touch the tips of all the fingers and thumbs to the same fingers on the opposite hand.
3. Hold the hands open and rounded as if holding a globe.
4. Relax the shoulders back and down, with the elbows held slightly away from the body, the forearms parallel to the earth and the spine naturally aligned.

Hakini is the goddess associated with the third eye, the center of inner wisdom, and Hakini mudra supports the unfolding of wisdom within all the dimensions of our being. This gesture facilitates Full Yogic Breathing, which naturally supports the integration of all areas of the body, enhancing our sense of embodiment. Hakini mudra opens both nostrils evenly, bringing equilibrium to the right and left sides of the body, as well as the active and receptive, masculine and feminine aspects of our being, naturally instilling a sense of integration and harmony.

The integration and harmony cultivated by Hakini mudra optimizes health and healing at all dimensions of being. At the physical level, this gesture enhances circulation to all of the systems of the body, supporting them in functioning harmoniously. This harmony within the body is further enhanced by the balance of all five elements cultivated by this gesture. At the subtle level, this gesture activates and integrates all five *prana vayus* while opening and balancing the first six *chakras*. At the spiritual level, this gesture naturally draws our awareness to the third eye, *Ajna chakra*, which is the command center for the integration of all the dimensions of our being. This overall integration at physical and subtle levels is symbolized by the global shape of the hands in Hakini mudra, representing our inherent wholeness and unity.

Systems Balanced:

Elements Activated:

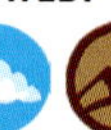
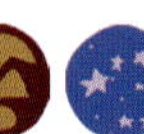
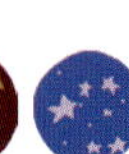
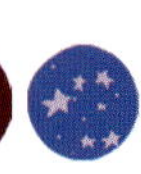

Doshas Balanced:

Prana Vayus Nourished:

Chakras Balanced:

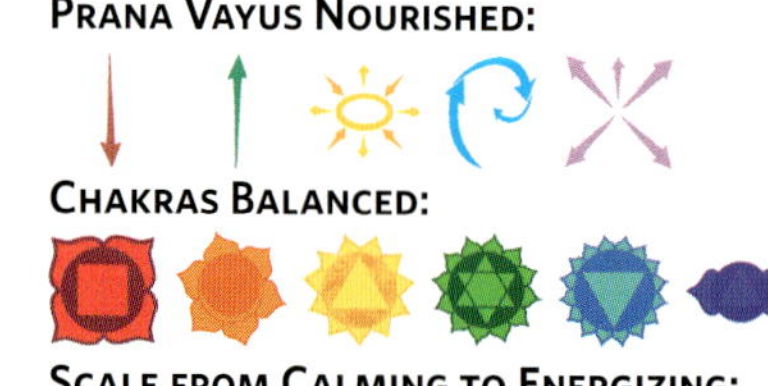

Scale from Calming to Energizing:

0 1 2 3 4 [5] 6 7 8 9 10

Guided Meditation: **Integrating All Areas of your Being**

- As you hold Hakini mudra, take several natural breaths to attune to all the feelings and sensations awakened by this gesture.
- Notice how each inhaling breath flows upward from the base of your body to your collar bones, and how each exhalation smoothly descends, instilling a sense of relaxation and release throughout your entire being.
- Take several breaths to sense this whole body breathing naturally cultivating integration and harmony.
- You will enhance this integration by directing your breath into the various planes of your body individually, culminating in an experience of unity.
- Begin by directing three full breaths into the left side of your body, sensing how this left body breathing naturally awakens the receptive, intuitive aspect of your being.
- Next, direct three full breaths into the right side of your body, sensing how this right body breathing naturally awakens your active, dynamic polarity.
- Now, sense your breath flowing through both the left and right sides of your body evenly, integrating them as a harmonious unity.
- With left and right integrated completely, now divide your body into front and back. Begin by directing three full breaths into the back of your body.
- Sense how this back body breathing allows you to attune to the subconscious dimension of your being, which holds the deep beliefs that underlie your thoughts and feelings.
- Next, direct three full breaths along the front of your body, attuning to the conscious aspects of your being, the habits and qualities that make up your personality.
- Now, breathe into the back and front of your body evenly, integrating subconscious and conscious as a seamless unity.
- With the left and right, back and front planes integrated completely, divide your body into a lower part, from the waist down, and an upper part, from the waist up.
- Begin by directing three full breaths into the lower part of your body, creating a sense of grounding and stability, allowing you to feel completely present in your physical being.
- Next, direct three full breaths into your upper body, allowing you to attune to the subtle dimensions of your being, opening a doorway to your inherent spiritual qualities.
- Now, breathe into your lower and upper body evenly, harmonizing the material and subtle dimensions of your being.
- Finally, breathe fully and freely throughout your entire body, sensing left and right, back and front, bottom and top, integrated as a harmonious unity.
- Affirm your integration as you repeat the following three times, aloud or silently: **"Through the integration of all areas of my body, I experience complete harmony."**
- Slowly, release the gesture, sensing complete integration.
- When you are ready, open your eyes, returning slowly and gently, with a greater sense of harmony.

Annamaya kosha (physical body)

• Directs breath and awareness to the entire body, balancing and integrating all systems of the body as well as the five elements.
• Creates an ideal balance between alertness and relaxation.
• The balancing effects cultivated by this gesture are generally helpful for Vata, Pitta and Kapha imbalances.

Pranamaya kosha (energy body)

• Balances all five prana vayus.
• Opens and balances the first six chakras.
• Balances Ida and Pingala nadis.

Manomaya kosha (psycho-emotional body)

• Cultivates an overall sense of integration and harmony.
• Builds self-esteem.
• Instills equanimity.

Vijnanamaya kosha (wisdom body)

• As we sense greater integration, we naturally connect with our true Self, whose essence is wholeness.

Anandamaya kosha (bliss body)

• As we attune to our inherent wholeness, sensations of joy and deep well-being awaken naturally.

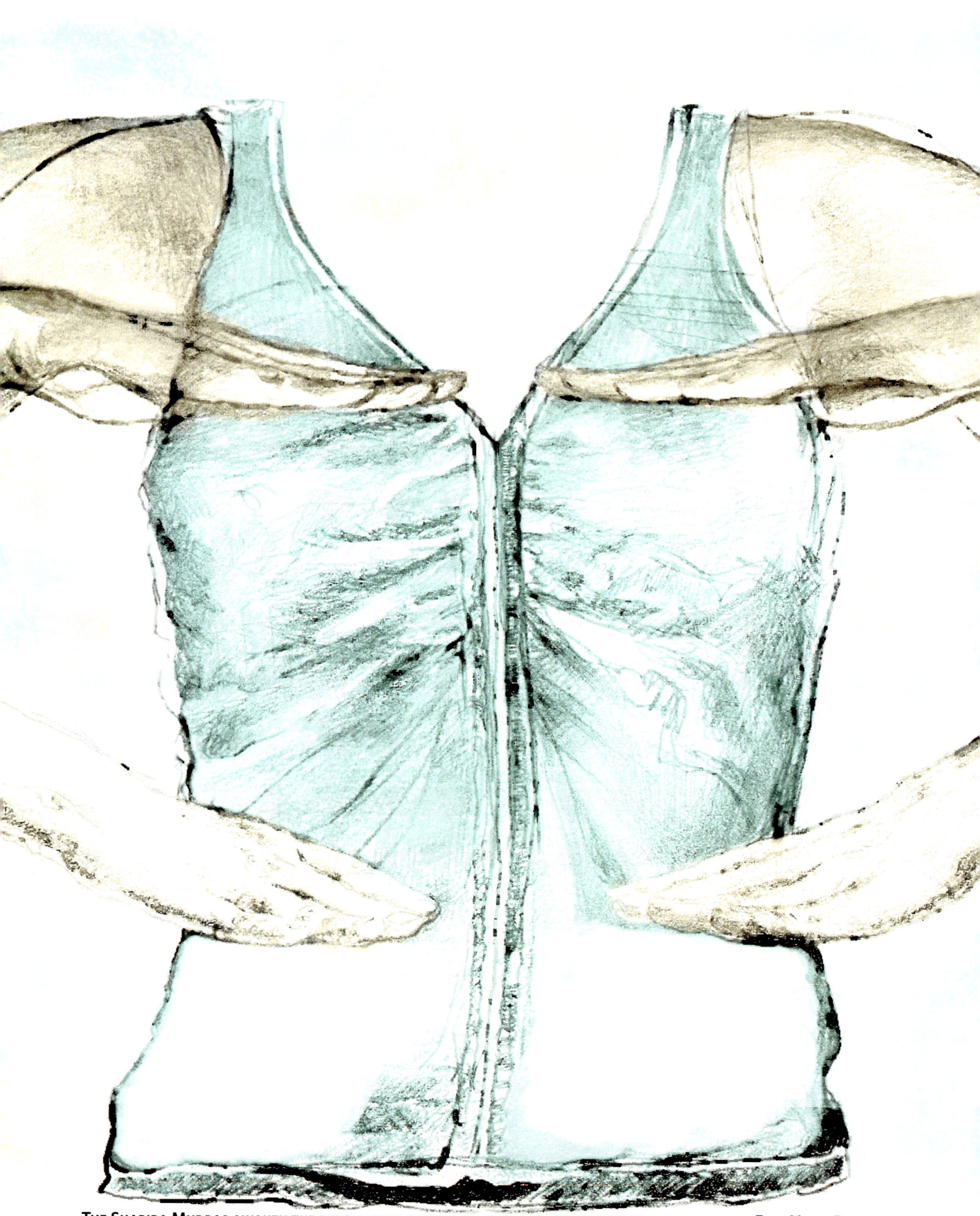

The Sharira Mudras awaken the breath in each area of the torso individually, preparing for Full Yogic Breathing.

Chapter Three

Awakening the Breath

THE SHARIRA MUDRAS

Sharira means "body," and the *Sharira Mudras* enhance awareness of the three main regions of the torso, while awakening the breath in the three main parts of the lungs: lower, middle and upper. The three Sharira mudras awaken each of these areas individually, while the final gesture of this family, Purna Svara mudra, facilitates Full Yogic Breathing, integrating all areas of the torso and lungs. At a symbolic level, each of the Sharira mudras is related to one of the three shariras, the three dimensions of our being, described in Yoga psychology. These are the *Sthula sharira*, the physical body; the *Sukshma sharira*, the subtle body; and the *Karana sharira*, the causal body. The first three mudras of this family awaken each of these bodies individually while the final gesture integrates them.

Kanishtha Sharira Mudra

This gesture activates abdominal breathing, directing breath, awareness and energy into the lowest portion of the torso while expanding the breath at the base of the lungs. This gesture supports our connection with the Sthula sharira, our physical body.

Madhyama Sharira Mudra

This mudra activates thoracic breathing, directing breath, awareness and energy into the middle of the chest while expanding the breath in the middle portion of the lungs. This gesture supports our connection with the Sukshma sharira, our subtle body, composed of energy, thoughts and feelings.

Jyeshtha Sharira Mudra

This gesture activates clavicular breathing, directing breath, awareness and energy into the uppermost parts of the chest and collarbones while expanding the breath in the uppermost portion of the lungs. This gesture supports our connection with the Karana sharira, the causal body, storehouse of our karmic patterns.

Purna Svara Mudra

This gesture activates Full Yogic Breathing, integrating all areas of the torso and lungs and all three bodies or shariras.

Mudra	Body Area / Breath Focus	Sharira Awakened
Kanishtha Sharira	Pelvis, abdomen, solar plexus & mid back Abdominal breathing	Sthula sharira The physical body, including all of the physiological systems & the 5 elements.
Madhyama Sharira	Chest, rib cage & upper back Thoracic breathing	Sukshma sharira The energy body, including our subtle anatomy (chakras, prana vayus & nadis), as well as our thoughts and emotions.
Jyeshtha Sharira	Upper chest, collarbones, neck & cervical spine Clavicular breathing	Karana sharira The causal body, our storehouse of karmic patterns & deep beliefs, which are transformed through spiritual awakening.
Purna Svara	Entire torso Full Yogic Breathing	The integration of all three bodies: Sthula, Sukshma, & Karana, leading to our true being that encompasses & transcends all three.

7 Kanishtha Sharira Mudra

Gesture of the Lower Body

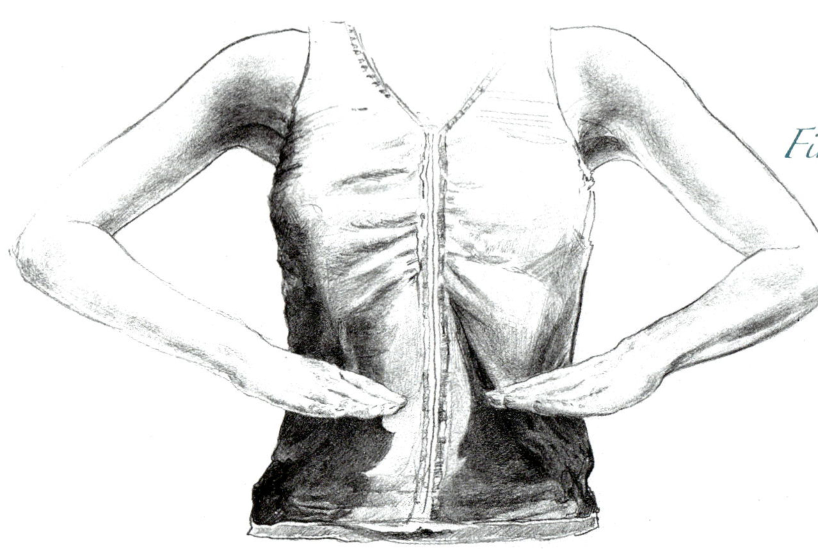

Firmly supported by body and breath,
I move forward in life
With complete confidence.

Core Quality

Lower Body Breathing

Especially helpful for

- Connecting to the lower body.
- Activating the diaphragm, the main muscle of respiration, supporting fuller abdominal breathing.
- Optimizing digestion.
- Releasing tension from the low back.
- Instilling equanimity and centering.
- Building a sense of confidence.

Mudras with similar effects

Bhu, Adhi, Gupta

Cautions

None

Instructions

1. Place the web between your thumbs and index fingers on either side of your waist, just below the ribs, with the thumbs facing backward and the fingers pointing forward.
2. Keep the fingers together with the palms and forearms parallel to the earth.
3. Hold the elbows out and away from the body, with the shoulders relaxed back and down and the spine naturally aligned.

Kanishtha means "lowest," and *sharira* means "body." Kanishtha Sharira mudra directs breath and energy into the lower body, enhancing our awareness of the pelvis, abdomen and solar plexus. The position of the hands, just below the rib cage, facilitates enhanced movement of the diaphragm, strengthening this main muscle of respiration, thereby increasing breath capacity. The breath is especially activated at the base of the lungs, the area with the greatest surface for the exchange of oxygen and carbon dioxide. The movement of the diaphragm and abdomen creates a massaging effect for the abdominal organs that optimizes digestion and elimination. This rhythmic movement also creates a pumping effect that assists in the return of venous blood to the heart and the circulation of lymphatic fluid. Additionally, the movement of the hands and breath creates a massaging effect for the low back, kidneys and adrenal glands.

Kanishtha Sharira mudra lengthens the exhaling breath, enhancing our connection to the earth and to the lower body, creating a sense of support and grounding. This deepening connection to the lower body naturally opens and balances *Muladhara chakra*, cultivating safety and security at all times and places along our life journey. This gesture enhances our awareness of the rhythmic movement of our hands in synchrony with the breath. This rhythmic movement gives the mind a point of focus, naturally cultivating calm and relaxation. Kanishtha Sharira mudra also gently activates the fire element at the solar plexus, instilling a sense of energy, allowing us to participate in all activities with both ease and vitality.

Systems Balanced:

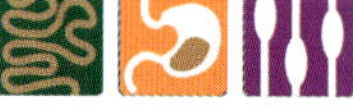

Elements Activated:

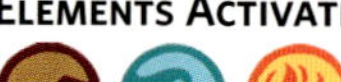

Doshas Balanced:

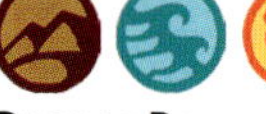

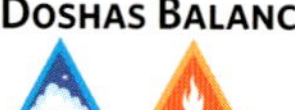

Prana Vayus Nourished:

Chakras Balanced:

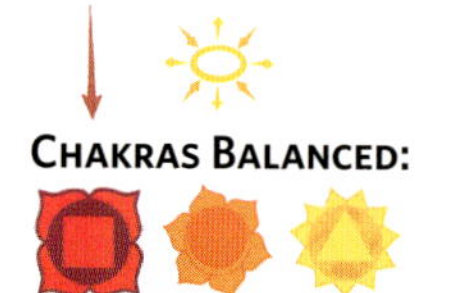

Scale from Calming to Energizing:

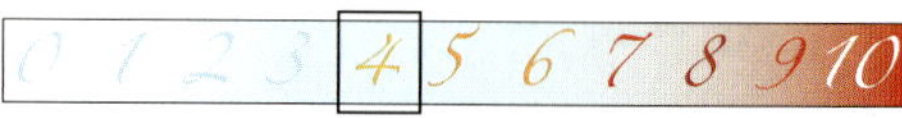

Guided Meditation: **Awakening the Breath in the Lower Body**

- As you hold Kanishtha Sharira mudra, take several natural breaths to attune to all the feelings and sensations evoked by this gesture.
- Notice how your hands naturally glide away from each other with each inhaling breath, and rest toward each other with each exhalation.
- Take several breaths to sense how the movement of your hands, in synchrony with your breathing, activates the diaphragm, allowing you to breathe more fully.
- Notice how your exhalation is lengthened naturally and directed downward toward the base of your body, instilling a sense of support and grounding.
- As your sense of grounding naturally deepens, take several breaths to fully inhabit your lower body, creating a firm, supportive foundation.
- With greater support at the base of your body, notice how your breath is naturally directed into the base of your lungs, allowing for maximum exchange of carbon dioxide and oxygen.
- As your breath expands at the base of your lungs, sense how your rhythmic abdominal breathing is increased, naturally massaging your organs of digestion and supporting their balanced functioning.
- Also sense how this rhythmic movement of your diaphragm creates a pumping effect, allowing fluids from your lower body to be drawn upward more efficiently.
- As you attune to your abdominal breathing even more deeply, you feel the massaging effect on your adrenal glands and kidneys, supporting their optimal functioning.
- Now, sense how your lengthened exhaling breath naturally releases tension from your low back, massaging your lumbar area internally, cultivating relaxation and ease throughout your entire lower body.
- As tension is released from your lower body, the rhythmic movement of your hands, belly and breath create a natural place for your mind to rest, instilling a sense of comfort and serenity.
- Fully attuned to your lower body breathing, with a firm foundation and enhanced serenity, you are fully supported along your journey.
- Affirm your sense of support as you repeat the following three times, aloud or silently: **"Attuned to my lower body breathing, I am fully supported along my journey."**
- Slowly release the gesture, taking several breaths to integrate completely the effects of your lower body breathing.
- When you are ready, open your eyes, returning slowly and gently, with a deeper sense of support and grounding.

Annamaya kosha (physical body)

• Directs breath and awareness to the abdominal area, creating a massaging effect that improves circulation to the eliminatory and digestive systems.
• The enhanced movement of the diaphragm releases tension from the lower back, improving circulation to the area of the kidneys and adrenal glands.
• Lengthens the exhalation, which helps remove residual air from the lungs.
• Improves venous blood return to the heart and lymphatic drainage through increased diaphragmatic movement.
• The grounding effects cultivated by this gesture are generally helpful for Vata imbalance.
• The calming effects are generally helpful for Pitta imbalance.

Pranamaya kosha (energy body)

• Activates the downward moving current of Apana vayu.
• Gently activates the horizontal current of Samana vayu.
• Opens and balances the first, second and third chakras, centers of safety, self-nourishment and personal power.

Manomaya kosha (psycho-emotional body)

• Instills a sense of support and grounding.
• Builds confidence.

Vijnanamaya kosha (wisdom body)

• Creates a point of focus that calms the mind and brings it into the present moment, allowing for greater clarity.

Anandamaya kosha (bliss body)

• Awakens feelings of fullness, wholeness and well-being within the abdomen.

8

Madhyama Sharira Mudra

Gesture of the Middle Body

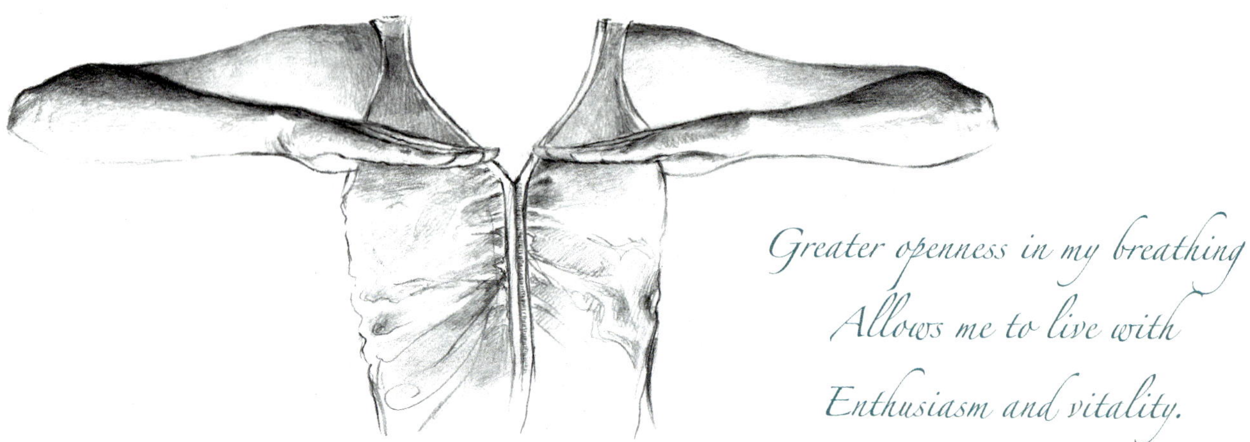

Core Quality

Middle Body Breathing

Especially helpful for

- Connecting to the middle body.
- Enhancing breath capacity, especially in the middle lungs.
- Releasing tension from the middle back.
- Supporting immune function.
- Instilling a sense of openness.

Mudras with similar effects

Tarjani, Urdhvam Merudanda, Dirgha Svara

Cautions

Physical pressure to the lymph nodes is not recommended for breast or lymphatic cancers.

Instructions

1. With the fingers together, stretch the thumbs away from the fingers as much as possible.
2. Gently press the thumbs into the centers of the armpits and rest the inner borders of the index fingers on the upper chest.
3. Keep the forearms and palms parallel to the earth.
4. Relax the shoulders back and down, with the spine naturally aligned.

Madhyama means "middle," and *sharira* means "body." Madhyama Sharira mudra directs breath, awareness and energy to the chest, side ribs and upper back. This gesture cultivates a rhythmic expansion and relaxation of the rib cage, creating a massaging effect that releases muscular tension from the middle body, optimizing thoracic breathing. This mudra lengthens the inhaling breath, which increases energy and vitality while each exhalation instills a sense of lightness and release. The steady pressure of the thumbs under the armpits together with the rhythmic movement of the rib cage massages the lymph nodes, supporting the health of the lymphatic system. This rhythmic movement also enhances circulation to the area of the thymus gland behind the upper sternum, supporting the health of the immune system.

At a psycho-emotional level, Madhyama Sharira mudra instills a sense of lightness and vitality, evoking the image of a bird in flight that remains airborne effortlessly. This gesture cultivates a feeling of uplifting energy, creating enthusiasm and motivation, allowing us to live life more vibrantly. This sense of enthusiasm is further enhanced by the opening of *Anahata chakra*, facilitated by this gesture. As the heart chakra opens, we are able to honor our feelings more completely, developing acceptance and compassion toward ourselves and others, allowing us to embrace our entire life journey more completely.

Systems Balanced:

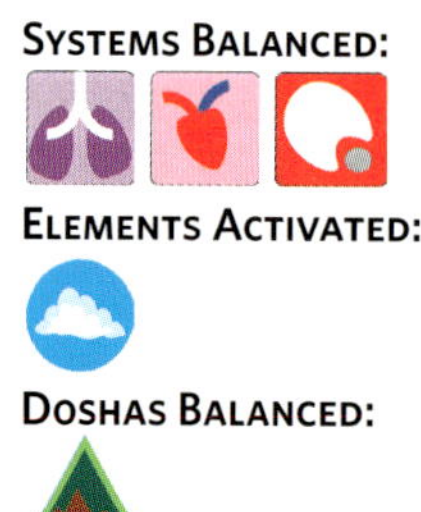

Elements Activated:

Doshas Balanced:

Prana Vayus Nourished:

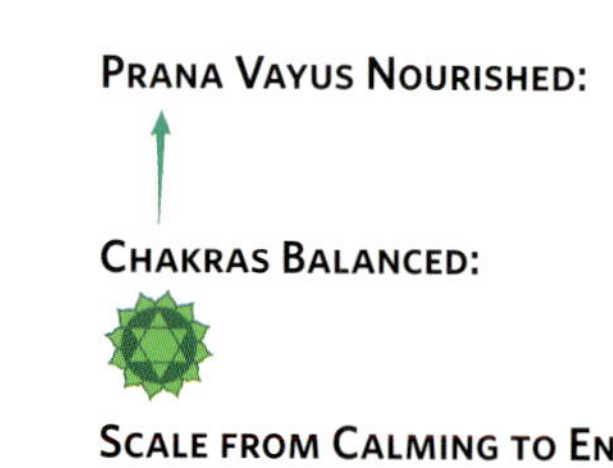

Chakras Balanced:

Scale from Calming to Energizing:

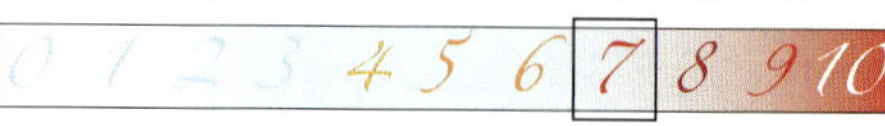

Guided Meditation: Awakening the Breath in the Middle Body

- ॐ As you hold Madhyama Sharira mudra, take several natural breaths to attune to all the feelings and sensations awakened by this gesture.
- ॐ Notice how your hands glide gently away from each other with each inhaling breath, and rest toward each other with each exhalation.
- ॐ Take several breaths to sense how each inhalation expands your rib cage evenly, and how each exhalation allows your chest and upper back to soften and relax completely.
- ॐ As you attune more deeply to your thoracic breathing, notice how tension is naturally released from your rib cage, allowing your shoulder blades to move more freely.
- ॐ Sense how this rhythmic movement of your hands and breath gently massages the area of the lymph nodes under your armpits, supporting the functioning of your lymphatic system.
- ॐ As you deepen your awareness of your middle body breathing, sense the release of tension from the area of your sternum naturally increasing circulation to your thymus gland, supporting the functioning of your immune system.
- ॐ As your entire rib cage breathes more freely, space is created in which your heart opens naturally.
- ॐ Take several breaths to sense your heart breathing, allowing all feelings to arise and pass away more easily.
- ॐ As your feelings are welcomed, you expand your ability to embrace yourself, others and your entire life journey more openly.
- ॐ With greater openness and ease, repeat the following three times, aloud or silently: **"Attuned to my middle body breathing, I naturally embrace life more completely."**
- ॐ Slowly release the gesture, taking several breaths to integrate completely the effects of your middle body breathing.
- ॐ When you are ready, open your eyes, returning slowly and gently, with a greater sense of openness.

Annamaya kosha (physical body)

• Opens the front, back and sides of the rib cage, releasing tension and enhancing breath capacity.
• The opening of the chest may be helpful for asthma when not in an acute phase.
• The pressure of the hands under the armpits creates a massaging effect that improves circulation to the lymph nodes.
• Directs breath and awareness to the area of the thymus gland.
• The energizing effects of this gesture are generally helpful for Kapha imbalance.

Pranamaya kosha (energy body)

• Activates Prana vayu, the upward moving current of energy.
• Expands and opens the heart chakra, center of unconditional love.

Manomaya kosha (psycho-emotional body)

• Enhances vitality while cultivating a sense of openness and enthusiasm.
• Builds trust and confidence.

Vijnanamaya kosha (wisdom body)

• The opening of the heart helps release emotional constriction, revealing the subtle heart's inherent lightness and openness.

Anandamaya kosha (bliss body)

• As tension is released from the chest, feelings of joy and contentment naturally radiate out from the heart center.

9

Jyeshtha Sharira Mudra

Gesture of the Upper Body

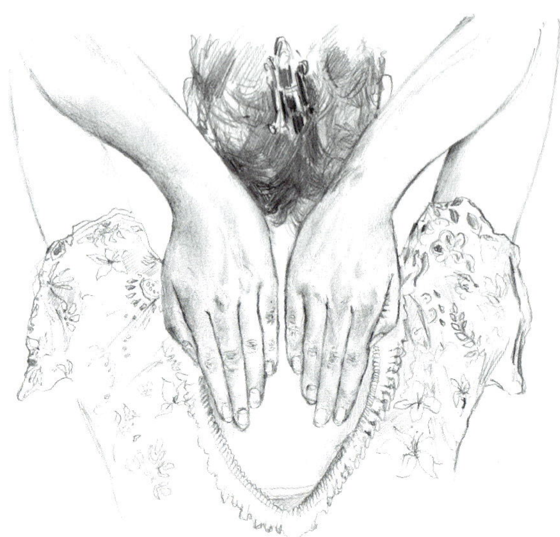

With a growing sense of expansiveness, I look at life from a wider perspective.

Core Quality

Upper Body Breathing

Especially helpful for

- Connecting to the upper body.
- Increasing energy and vitality.
- Bringing circulation to the area of the thyroid gland.
- Stimulating the senses.
- Enhancing enthusiasm and creativity.
- Awakening to our infinite possibilities.

Mudras with similar effects

Angushtha, Linga, Kali, Vishuddha

Cautions

Contraindicated for those with high blood pressure, cardiac conditions, migraine, glaucoma and hyperthyroid conditions. Those with shoulder or neck issues may use Angushtha mudra as a substitute.

Instructions

1. Raise the arms directly overhead while drawing the shoulders downward.
2. Bend the elbows and place the palms onto the shoulder blades, with the elbows angled out to the sides.
3. Relax the shoulders down as the crown of the head lifts and the sides of the neck reach slightly backward.
4. Maintain the spine naturally aligned.

Jyeshtha means "eldest" or "highest," and *sharira* means "body." Jyeshtha Sharira mudra directs breath, awareness and energy into the uppermost portions of the chest, collarbones, neck and throat. This gesture powerfully lengthens the inhalation, increasing heart rate and blood pressure, thereby enhancing energy and vitality. This mudra increases circulation to the area of the thyroid gland, located at the throat, stimulating metabolism. Jyeshtha Sharira mudra creates space between the shoulder blades, supporting the alignment of the cervical spine, allowing the head to rest evenly over the torso.

Jyeshtha Sharira mudra activates the qualities of the space element, including a sense of expansiveness that allows us to access the subtle dimensions of our being. This wider perspective can be helpful in allowing us to recognize our own possibilities beyond the limitations of the personality. This gesture activates *Vishuddha chakra*, located at the throat, supporting the process of spiritual purification. Through this process, limiting beliefs come to the surface to be seen and gradually released, further enhancing our ability to open to our limitless possibilities. As Jyeshtha Sharira mudra opens us to new possibilities, creativity is naturally enhanced, especially through speaking and singing.

For greater comfort in this gesture, we recommend the seated position using the support of a wall or the restorative position, lying on the back with the arms resting on a cushion, with a bolster under the knees.

Systems Balanced:

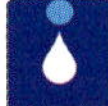

Elements Activated:

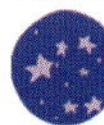

Doshas Balanced:

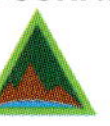

Prana Vayus Nourished:

Chakras Balanced:

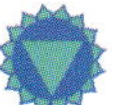

Scale from Calming to Energizing:

Guided Meditation: Awakening the Breath in the Upper Body

- ॐ As you hold Jyeshtha Sharira mudra, take several natural breaths to attune to all the feelings and sensations awakened by this gesture.
- ॐ Notice how your breath is naturally directed into the uppermost parts of your chest, collarbones, throat and neck, instilling a sense of expansiveness.
- ॐ With each inhalation, sense your spine lengthening naturally, creating space between each vertebra.
- ॐ With each exhaling breath, all tension is released, allowing your shoulders and collarbones to soften downward naturally.
- ॐ As your breath flows more easily through your upper chest, throat and neck, take several breaths to sense the increased circulation to your thyroid gland, enhancing your level of energy and vitality.
- ॐ As your breath flows more freely throughout the uppermost areas of your body, you naturally widen your horizons, gaining a more open perspective of your life journey.
- ॐ Viewing life more openly, take several breaths to sense greater expansiveness and clarity, allowing you to envision your own infinite possibilities.
- ॐ Affirm your expansiveness as you repeat the following three times, aloud or silently: **"As I expand my upper body breathing, I awaken to my infinite possibilities."**
- ॐ Now, slowly release the gesture, taking several breaths to integrate completely the effects of your upper body breathing.
- ॐ When you are ready, open your eyes, returning slowly and gently, with a greater awareness of your limitless possibilities.

Annamaya kosha (physical body)

• Expands the breath in the uppermost portions of the lungs.
• Increases heart rate and blood pressure, providing exercise for the cardiovascular system.
• Increases circulation to the area of the thyroid gland.
• Supports the alignment of the cervical spine.
• The energizing effects of this gesture are generally helpful for Kapha imbalance when practiced within the range of physical comfort.

Pranamaya kosha (energy body)

• Activates Udana vayu, the uppermost current of energy.
• Opens and balances the fifth chakra, center of spiritual purification.

Manomaya kosha (psycho-emotional body)

• Instills energy and enthusiasm.
• Increases concentration and alertness.
• Cultivates a feeling of expansiveness and uplifting energy.

Vijnanamaya kosha (wisdom body)

• The sense of expansiveness allows us to open to our own limitless possibilities.

Anandamaya kosha (bliss body)

• As we attune to the subtle realms of our being, sensations of limitlessness and freedom arise naturally.

10

Purna Svara Mudra

Gesture of the Complete Breath

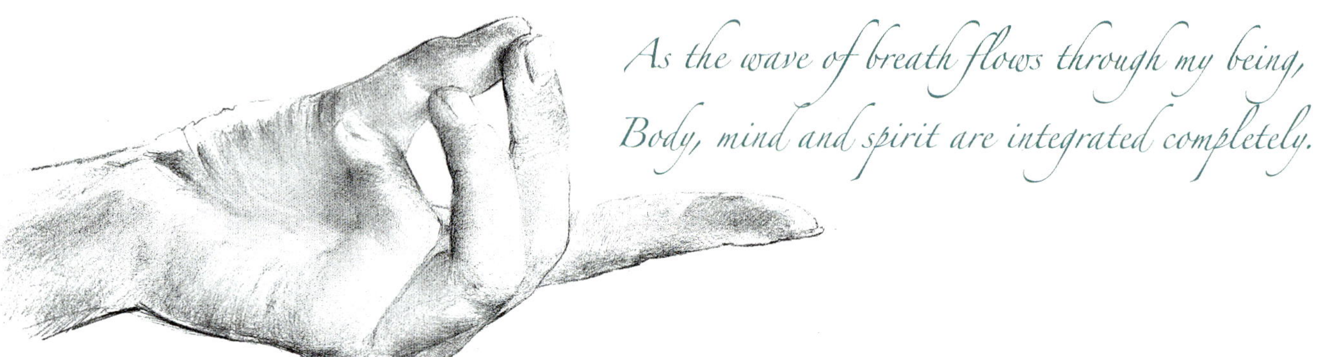

Core Quality

Complete Breathing

Especially Helpful For

- Facilitating Full Yogic Breathing, which may be helpful for respiratory conditions.
- Releasing tension from the entire torso.
- Supporting health and healing in all systems of the body.
- Integrating body, mind and spirit.

Mudras with Similar Effects

Hakini, Dharma Pravartana, Mandala, Dharma Chakra

Cautions

None

Instructions

1. Touch the tip of the little finger of each hand to the base joint of the thumb.
2. Touch the tip of the ring finger to the middle joint of the thumb.
3. Touch the tip of the middle finger to the tip of the thumb.
4. Rest the backs of the hands on the thighs or knees.
5. Relax the shoulders back and down, with the spine naturally aligned.

Purna means "full" or "whole," and *svara* means "breath." Purna Svara refers to *Dirgha Pranayama*, Full Yogic Breathing. Purna Svara mudra naturally cultivates Full Yogic Breathing, which we experience as a wave of energy flowing throughout our entire torso. This complete breathing integrates the three areas of the torso (base, middle and top) and the three portions of the lungs (lower, middle and upper). This gesture releases tension from the abdomen, diaphragm, rib cage and the auxiliary muscles of respiration in the shoulders and neck, permitting freer breathing and enhanced lung capacity. The Full Yogic Breathing facilitated by Purna Svara mudra supports the health of all of the systems of the body.

Purna Svara mudra instills a sense of integration and harmony throughout our entire being. This integration is activated by the placement of the fingers along the thumb. The little fingertip pressed into the base of the thumb activates the breath in the lower body and the base of the lungs, and is associated with the *Sthula sharira*, the physical body. The ring fingertip pressed into the middle joint of the thumb activates the breath in the middle body and middle portion of the lungs, and is associated with the *Sukshma sharira*, the energy body. The middle fingertip, which touches the top of the thumb, activates the breath in the upper body and top of the lungs, and is associated with the *Karana sharira*, the causal body. The position of the fingers pressed against the thumb integrates the three bodies simultaneously while the extended index finger serves as a pointer to our true being, which encompasses and transcends all of them.

Systems Balanced:

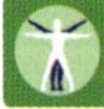

Elements Activated:

Doshas Balanced:

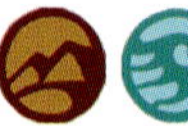

Prana Vayus Nourished:

Chakras Balanced:

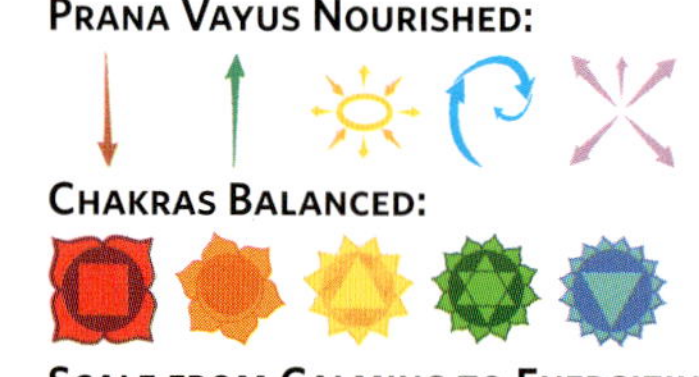

Scale from Calming to Energizing:

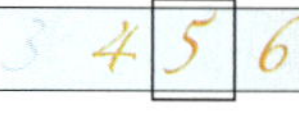
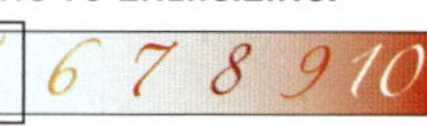

Guided Meditation: Awakening all Areas of Breathing

- As you hold Purna Svara mudra, take several natural breaths to attune to all the feelings and sensations awakened by this gesture.
- Notice how your breath flows freely from the base of your body all the way to your neck, and then smoothly back down again.
- Sense your inhalation awakening each area of your body sequentially, beginning with your lower body, then flowing up into your chest, finally filling your collarbones, shoulders and neck.
- As you exhale, sense your wave of breath flowing downward, instilling a sense of deep release in your collarbones and chest, and finally allowing your abdomen to be drawn inward completely.
- Take some time to attune to the soft wavelike motion of your breath flowing throughout your entire being, naturally cultivating a sense of integration and harmony.
- As your wave of breathing flows more freely, you naturally become more sensitive to the expansion of the breath in each part of your lungs.
- As you inhale, sense the base of your lungs expanding, followed by the middle lungs, and finally filling the very top of your lungs.
- Sense your exhalation releasing the air gradually, beginning at the top, emptying the middle lungs, and finally releasing the air from the base of your lungs completely.
- Take several breaths to sense your wave of breath nourishing the back, front and sides of your lungs evenly, instilling an overall feeling of fullness and vitality.
- As your wave of breath flows more easily, any blockages in your breathing are released naturally, allowing vital energy to flow freely throughout your entire being.
- Take some time to sense your complete breathing, instilling integration and harmony throughout all areas of your lungs and all parts of your body.
- Affirm your free breathing, repeating the following three times, aloud or silently: **"Attuned to my complete breathing, I experience greater integration and harmony."**
- Slowly release the gesture, taking several breaths to integrate completely the effects of your full body breathing.
- When you are ready, open your eyes, returning slowly and gently, with a greater sense of integration and harmony.

Annamaya kosha
(physical body)

• Naturally activates Full Yogic Breathing, expanding lung capacity.
• Balances the nervous system, supporting the optimal functioning of all systems of the body.
• The balancing effects of this gesture are generally helpful for Vata, Pitta and Kapha imbalances.

Pranamaya kosha
(energy body)

• Activates all five prana vayus.
• Opens and balances the first through the fifth chakras.

Manomaya kosha
(psycho-emotional body)

• Integrates body, mind and spirit, resulting in a global sense of wholeness and harmony.

Vijnanamaya kosha
(wisdom body)

• The integration of all areas of our being naturally opens a doorway that allows us to perceive our essential nature as unity.

Anandamaya kosha
(bliss body)

• As Full Yogic Breathing becomes fluid and natural, it is experienced as a wave of well-being that flows throughout the entire body.

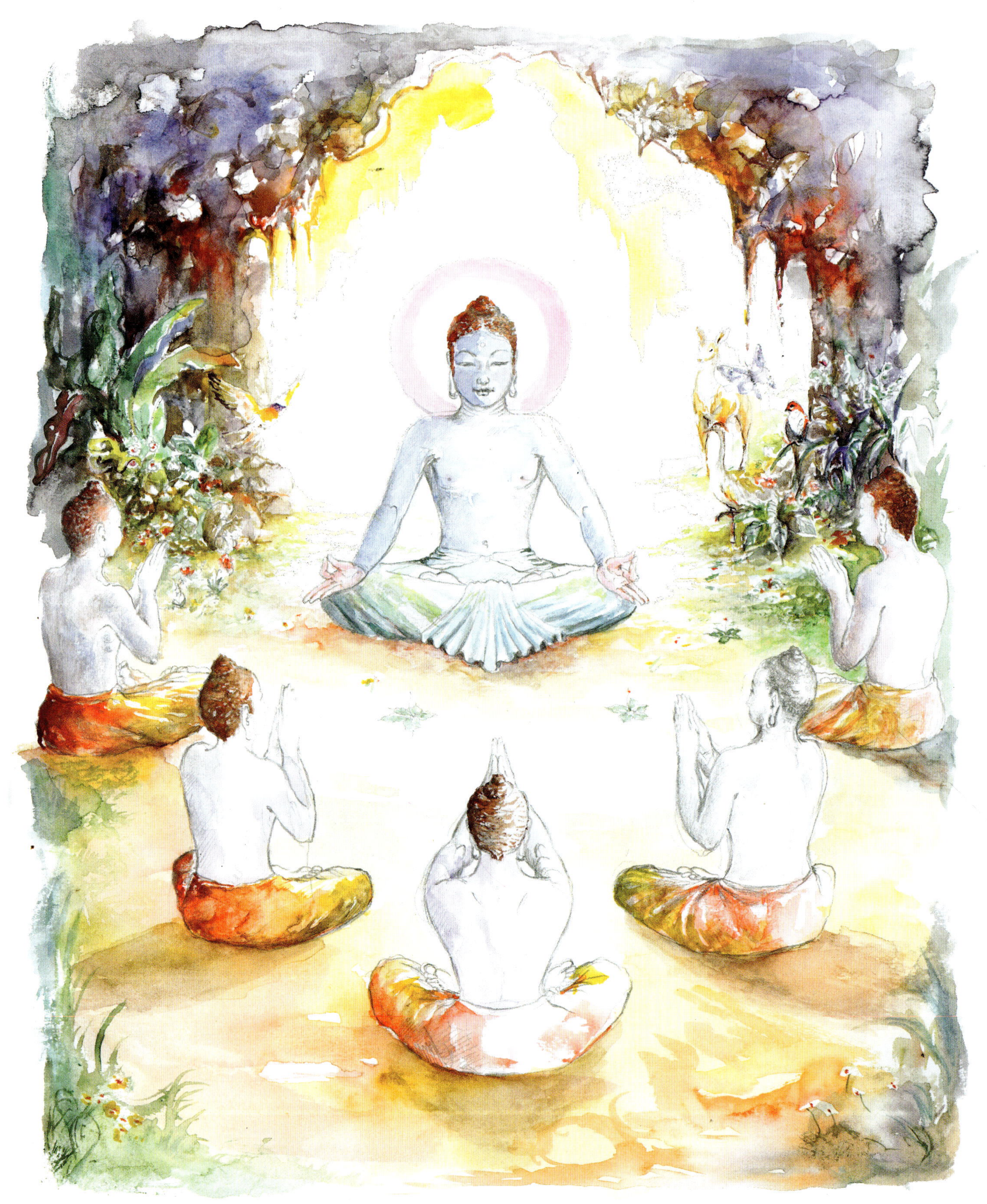

Balanced energy is a foundation for spiritual awakening.

Chapter Four

Balancing your Level of Energy

THE MERUDANDA MUDRAS

The practice of the *Merudanda Mudra* family demonstrates how the use of mudras can support us in balancing our level of energy. Every mudra has an energetic effect, either calming, balancing or energizing. Each mudra in this book is accompanied by an energy scale that reflects each gesture's energetic effects. The Merudanda Mudras are especially helpful for understanding how to use gestures to adjust our level of energy quickly and easily.

Each gesture in the Merudanda Mudra family directs breath and awareness to a specific area of the body, beginning at the pelvic floor, then continuing progressively upward to the top of the chest. The first gesture, Adhi mudra, directs breath and awareness to the base of the body while the second one, Adho Merudanda mudra, brings breath and awareness into the pelvis, and so on, with each of the following gestures increasing energy, alertness and vitality. This family of mudras works somewhat like the gears of a car, beginning with a low speed that is slow, calming and grounding, then moving sequentially toward a high speed that is more vitalizing and energizing. The practice of the entire Merudanda Mudra family has an overall balancing effect on our level of energy while the individual gestures can be used to adjust our energy level as needed.

At a physiological level, the Merudanda Mudras create an awareness of the autonomic nervous system (ANS), which is made up of two complementary branches. The sympathetic branch initiates excitation, making energy reserves available in times of need. The parasympathetic branch is responsible for restorative and regenerative functions, storing potential energy. These two complementary branches work together like the gas pedal and brakes of a car to create a balance of activity and rest, providing optimal energy for all of our activities. As we practice the Merudanda Mudras, we develop the ability to support the dynamic balance of the autonomic nervous system.

Mudra	Area Where Breath is Directed	Level of Energy	Core Quality
• Adhi	Pelvic floor	Grounding, calming & relaxing. 1 2 3 4 5 6 7 8 9 10	Stillness
• Adho Merudanda	Center of the pelvis	Stabilizing, centering & nourishing. 1 2 3 4 5 6 7 8 9 10	Centering
• Merudanda	Solar plexus/along the spinal column	Energizing, instilling enthusiasm & vitality. 1 2 3 4 5 6 7 8 9 10	Alignment
• Urdhvam Merudanda	Upper chest, side ribs, upper back	Very energizing, cultivating expansiveness & openness. 1 2 3 4 5 6 7 8 9 10	Expansiveness

11

Adhi Mudra

Gesture of Primordial Stillness

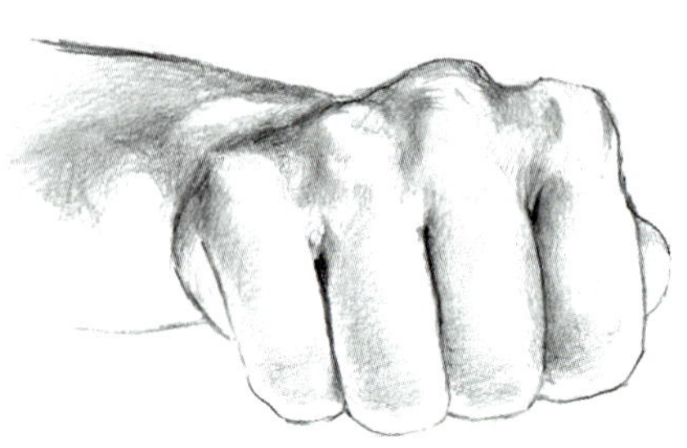
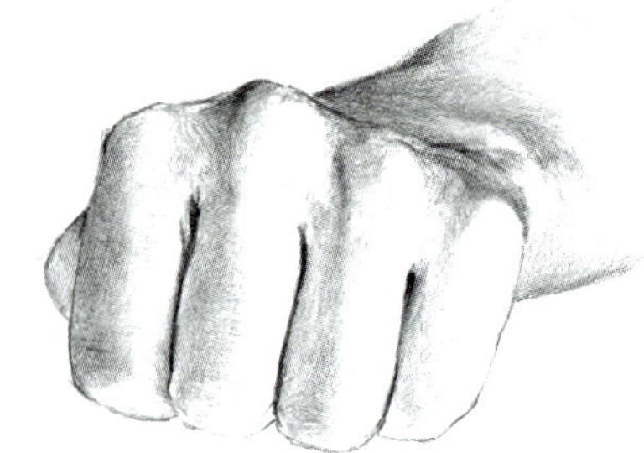

Like a statue softly breathing,
I rest in the perfect stillness of my being.

Core Quality

Stillness

Especially helpful for

- Connecting with the stillness of our essential being.
- Supporting the strength and density of the bones.
- Instilling a sense of grounding.
- Supporting the treatment of anxiety.
- Facilitating seated meditation.

Mudras with similar effects

Bhu, Murti, Chinmaya

Cautions

As this gesture can lower blood pressure, people with low blood pressure should carefully monitor the effects.

Instructions

1. Tuck the thumbs into the palms and curl the fingers loosely around the thumbs, forming soft fists with both hands.
2. Rest the hands onto the thighs or knees, with the palms facing down.
3. Relax the shoulders back and down, with the spine naturally aligned.

Adhi means "primordial," and refers to the stillness of our essential being that underlies all of our activities, thoughts and feelings. Adhi mudra directs breath, awareness and energy to the base of the body, instilling a sense of support and grounding. This gesture further enhances grounding by activating the earth element's qualities, including stability and immobility. This enhanced stability cultivates embodiment and a feeling that we are fully supported by the structure of the body. This gesture lengthens the exhaling breath, activating the parasympathetic nervous system and initiating the relaxation response. Adhi mudra also expands the pause after the exhalation, creating a space in which we can experience the stillness of our essential being even more deeply. The grounding, relaxation and stillness cultivated by this gesture create an experience of absolute peace and tranquility.

With a rating of zero on the energy scale, Adhi mudra is one of the most calming of all the gestures. The experience of calm and relaxation facilitated by this gesture can become so profound that it feels as though we are entering a state of hibernation in which the breath becomes almost completely still. This deep relaxation allows for the restoration of all of the bodily systems, especially the nervous system and senses. As the physical body is relaxed and restored, the mind naturally becomes calm and serene, making this gesture especially helpful for anxiety. This serenity naturally opens a doorway to an experience of inner peace always present as the background of all of our activities.

Systems Balanced:

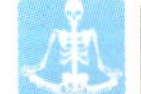
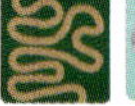
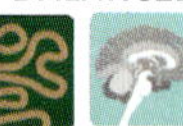

Elements Activated:

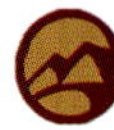

Doshas Balanced:

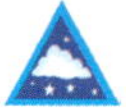

Prana Vayus Nourished:

Chakras Balanced:

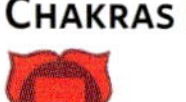

Scale from Calming to Energizing:

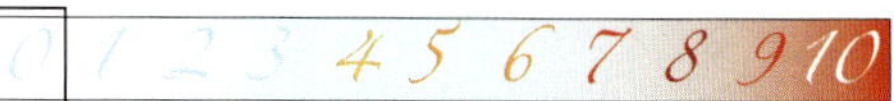

Guided Meditation: **Statue of Stillness**

- As you hold Adhi mudra, take several natural breaths to attune to all the feelings and sensations evoked by this gesture.
- Notice how your breath is gently directed downward, toward the base of your body, instilling a sense of stability and grounding.
- Take some time to sense the natural pause at the end of each exhaling breath, cultivating a space of silence in which your body and mind can deeply rest.
- For your next few breaths, attune to these pauses even more deeply, experiencing a sense of serenity that allows you to become completely still, like a statue softly breathing.
- As stillness encompasses each area of your body, you experience the absolute peace and harmony that is a reflection of your true being.
- Begin by taking several breaths to allow stillness to permeate your pelvis, legs and feet, creating a firm foundation for your statue of serenity.
- Now, allow your abdomen, solar plexus, low and mid back to enter into stillness and completely relax.
- With your lower body still and serene, take several breaths to sense your heart, lungs, chest and upper back merging with your statue of serenity.
- Serenity now fills your shoulders, arms and hands, all the way to your fingertips, integrating these areas into your statue of stillness.
- Finally, stillness permeates your neck and head, inviting all of your senses to naturally turn inward and gently rest.
- Now, take some time to sense your entire being as a statue of stillness softly breathing.
- Affirm your essential stillness, repeating the following three times, aloud or silently: **"In absolute stillness of being, I experience complete peace and serenity."**
- Now, slowly release the gesture, taking several breaths to rest in absolute stillness.
- When you are ready, open your eyes, returning slowly and gently, while remaining aligned with the stillness of your true being.

Annamaya kosha (physical body)

• Directs breath and awareness to the base of the body, helping to release tension from this area, supporting the health of the eliminatory system.
• Enhances embodiment and a sense of inner stability, which may help improve balance and decrease falls, especially in seniors.
• The enhanced sense of stability creates a feeling of support within the musculo-skeletal system.
• Slows the breath and lengthens the exhalation, which reduces heart rate and blood pressure.
• The grounding effects cultivated by this gesture are generally helpful for Vata imbalance.
• The calming effects are generally helpful for Pitta imbalance.

Pranamaya kosha (energy body)

• Activates Apana vayu, the downward moving current of energy.
• Opens and balances the first chakra, center of safety.

Manomaya kosha (psycho-emotional body)

• Instills a sense of grounding and security, helping to reduce stress and anxiety.
• Cultivates space between thoughts, allowing us to experience stillness and silence.

Vijnanamaya kosha (wisdom body)

• As the body, breath and mind enter into stillness, we experience the absolute serenity of our true being.

Anandamaya kosha (bliss body)

• In stillness, a sense of deep contentment and harmony permeates our being.

12 Adho Merudanda Mudra

Gesture of the Base of the Spine

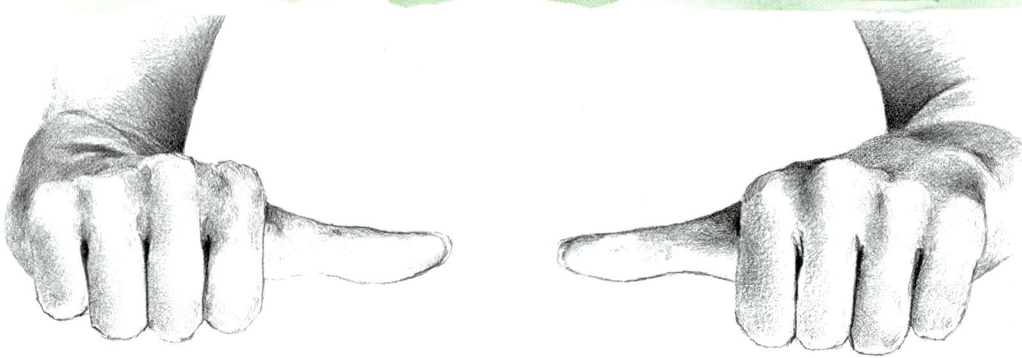

With a deeper sense of centering,
I experience perfect equanimity.

Core Quality
Centering

Especially Helpful For
- Instilling a sense of centering.
- Facilitating pelvic stabilization.
- Optimizing the health of the reproductive and urinary systems.
- Enhancing emotional equanimity.

Mudras with Similar Effects
Shankha, Svadhisthana, Jalashaya, Varuna

Cautions
None

Instructions
1. Curl the fingers into the palms with the thumbs to the outside.
2. Extend the thumbs straight out.
3. Place the fists on the thighs with the palms facing downward and the thumb tips pointing directly toward each other.
4. Relax the shoulders back and down, with the spine naturally aligned.

Adho means "lower" or "downward," and *merudanda* refers to the "spinal column." Adho Merudanda mudra directs breath, awareness and energy into the pelvis and sacrum, our body's center of gravity. As we deepen our connection to this area, we naturally enhance our sense of inner balance and centering. As awareness is drawn to the center of the pelvis, abdominal breathing is naturally activated, creating a massaging effect that enhances circulation to the urinary and reproductive systems. This gesture cultivates a sense of centering that allows us to inhabit our pelvic area with greater ease, naturally enhancing our level of comfort with our own sexuality. The enhanced sense of centering cultivates a feeling of stability and integrity throughout the structure of the physical body.

With a rating of three on the energy scale, Adho Merudanda mudra is a calming and centering gesture, with some energizing qualities. This mudra deepens our connection to the pelvis, the seat of the water element, cultivating an experience of a vast inner sea that holds tremendous potential energy. As we attune to our center more deeply, we are able to channel its energy outward to nourish our entire being. As Adho Merudanda mudra deepens our sense of centering, it naturally cultivates an experience of equanimity, enhancing our ability to rest within our center, our deep sea of inner peace, no matter what is happening in our surroundings.

Systems Balanced:

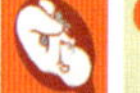 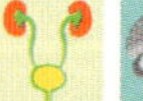 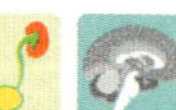

Elements Activated:

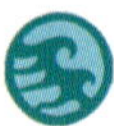

Doshas Balanced:

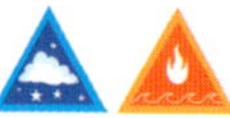

Prana Vayus Nourished:

↓

Chakras Balanced:

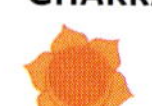

Scale from Calming to Energizing:

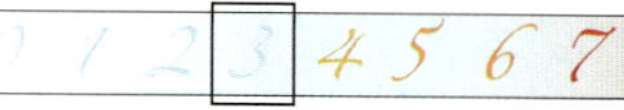

Guided Meditation: Circle of Centering

- As you hold Adho Merudanda mudra, take several natural breaths to attune to all the feelings and sensations evoked by this gesture.
- Notice how each exhaling breath is directed inward, toward the center of your pelvis, and how each inhaling breath radiates outward from the core of your being toward your extremities.
- Take several breaths to attune to this inward and outward flow of breath and energy, allowing you to naturally deepen your sense of centering.
- With your next exhalation, attune to the center of your pelvis, and as you inhale, visualize a circle of energy encompassing the area from your solar plexus to your buttocks.
- Take several breaths to experience this circle of energy nourishing your pelvis, abdomen and the base of your body while naturally deepening your sense of centering.
- With your next exhalation, concentrate energy at the core of your being, and as you inhale, visualize your circle expanding to encompass the area from your chest to your knees.
- Take several breaths to allow this expanding circle of energy to nourish your heart, lungs and organs of digestion completely.
- With your next exhaling breath, attune to the center of your pelvis, and as you inhale, allow your circle of energy to expand outward to encompass your entire body up to the crown of your head and down to the soles of your feet, including your upper extremities.
- Take several breaths to sense your circle of energy radiating outward from the center of your pelvis toward your extremities, and then inward to the core of your being, naturally deepening your sense of centering.
- With a deeper sense of centering, you naturally remain calm and serene in the depths of your being at all moments along your life journey.
- Affirm your centering as you repeat the following three times, aloud or silently: **"Centered in my being, I continue my journey with complete equanimity."**
- Slowly release the gesture, taking several breaths to rest within your center.
- When you are ready, open your eyes, returning slowly and gently, with a deeper sense of centering.

Annamaya kosha (physical body)

• Directs breath and awareness to the center of the pelvis, creating a massaging effect that releases muscular tension form the pelvic area.
• The massaging effect within the pelvis enhances circulation to the urinary and reproductive systems.
• Improves our sense of postural balance.
• The engagement of the pelvic muscles may be helpful for urinary incontinence.
• The centering effects of this gesture are generally helpful for Vata imbalance.
• The enhanced equanimity is generally helpful for Pitta imbalance.

Pranamaya kosha (energy body)

• Activates Apana vayu, the downward moving current of energy.
• Opens and balances the second chakra, center of self-nourishment.

Manomaya kosha (psycho-emotional body)

• Calms the mind.
• Cultivates emotional balance.

Vijnanamaya kosha (wisdom body)

• As we deepen our sense of centering, we naturally align with our true being, whose very essence is equanimity.

Anandamaya kosha (bliss body)

• As we rest in equanimity, a sense of fullness and wholeness arises natural.

13

Merudanda Mudra

Gesture of the Spine

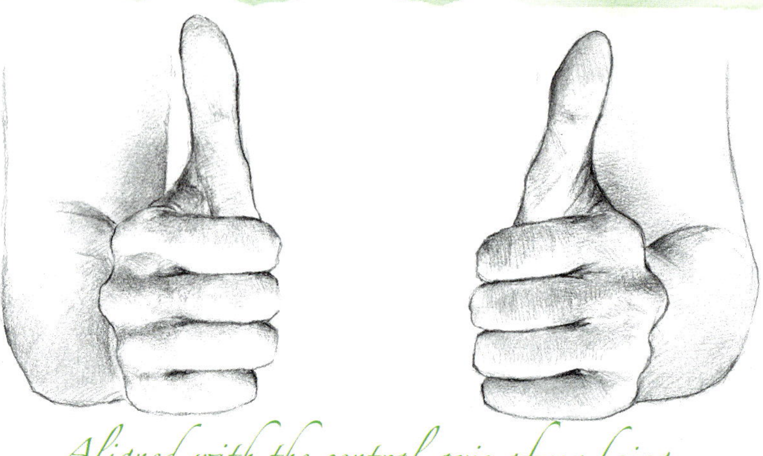

*Aligned with the central axis of my being,
I live with complete integrity.*

Core Quality
Alignment

Especially helpful for
- Aligning with our earth-sky axis of energy.
- Supporting alignment of the spine, creating optimal space for the functioning of all organs and systems.
- Integrating the material and spiritual aspects of our being.
- Cultivating an ideal balance of vitality and grounding.

Mudras with similar effects
Shivalingam, Shakata, Anudandi

Cautions
None

Instructions
1. Make your hands into fists with the thumbs to the outside.
2. Point the thumbs straight up, maintaining a gentle pressure of the fingernails into the palms.
3. Rest the hands on the thighs or knees.
4. Relax the shoulders back and down, with the spine naturally aligned.

Within Hindu mythology, ***Meru*** is a sacred mountain considered to be the center of the universe, and *danda* means "staff." *Merudanda* is therefore the central axis or staff along which all of creation is aligned and supported. Merudanda is also the name for "the spinal column," the central axis of support for our physical body. Merudanda mudra directs breath and awareness along the central channel of energy that runs through the center of the body from earth to sky. As it awakens awareness of our energetic axis, Merudanda mudra lengthens the spine, creating space between each of the vertebrae, facilitating optimal posture, which subsequently supports the functioning of all the systems of the body.

With a rating of six on the energy scale, Merudanda mudra is moderately energizing. This gesture instills optimism and vitality with each inhalation, and with each exhalation, it cultivates a greater sense of stability and grounding. This combination of vitality and grounding supports us in maintaining a balanced level of energy throughout all of our activities. As this gesture enhances awareness of the earth-sky axis, it balances the upward and downward moving currents of *Prana* and *Apana vayus.* Merudanda mudra also activates *Samana vayu*, the horizontal current, located at the solar plexus, where Prana and Apana vayus meet. The free flow of energy along the earth-sky axis nourishes and harmonizes the entire *chakra* system. At a psycho-emotional level, Merudanda mudra cultivates an enhanced sense of integrity in which thought, feeling, word and deed become a natural reflection of our deepest values and beliefs.

Systems Balanced:

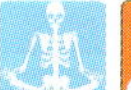 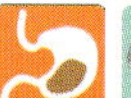 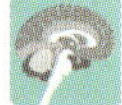

Prana Vayus Nourished:

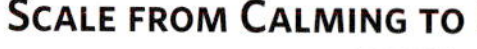

Elements Activated:

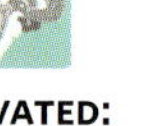   

Chakras Balanced:

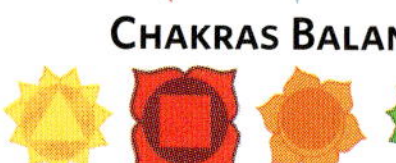 

Doshas Balanced:

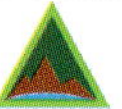

Scale from Calming to Energizing:

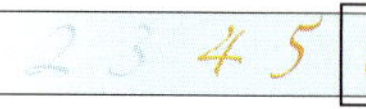 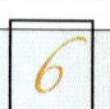 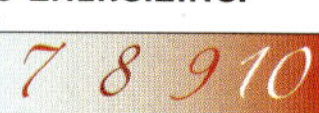

Guided Meditation: Aligning with your Earth-Sky Axis

ॐ As you hold Merudanda mudra, take several natural breaths to attune to all the feelings and sensations awakened by this gesture.

ॐ Sense each inhaling breath ascending from the base of your body to the crown of your head, instilling a feeling of uplifting energy.

ॐ Sense each exhaling breath descending smoothly from the crown of your head to the base of your body, cultivating relaxation and grounding.

ॐ Take some time to attune to your rhythmic breathing, sensing the earth-sky axis of energy that runs through the center of your being.

ॐ Begin by experiencing this axis of energy within your physical body. Notice how each inhalation lengthens and aligns your spine, while each exhalation allows its curves to relax naturally.

ॐ As your spine is aligned, take several breaths to sense how space is created for the nerve pathways to exit your spinal column more easily, nourishing your entire body.

ॐ As your physical body is aligned from earth to sky, you become more sensitive to the axis of energy within your subtle body.

ॐ With each inhalation, sense energy ascending along the subtle channel from the base of your body to the crown of your head.

ॐ With each exhaling breath, sense the energetic release from the crown of your head to the base of your body, dissolving all blockages in the flow of subtle energy.

ॐ Take several breaths to experience this flow along the earth-sky axis of energy, integrating and harmonizing your entire subtle anatomy.

ॐ With your physical and energetic dimensions aligned completely, you naturally experience integration and harmony within your psycho-emotional being.

ॐ As you breathe along your earth-sky axis, sense a natural integrity within your thoughts, feelings, words and deeds, allowing you to align with your deepest values and beliefs.

ॐ Attuned to the earth-sky axis, sense complete alignment at all levels of your being, allowing you to live in harmony at each moment along your journey.

ॐ Affirm your earth-sky alignment, repeating the following three times, aloud or silently: **"Aligned from earth to sky, I sense complete integration of body, breath and mind."**

ॐ Slowly release the gesture, taking several breaths to rest within your earth-sky axis.

ॐ When you are ready, open your eyes, returning slowly and gently, fully aligned at all levels of your being.

Annamaya kosha (physical body)

• Directs breath and awareness into the spinal column, naturally supporting correct alignment of the spine.
• The enhanced rhythmic movement of the breath in the abdomen and solar plexus creates a massaging effect that improves circulation to the digestive system.
• The energizing effects cultivated by this gesture are generally helpful for Kapha imbalance.

Pranamaya kosha (energy body)

• Balances the flow of Prana and Apana vayus while activating Samana vayu, the horizontal current of energy.
• Brings awareness to the entire chakra system, with a special focus on the third chakra, center of personal power.

Manomaya kosha (psycho-emotional body)

• Cultivates determination and willpower.
• Instills optimism and confidence.

Vijnanamaya kosha (wisdom body)

• Aligning with the earth-sky axis cultivates a natural sense of integrity, which is a reflection of the inherent authenticity of our true being.

Anandamaya kosha (bliss body)

• The free flow of breath and energy along the spine is accompanied by feelings of harmony and alignment with our source energy.

14 Urdhvam Merudanda Mudra

Gesture of the Upper Spine

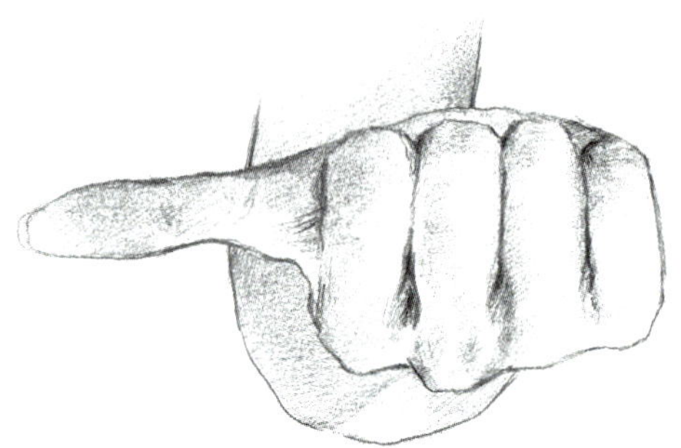
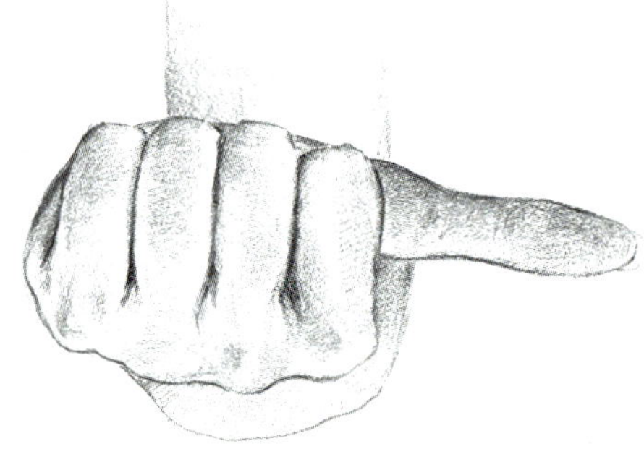

Openness to new ways of seeing
Allows me to live with enthusiasm and energy.

Core Quality

Expansiveness

Especially Helpful For

- Cultivating openness, optimism and enthusiasm, allowing us to widen our horizons.
- Releasing tension from the upper back, especially between the shoulder blades.
- Enhancing breath capacity, especially at the back of the lungs.

Mudras with Similar Effects

Kaleshvara, Purna Hridaya, Jyeshtha Sharira

Cautions

Because this mudra is energizing, monitor your condition if you have hypertension, heart disease or migraines.

Instructions

1. Curl the fingers into the palms of the hands, with the thumbs outside, maintaining a gentle pressure of the fingernails into the palms.
2. Rest the backs of the hands on the thighs or knees.
3. Straighten the thumbs and point them outward, away from each other.
4. Relax the shoulders back and down, with the spine naturally aligned.

Urdhvam means "upper" or "higher," and in this context, refers to the upper torso. *Merudanda* is the "spinal column." *Urdhvam Merudanda* refers to the upper portion of the torso and spinal column. Urdhvam Merudanda mudra directs breath, awareness and energy into the top of the chest, side ribs and upper back, expanding the rib cage and increasing breath capacity in the middle and upper lungs. This gesture helps to release tension from the area between the shoulder blades, creating space between the thoracic vertebrae, an area that can often chronically hold tension. This mudra also brings breath and energy to the uppermost part of the chest, enhancing circulation to the thymus gland.

With a rating of eight on the energy scale, Urdhvam Merudanda mudra is highly energizing, instilling a sense of enthusiasm, optimism and vitality. This gesture releases muscular constriction from the side ribs and upper back. This release of tension allows sensations and feelings held in the back of the body to come to the surface naturally. This mudra supports us in welcoming these sensations and feelings without judging or analyzing, allowing for their gradual release. Through this release, we experience a growing sense of enthusiasm along with the ability to expand our horizons and glimpse our infinite possibilities. Urdhvam Merudanda mudra also provides the energy and vitality to transform our new, more open vision into a lived reality.

Systems Balanced:

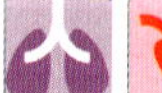

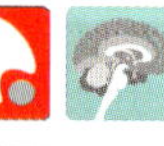
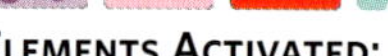

Elements Activated:

Doshas Balanced:

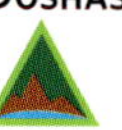

Prana Vayus Nourished:

Chakras Balanced:

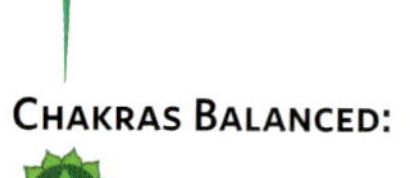

Scale from Calming to Energizing:

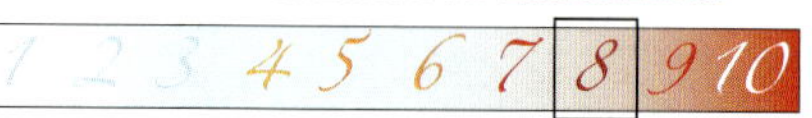

Guided Meditation: Expanding the Breath in the Back Body

- As you hold Urdhvam Merudanda mudra, take several natural breaths to attune to all the feelings and sensations awakened by this gesture.
- Notice how your breath is naturally directed into the top of your chest, side ribs and upper back, instilling a sense of expansiveness.
- Take several breaths to notice how each inhalation expands your rib cage horizontally, enhancing breath capacity while each exhalation allows your upper torso to soften and relax completely.
- As your rib cage expands and relaxes with your breathing, sense your shoulders widen away from each other with each inhalation and soften inward with each exhaling breath, naturally releasing tension from your upper back.
- As tension is released, space is created between your shoulder blades, allowing your breath to flow more freely throughout your entire upper body.
- As breath flows freely, you naturally attune more easily to any sensations arising in the back of your body.
- Take several breaths to welcome these sensations, allowing them to simply be, with no need to judge or analyze them in any way.
- As you breathe more freely, you may also notice emotions or feelings that come to the surface asking to be seen and released.
- By embracing all that arises in your back body, these sensations and feelings gradually soften and begin to dissolve with your breathing.
- With greater lightness and ease throughout your upper body, your entire rib cage expands naturally as if spreading your wings to perceive your own limitless possibilities.
- Take several breaths to glide freely, experiencing more open breathing and a sense of expansiveness throughout your entire being.
- Affirm expansiveness in your breath and being, repeating the following three times, aloud or silently: **"Breathing freely in the back of my body, I open to my infinite possibilities."**
- Now, slowly release the gesture, taking several breaths to rest in complete openness.
- When you are ready, open your eyes, returning slowly and gently, with a greater sense of expansiveness at all levels of your being.

Annamaya kosha (physical body)

• Expands the top of the chest, side ribs, and upper back, enhancing breath capacity in the upper lungs.
• Creates space between the shoulder blades and between the thoracic vertebrae, releasing tension from the upper back.
• The opening of the lungs and the energizing effects cultivated by this gesture are generally helpful for Kapha imbalance.

Pranamaya kosha (energy body)

• Activates Prana vayu, the upward moving current of energy.
• Opens and balances the heart chakra, center of unconditional love.

Manomaya kosha (psycho-emotional body)

• Instills a sense of openness.
• Enhances optimism and self-confidence.
• Cultivates vitality and energy.

Vijnanamaya kosha (wisdom body)

• As tension is released from the back body, we open to new possibilities, reflecting the essential limitlessness of our true being.

Anandamaya kosha (bliss body)

• As openness is created, sensations of limitlessness and freedom arise naturally from the back of the body.

Chapter Five

Awareness of the Dimensions of Being

MUDRAS FOR THE FIVE KOSHAS

The model of the *Koshas* from the *Taittiriya Upanishad* is a map of the human being that serves as a guide for the spiritual journey. *Kosha* can be translated as "sheath" or "layer," and refers to the multiple dimensions of our being, our five "bodies:" physical, energetic, psycho-emotional, wisdom and bliss. A less frequently used but equally important translation of the word kosha is "treasure," referring to all of the dimensions of our being as treasures waiting to be revealed. Each of the names of the koshas is followed by the word *maya*, which, in this context, means "consisting of."

1. Annamaya Kosha: Physical Body

Anna means "food," and the *Annamaya kosha* is the material dimension of our being that is sustained by food. It encompasses the anatomy and physiology of the body, as well as the five elements - earth, water, fire, air and space - that form the matrix of our body as well as all of creation. By deepening awareness of our physical being, the bodily systems and the five elements come into balance more easily. This balance lays a firm foundation for awakening and integrating the other dimensions of our being.

2. Pranamaya Kosha: Energy Body

Prana is the life force energy that permeates all of creation, including our bodies. The *Pranamaya kosha* is that aspect of our being composed of vital energy. The breath is a primary vehicle for receiving and distributing prana throughout our subtle anatomy, which includes the *chakras*, energy centers; the *prana vayus*, energy currents; and the *nadis*, energy channels. The free flow of prana is essential for the nourishment of the physical systems as well as for cultivating balance in the mind and emotions. Awakening the body of energy allows us to see that we are more than our physical body, thereby opening a doorway to the more subtle dimensions of our being.

3. Manomaya Kosha: Psycho-Emotional Body

Manas means "mind," and the *Manomaya kosha* is the psycho-emotional dimension of our being, made up of thoughts and feelings that compose the personality. This kosha tends to be one of the most challenging facets of our being because it is the field in which we experience the full range of feelings from happiness to suffering. As we embrace our psycho-emotional being without judging or rejecting our thoughts and feelings, we naturally live with greater lightness and ease.

4. Vijnanamaya Kosha: Wisdom Body

Vijnana means "higher wisdom," and the *Vijnanamaya kosha* is the dimension of our being that allows us to witness, understand and eventually release limiting beliefs. As these beliefs are released, patterns of thought and emotion associated with them dissolve naturally, allowing us to continue our journey with a greater sense of freedom and clarity.

5. Anandamaya Kosha: Bliss Body

Ananda means "bliss," and the *Anandamaya kosha* encompasses our inherent positive qualities, which unfold naturally as limiting beliefs are released. These essential qualities include equanimity, contentment, joy, limitlessness, wholeness and inner peace. The blissful experiences awakened during meditation and other spiritual practices are expressions of the Anandamaya kosha.

Brahman: The Destination of the Journey

The exploration and integration of the five koshas naturally leads us to the recognition of our own true being whose nature is freedom and unity. Within many Indian spiritual traditions, this all-pervading oneness is called *Brahman*. Brahman both encompasses and transcends all of the koshas.

Mudra	Kosha
Prithivi	Annamaya kosha - the physical body
Vittam	Pranamaya kosha - the energy body
Purna Hridaya	Manomaya kosha - the psycho-emotional body
Citta	Vijnanamaya kosha - the wisdom body
Hansi	Anandamaya kosha - the bliss body

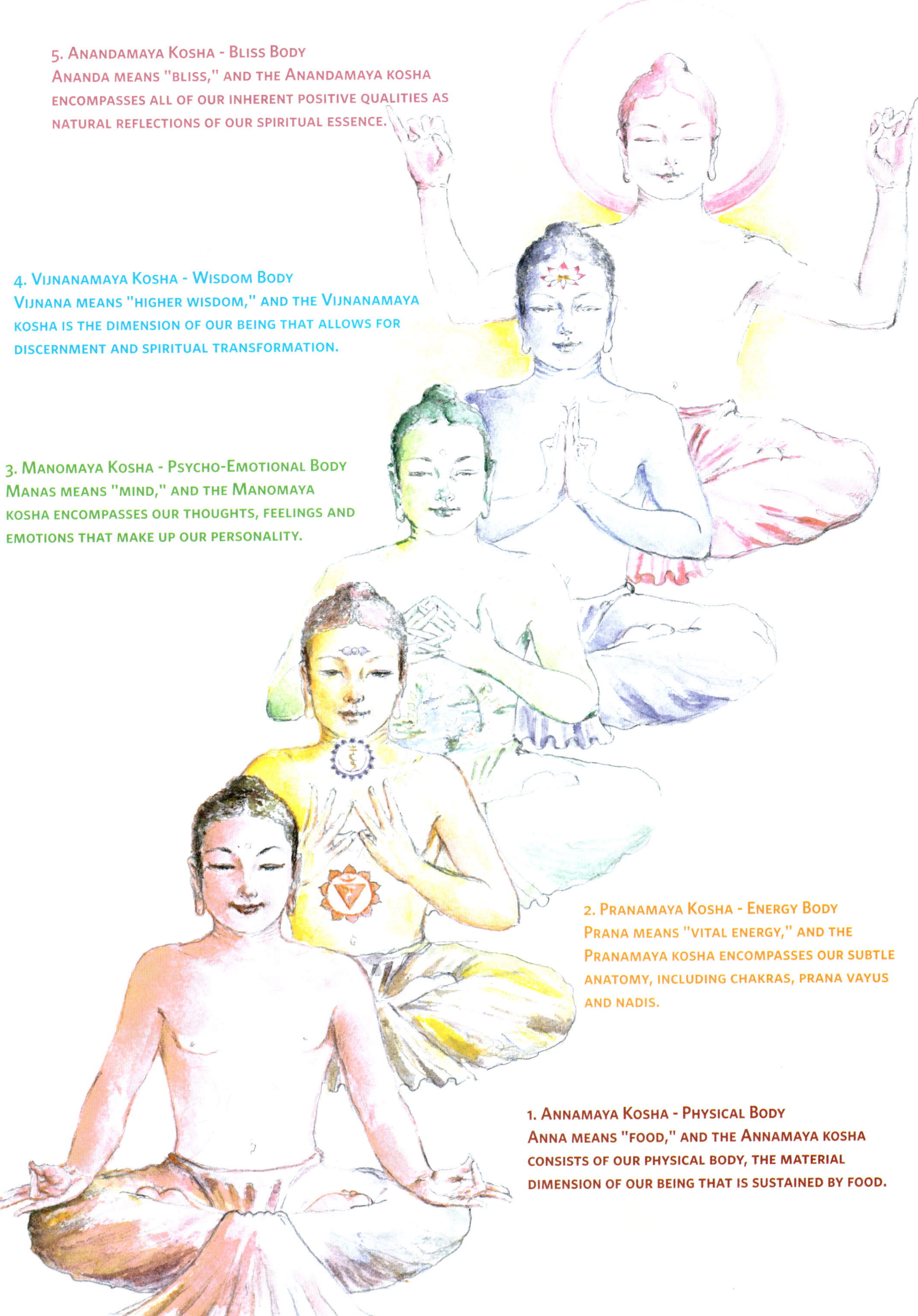
5. Anandamaya Kosha - Bliss Body
Ananda means "bliss," and the Anandamaya kosha encompasses all of our inherent positive qualities as natural reflections of our spiritual essence.
4. Vijnanamaya Kosha - Wisdom Body
Vijnana means "higher wisdom," and the Vijnanamaya kosha is the dimension of our being that allows for discernment and spiritual transformation.
3. Manomaya Kosha - Psycho-Emotional Body
Manas means "mind," and the Manomaya kosha encompasses our thoughts, feelings and emotions that make up our personality.
2. Pranamaya Kosha - Energy Body
Prana means "vital energy," and the Pranamaya kosha encompasses our subtle anatomy, including chakras, prana vayus and nadis.
1. Annamaya Kosha - Physical Body
Anna means "food," and the Annamaya kosha consists of our physical body, the material dimension of our being that is sustained by food.

15

Prithivi Mudra

Gesture of the Earth

For Annamaya Kosha - the Physical Body

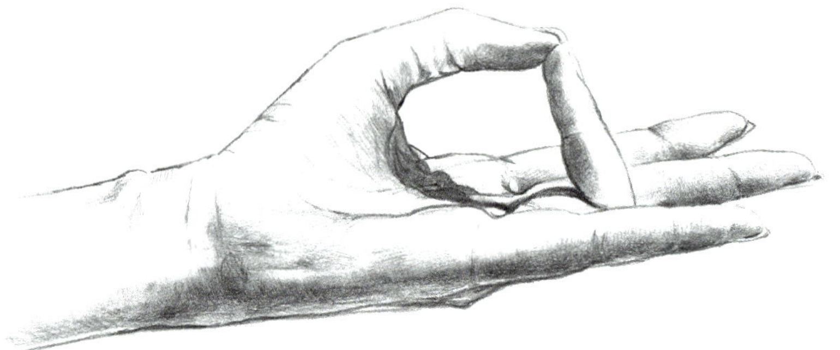

*Completely at home in my physical being,
I step forward in life confidently.*

Core Quality

Embodiment

Especially helpful for

- Enhancing embodiment.
- Supporting optimal posture.
- Reducing stress and blood pressure.
- Improving eliminatory health.
- Instilling a sense of security.

Mudras with similar effects

Bhu, Adhi, Rupa, Chinmaya

Cautions

None

Instructions

1. Touch the tips of the thumbs to the tips of the ring fingers of each hand while extending the other fingers straight out.
2. Rest the backs of the hands on the thighs or knees.
3. Relax the shoulders back and down, with the spine naturally aligned.

Anna means "food" or "matter," and the *Annamaya kosha* refers to the physical body, the dimension of our being that is nourished by food. This dimension includes our anatomy and physiology as well as the five elements that form the matrix of the body. A key to health and healing within our physical being is becoming completely present with our physical bodies. By cultivating embodiment, we naturally increase our sensitivity to the body's messages, helping us to perceive early signs of imbalance. Increased body awareness also gives us a greater sense of which dietary and lifestyle habits genuinely support our physical being. In addition, enhanced body awareness allows us to use our bodies with the least strain and maximum ease and efficiency, reducing the risk of injury. As we inhabit our bodies more fully, we develop greater respect for the intelligence that orchestrates its miraculous functioning. With greater presence and appreciation, self-love and self-care develop naturally, allowing us to live in complete harmony within our bodies.

Prithivi means "earth," and Prithivi mudra directs breath, awareness and energy down into the base of the body, cultivating a sense of grounding, stability and safety that allows us to inhabit our bodies more completely. This gesture deepens our connection with the natural world, instilling a sense of confidence and trust in our surroundings. This gesture also cultivates a greater sense of support within the structure of the physical body, making this an excellent gesture for the health of the skeletal system. The combination of grounding and embodiment, cultivated by this mudra, supports us in moving forward in life securely, laying a firm foundation for exploring and integrating our more subtle dimensions.

Systems Balanced:

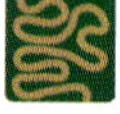

Elements Activated:

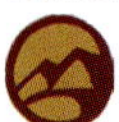

Doshas Balanced:

Prana Vayus Nourished:

Chakras Balanced:

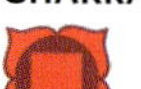

Scale from Calming to Energizing:

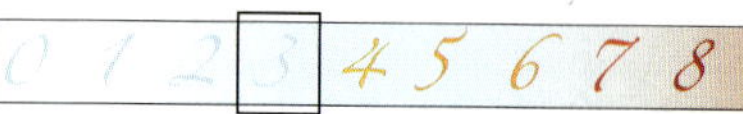

Guided Meditation: Coming Home to Your Body

ॐ As you hold Prithivi mudra, take several natural breaths to attune to all the feelings and sensations evoked by this gesture.

ॐ Notice how your breath is gently directed toward the base of your body, cultivating a sense of stability and grounding.

ॐ Sense how your exhalation is lengthened naturally, instilling a feeling of calm and tranquility that allows you to rest more comfortably within your physical body.

ॐ As you explore your body part by part, you naturally enhance your sensitivity to the contours, shape, volume and density of each area of your physical being.

ॐ Begin by bringing your awareness into your toes, feet and ankles, taking some time to become fully present in these areas of your body.

ॐ Now, focus your awareness into your lower legs and knees, sensing their contours, volume and density, taking several breaths to inhabit these areas completely.

ॐ Next, allow your awareness to rest in your thighs, becoming present to all sensations and feelings, allowing you to come home to this area of your being.

ॐ For your next few breaths, bring your awareness into your hips, pelvis and buttocks, experiencing greater grounding and stability as you sense the contact of these areas with the earth beneath.

ॐ Firmly grounded, direct your awareness into your abdomen, waist and low back, becoming more present within these areas of your being as you attune to their movement in synchrony with your rhythmic breathing.

ॐ For your next few breaths, direct awareness into your solar plexus and mid back, sensing the contours, volume and density, allowing you to fully inhabit the middle region of your body.

ॐ Now, bring your awareness into your chest, side ribs and upper back, taking several breaths to experience all sensations and feelings, allowing you to naturally come home to this area of your being.

ॐ Your awareness now encompasses your shoulders, arms, elbows and hands, taking all the time you need to become fully present in your upper extremities.

ॐ Now, fully inhabit your neck, throat and head, taking several breaths to sense your enhanced awareness within theses areas of your being, allowing them to soften and relax completely.

ॐ Complete your journey by inhabiting all the areas of your physical being simultaneously, sensing yourself completely at home within your body.

ॐ Inhabiting your entire body, repeat the following three times, aloud or silently: **"Fully present in my physical being, I experience complete ease and harmony."**

ॐ Slowly release the gesture, taking several breaths to experience complete embodiment.

ॐ When you are ready, open your eyes, returning slowly and gently, fully present within your physical body, the Annamaya kosha.

Annamaya kosha (Physical Body)

• Directs breath and awareness to the pelvic floor, releasing muscular tension and optimizing circulation to this area.
• Cultivates a sense of embodiment that allows us to become aware of the first signals of imbalance.
• Brings the breath into the base of the body and lengthens the exhalation, which is helpful for stress reduction and lowering blood pressure.
• Lengthens the spine, supporting optimal posture.
• The grounding and relaxing effects cultivated by this gesture are generally helpful for Vata imbalance.

Pranamaya kosha (Energy Body)

• Activates Apana vayu, the downward moving current of energy.
• Opens and balances the first chakra, center of safety.

Manomaya kosha (Psycho-Emotional Body)

• Facilitates a state of deep calm.
• Cultivates stability, continuity and patience.
• Enhances our trust in the support of the earth.

Vijnanamaya kosha (Wisdom Body)

• As we become more present within our physical being, we are able to deepen our exploration to the more subtle dimensions of our being.

Anandamaya kosha (Bliss Body)

• As we inhabit our bodies completely, an experience of oneness and unity arises naturally.

16 VITTAM MUDRA

Gesture of Vital Energy

For Pranamaya Kosha - the Energy Body

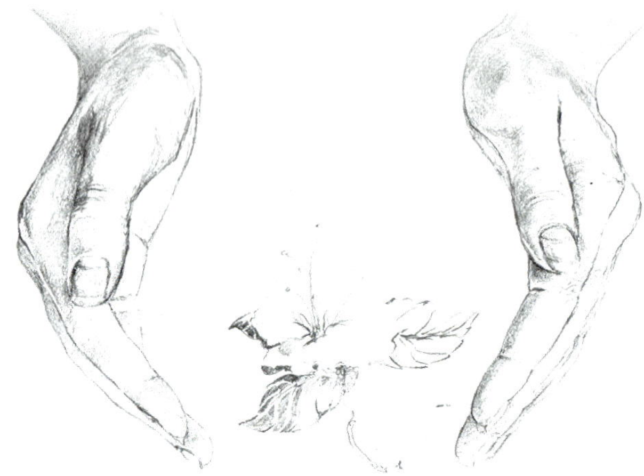

Attuned to the free flow of vital energy,
I move with the rhythms of life
Smoothly and easily.

CORE QUALITY
Free Flow of Vital Energy

ESPECIALLY HELPFUL FOR
- Reestablishing the free flow of subtle energy.
- Nourishing the reproductive and urinary systems.
- Relaxing the lower back.
- Awakening vitality.

MUDRAS WITH SIMILAR EFFECTS
Svadhisthana, Shakti, Mira, Yoni

CAUTIONS
None

INSTRUCTIONS
1. Hold the hands slightly cupped in front of the lower abdomen with the palms facing each other about twelve inches apart.
2. Allow the hands to naturally expand away from each other on the inhalation and to rest gently back toward each other on the exhalation.
3. Relax the shoulders back and down, with the spine naturally aligned.

Prana is the "life force energy" that sustains all of creation, including our physical bodies. The *Pranamaya kosha* is our dimension of vital energy, the manifestation of the life force within our own being. It encompasses the three facets of our subtle anatomy: the *chakras*, energy centers; the *prana vayus*, energy currents; and the *nadis*, energy channels. The health of our subtle anatomy depends on the quantity and quality of the life force energy we receive, as well as the extent to which it flows freely. We receive prana in the form of fresh air and water; fresh, natural food; natural surroundings and sunlight. The health of our subtle anatomy is also influenced by our environment and interactions. For this reason, regular participation in spiritual activities is recommended. The breath is our most essential source of prana; the way we breathe affects the quantity and quality of prana and, subsequently, our overall health and vitality. Mudra practice directs prana to specific areas of the body, releasing energetic blockages and reestablishing the free flow of prana to both our subtle and physical anatomy.

Vittam means "vital energy," and Vittam mudra directs breath, awareness and energy into the pelvis and abdomen. As we deepen our awareness of these areas, we experience them as an inner spring of vitality whose energy can be channeled throughout our entire being as a vehicle for health, healing and awakening. Vittam mudra activates the qualities of the water element, including fluidity and flexibility, supporting the free flow of vital energy within both the subtle and the physical bodies. The rhythmic abdominal breathing cultivated by this gesture, together with the activation of the water element, support the health of the reproductive and urinary systems.

SYSTEMS BALANCED:

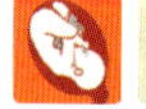 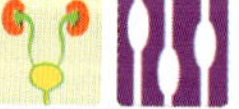

ELEMENTS ACTIVATED:

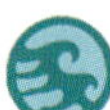

DOSHAS BALANCED:

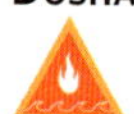 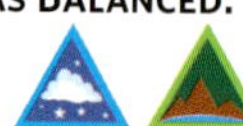

PRANA VAYUS NOURISHED

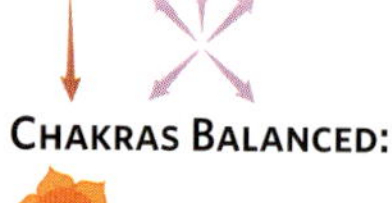

CHAKRAS BALANCED:

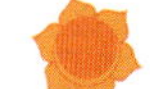

SCALE FROM CALMING TO ENERGIZING:

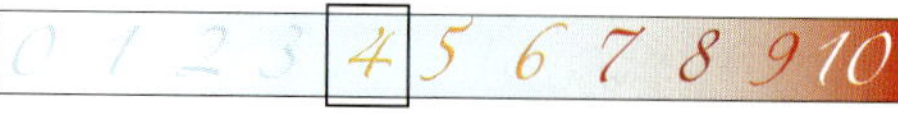

Guided Meditation: Expanding Vital Energy

- ॐ As you hold Vittam mudra, take several natural breaths to attune to all the feelings and sensations awakened by this gesture.
- ॐ Notice how your breath is gently directed into your pelvis and abdomen, allowing you to experience this area of your being as an inner spring of vital energy.
- ॐ Take several breaths to sense how your abdomen rises and falls in synchrony with your breathing, naturally deepening your connection to your own inner spring.
- ॐ Experience your hands as an extension of your rhythmic breathing, expanding away from each other with each inhalation, and softening toward each other with each exhaling breath.
- ॐ As your hands, breath and abdomen move in synchrony, take some time to sense vibrant energy awakening within your inner spring.
- ॐ As this energy expands naturally, you are able to channel it into each area of your being, reestablishing the free flow of prana, the life force energy, optimizing your level of health and vitality.
- ॐ As you inhale, rest your awareness within your inner spring, and as you exhale, channel prana down into your legs and feet, nourishing these areas with vital energy.
- ॐ Take several breaths to sense your legs and feet expanding and softening energetically in synchrony with your abdominal breathing.
- ॐ Now, with your next inhaling breath, return to the comfort of your inner spring, and as you exhale, sense vital energy infusing your buttocks and lower back completely.
- ॐ Sense these areas pulsing in synchrony with your rhythmic breathing, allowing them to be nourished with vital energy.
- ॐ Now, as you inhale, return to your inner spring, and with your exhaling breath, allow prana to naturally infuse your solar plexus, chest, mid and upper back.
- ॐ Experience these areas expanding and releasing in synchrony with your rhythmic abdominal breathing, bathing them with vital energy.
- ॐ With your legs and torso nourished completely, now allow the life force energy to be channelled into your shoulders, arms and hands, filling your upper extremities.
- ॐ Take several natural breaths to sense these areas expanding and releasing in synchrony with your rhythmic breathing, infusing them with vital energy.
- ॐ Now, with your next inhalation, return to the vitality of your inner spring, and as you exhale, allow your neck and head to be bathed in life force energy.
- ॐ Experience these areas gently expanding and releasing in synchrony with your rhythmic breathing, nourishing them with prana.
- ॐ Now, take some time to allow the life force energy to radiate outward from your inner spring, sensing your entire being expanding and softening energetically in synchrony with your rhythmic breathing.
- ॐ Attuned to your energetic body, repeat the following three times, aloud or silently: **"As life force energy flows freely throughout my being, I experience optimal vitality."**
- ॐ Release the gesture, taking several breaths to experience energetic nourishment.
- ॐ When you are ready, open your eyes, returning slowly and gently, with your body of energy, the Pranamaya kosha, nourished completely.

Annamaya kosha (physical body)

• Directs breath and awareness into the pelvic and abdominal areas, creating a massaging effect that improves circulation to the reproductive and urinary systems.
• The enhanced abdominal breathing gently massages the lower back, releasing tension and tightness.
• The abdominal breathing supports the return of venous blood and lymphatic fluid from the lower extremities.
• The enhanced vital energy cultivated by this gesture is generally helpful for Kapha imbalance.
• The centering is generally helpful for Vata imbalance.
• The enhanced connection to subtle energy is generally helpful for Pitta imbalance.

Pranamaya kosha (energy body)

• Activates Apana vayu, the downward moving current of energy, as well as Vyana vayu, the all-pervading energy, moving from center to extremities.
• Opens and balances the second chakra, center of self-nourishment.

Manomaya kosha (psycho-emotional body)

• Instills a sense of fluidity and adaptability.
• Cultivates emotional balance.

Vijnanamaya kosha (wisdom body)

• Awareness of the energy body helps us to loosen rigid identification with the personality.

Anandamaya kosha (bliss body)

• As prana flows more freely, we experience a deepening connection with the subtle realms of our being.

17

Purna Hridaya Mudra

Gesture of the Open Heart

For Manomaya Kosha - the Psycho-Emotional Body

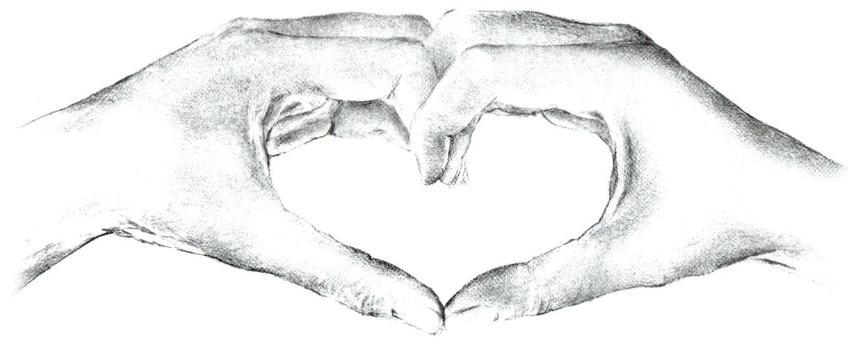

Through welcoming thoughts and feelings,
I fully embrace my psycho-emotional being.

Core Quality

Honoring Thoughts and Feelings

Especially helpful for

- Becoming comfortable with our psycho-emotional being.
- Releasing muscular constriction from the chest.
- Improving breath capacity.
- Enhancing immunity.
- Supporting treatment of depression.

Mudras with similar effects

Medha Prana Kriya, Tarjani, Urdhvam Merudanda, Vajrapradama

Cautions

None

Instructions

1. Hold the hands in front of the heart with the palms facing each other and the fingertips pointing upward.
2. Interlace the fingers inward so that they cross at the upper segment, with the right index finger closest to the heart.
3. Stretch the thumbs downward to touch at their tips so that a heart shape is formed.
4. Relax the shoulders back and down, with the elbows held away from the body and the spine naturally aligned.

Manas means "mind," and the *Manomaya kosha* is our psycho-emotional being, encompassing our thoughts and feelings. This dimension is often challenging, as it is the field in which we seek happiness and also experience suffering. It is natural to move toward that which we believe will make us happy and avoid that which causes suffering. This approach to living, however, creates a never ending cycle of loss and gain, happiness and pain, in which lasting contentment is elusive. The ultimate solution to psycho-emotional suffering is spiritual freedom. Recognizing our inherent freedom, however, is a lifetime journey, and one of the first steps is welcoming our thoughts and feelings as integral facets of our being. As we embrace our psycho-emotional being without identifying with it so completely, we come to see that the mind is not our "enemy," but a vehicle for creating trust and security as a foundation for gradually opening to the love that is the essence of our true being.

Purna means "full," and *hridaya* means "heart." Purna Hridaya mudra supports the opening of our subtle heart by expanding the breath in the chest, side ribs and upper back, expanding breath capacity. The heart-opening cultivated by this gesture enhances our ability to embrace thoughts and feelings, welcoming them more easily. The rhythmic flow of the breath cultivated by this gesture creates a point of focus for the mind to rest, allowing us to explore our psycho-emotional dimension more easily. Purna Hridaya mudra lengthens the inhaling breath, instilling a feeling of uplifting energy, cultivating energy and vitality that supports us in welcoming feelings. It also lengthens the exhaling breath, allowing us to release tension from the heart center.

Systems Balanced:

 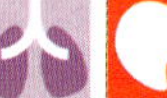 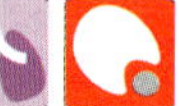

Elements Activated:

Doshas Balanced:

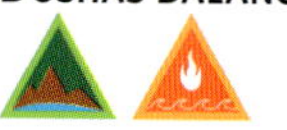

Prana Vayus Nourished:

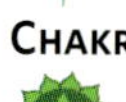

Chakras Balanced:

Scale from Calming to Energizing:

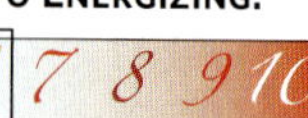

Guided Meditation: Riding the Wave of Feeling

- As you hold Purna Hridaya mudra, take several natural breaths to attune to all the feelings and sensations awakened by this gesture.
- With each inhalation, sense your rib cage expanding evenly, and with each exhalation, your chest, side ribs and upper back soften and relax completely.
- As your rib cage expands and softens with your breath, take some time to sense a growing openness within your heart center.
- As your heart center opens gradually, you embrace your psycho-emotional being more easily, welcoming thoughts and feelings, allowing them to arise and pass away freely.
- Begin by allowing a positive thought to arise while experiencing the feeling that naturally accompanies it.
- Allow this feeling to simply be, and as you embrace it without resistance, you will begin to sense it as a wave of pure energy that you ride easily in synchrony with your breathing.
- With each inhaling breath, you ride this feeling to its crest, and with each exhalation, you experience greater ease and release throughout your psycho-emotional being.
- As you ride your wave of positive feeling with greater ease, take several breaths to sense how your heart center is nourished with vital energy.
- As your heart opens more completely, you gradually develop the ability to welcome even challenging thoughts and feelings as waves of pure energy.
- To deepen this ability, invite a difficult thought to arise within your being, experiencing the feeling that accompanies it naturally.
- Take all the time you need to sense this challenging feeling as a wave of pure energy that you ride together with your breathing.
- With each inhaling breath, welcome any tension or resistance that arises, and with each exhalation, allow this tension to be released, riding your wave of feeling with greater lightness and ease.
- As you ride this wave of feeling with greater ease, take several breaths to sense how your heart center is naturally filled with serenity and peace.
- As your heart center is bathed in serenity, you naturally embrace your psycho-emotional being more easily and completely.
- Affirm your growing ease as you repeat the following three times, aloud or silently: **"Riding my wave of feeling, I sense greater ease in my psycho-emotional being."**
- Now, slowly release the gesture, taking several breaths to rest in the ease that arises through riding waves of feeling as pure energy.
- When you are ready, open your eyes, returning slowly and gently, more at ease within the Manomaya kosha, your psycho-emotional body.

Annamaya kosha (Physical body)

• Directs breath and awareness to the chest, side ribs and upper back, releasing tension and optimizing respiration.
• Directs breath and awareness to the upper sternum, increasing circulation to the area of the thymus gland.
• The mildly energizing effects and the expansion of the lungs cultivated by this gesture are generally helpful for Kapha imbalance.
• The heart-opening is generally helpful for Pitta imbalance.

Pranamaya kosha (Energy body)

• Activates Prana vayu, the upward moving current of energy.
• Opens and balances the fourth chakra, center of unconditional love.

Manomaya kosha (Psycho-emotional body)

• Calms the mind and creates space between thoughts.
• Instills compassion and self-acceptance.

Vijnanamaya kosha (Wisdom body)

• Through welcoming thoughts and emotions, they lose their heavy and dense quality, allowing us to witness them as waves of pure energy.

Anandamaya kosha (Bliss body)

• As we gain the ability to welcome and embrace thoughts and feelings, a sense of joy and radiance arise from deep within the heart.

18

Citta Mudra

Gesture of Witness Consciousness

For Vijnanamaya Kosha - the Wisdom Body

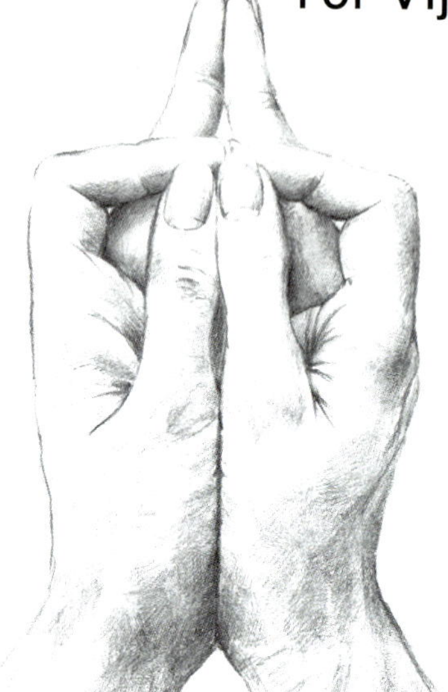

Through the gradual release of limiting beliefs, I continue my journey with greater clarity.

Core Quality

Awakening the Inner Witness

Especially helpful for

- Releasing limiting beliefs through witnessing.
- Releasing tension from the shoulders and neck.
- Improving mental clarity.

Mudras with similar effects

Uttarabodhi, Kali, Trishula, Jnana

Cautions

None

Instructions

1. Touch the pads of the index fingers to the tips of the thumbs of the same hand and extend the other fingers straight out.
2. Bring the hands together in front of the chest, slightly away from the body, with the pads of the middle, ring and little fingers touching the same fingers of the opposite hand.
3. The thumbs touch along their length, and the tips of the index fingers touch each other, forming a line parallel to the earth.
4. Relax the shoulders back and down, with the elbows held away from the body and the spine naturally aligned.

Vijnana means "higher wisdom," and the *Vijnanamaya kosha* is the dimension of our being that allows us to witness, honor and gradually release limiting beliefs. At the level of the *Manomaya* kosha, we learn to welcome our thoughts and feelings without resisting or judging. At the level of the Vijnanamaya kosha, we recognize that our challenging thoughts and feelings are reflections of deep conditioning in the form of limiting beliefs. By awakening the inner witness, we are able to observe these beliefs without identifying with them so completely. When seen more clearly, these beliefs lose their power to draw us into their "stories," and are gradually released. As we deepen our power of witnessing, we align with our true being more completely, allowing us to live with greater freedom and clarity.

Citta means "consciousness," and Citta mudra supports the awakening of witness consciousness in which thoughts, feelings and limiting beliefs are seen more clearly, without identifying with them so completely. This gesture directs breath, awareness and energy into the neck and head, with a special focus on the third eye point, our center of wisdom and clarity. As Citta mudra facilitates one-pointed concentration, it cultivates greater objectivity in which limiting beliefs can be seen and released more easily. The two eyes formed by the index fingers and thumbs represent our "eyes of clear seeing," symbolizing our ability to discern the true Self from the limited personality. The triangle formed by this mudra represents the harmony of body, mind and spirit that supports witnessing.

Systems Balanced:

 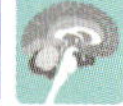

Elements Activated:

Doshas Balanced:

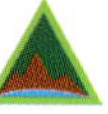

Prana Vayus Nourished:

Chakras Balanced:

Scale from Calming to Energizing:

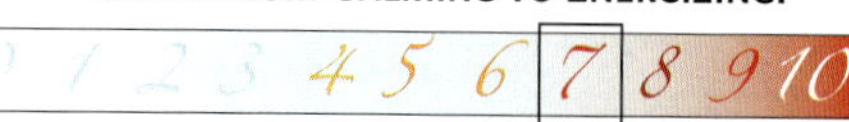

Guided Meditation: Awakening the Inner Witness

- As you hold Citta mudra, take several natural breaths to attune to all the feelings and sensations awakened by this gesture.
- Notice how your breath is gently directed into your upper chest, neck and head, instilling a sense of expansiveness.
- As you experience greater expansiveness, your awareness naturally rests at the third eye, your center of wisdom.
- As you attune to your center of wisdom, your inner witness awakens naturally, expanding your ability to see all that occurs in your mind and body with objectivity and clarity.
- To enhance your power of witnessing, take several breaths to envision a screen in front of your forehead on which thoughts, feelings, images and memories arise naturally.
- Begin by visualizing on your screen a time and place when you were very happy, noticing all the details of this scene while remaining the witness of everything you see.
- Emotions may arise along with these images; take several breaths to experience these feelings without identifying with them so closely.
- As you develop your ability to witness without identifying, notice how greater objectivity and clarity arise naturally.
- Now, allow images to arise on your screen of a time and place that was challenging, taking several breaths to choose an event that you feel comfortable exploring.
- As images related to this challenging time are projected onto your screen, allow all accompanying feelings to arise naturally without identifying with them so completely.
- As you deepen your ability to be present with these images and feelings without resisting, take several breaths to sense how any heaviness or density begins to dissolve naturally.
- As you experience greater lightness and ease , take some time to notice how greater objectivity and clarity arise naturally.
- Now, observe both the happy and challenging scenes on your screen simultaneously, taking several breaths to deepen your power of witnessing.
- As you hold both scenes, you recognize that you are neither the images on the screen nor their accompanying feelings, but the conscious presence that witnesses all that arises within your mind and body.
- Take several breaths to rest in witness consciousness, experiencing the inner silence, wisdom and clarity that unfold naturally through deepening your power of witnessing.
- Affirm the power of witnessing as you repeat the following three times, aloud or silently: **"I am the conscious presence that witnesses all that arises in the mind and body."**
- Slowly release the gesture, taking several breaths to rest within your inner witness.
- When you are ready, open your eyes, returning slowly and gently, more aligned with the Vijnanamaya kosha, your body of wisdom.

Annamaya kosha (physical body)

- **Directs breath and awareness to the neck and head, relaxing the muscles of the face while allowing the senses to rest.**
- **Releases tension from the shoulders, throat and vocal cords.**
- **Brings breath and awareness to the area of the pituitary gland.**
- **The energizing effects cultivated by this gesture are generally helpful for Kapha imbalance.**

Pranamaya kosha (energy body)

- **Activates Udana vayu, the uppermost current of energy.**
- **Opens and balances the sixth chakra, center of wisdom.**

Manomaya kosha (psycho-emotional body)

- **Creates space between thoughts, facilitating the process of witnessing.**

Vijnanamaya kosha (wisdom body)

- **Through awakening the inner witness, limiting beliefs are released, allowing us to discern between the true Self and the everyday personality more clearly.**

Anandamaya kosha (bliss body)

- **With greater clarity, a sense of freedom arises naturally.**

19

Hansi Mudra

Gesture of the Inner Smile

For Anandamaya Kosha - the Bliss Body

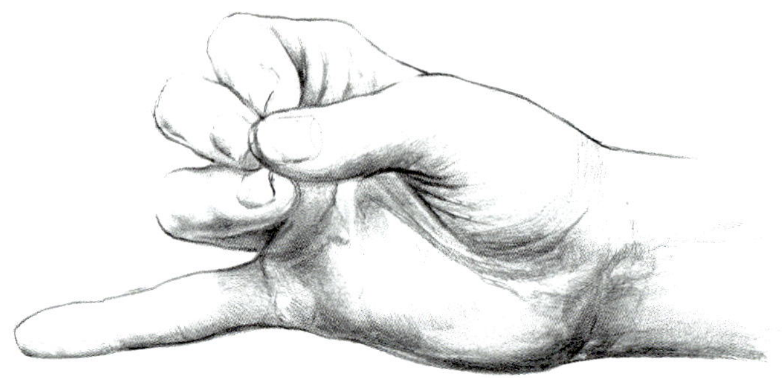

An inner smile radiates throughout my being,
Awakening all of my essential positive qualities

Core Quality

Unfolding Positive Qualities

Especially Helpful For

- Revealing our inherent positive qualities.
- Releasing tension from the jaw, which may be helpful for TMJ dysfunction.
- Enhancing immunity.

Mudras with Similar Effects

Bhairava, Ananta, Mandala, Bhramara

Cautions

None

Instructions

1. Touch the tips of the index, middle, and ring fingers to the tips of the thumbs of the same hand.
2. Extend the little fingers straight out.
3. Rest the backs of the hands on the thighs or knees.
4. Alternatively, the hands may be held out to the sides of the body, with the little fingers pointing upward.
5. Relax your shoulders back and down, with the spine naturally aligned.

Ananda means "bliss," and the *Anandamaya kosha*, the body of bliss, encompasses all of the inherent positive qualities of our true being that unfold as limiting beliefs are released. As we align with the clarity of our true being, we tap into a spring of wisdom and understanding from which joy, wholeness, limitlessness and bliss unfold naturally. Our dimension of bliss is closely related to spiritual freedom, but it is not yet complete liberation because these experiences may still be temporary. There is also the possibility of becoming attached to experiences of bliss, which becomes an obstacle to complete freedom. Meditation, especially when supported by the practice of mudras, allows these essential positive qualities to blossom naturally. We begin by cultivating these qualities consciously, and eventually come to see them as reflections of our true being.

Hansi refers to "smiling" or "laughter," and Hansi mudra directs breath, awareness and energy into the upper chest, neck and head, cultivating an experience of joy and lightness. This gesture brings a smile to our lips and as this smile spreads throughout our being, it naturally supports the awakening of all our inherent positive qualities. This mudra enhances circulation to the thymus gland in the upper sternum, supporting the health of the immune system. Hansi mudra also stimulates the release of endorphins and instills a sense of optimism.

Systems Balanced:

 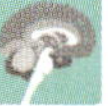 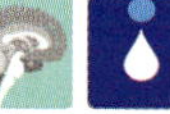

Elements Activated:

Doshas Balanced:

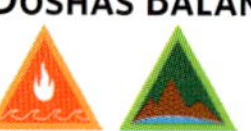

Prana Vayus Nourished:

Chakras Balanced:

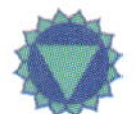 

Scale from Calming to Energizing:

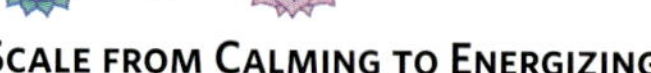

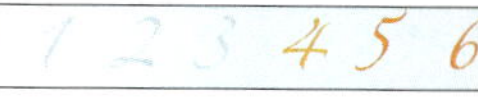

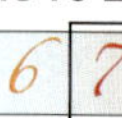

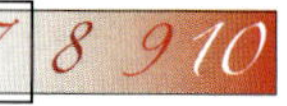

Guided Meditation: Awakening Your Essential Positive Qualities

- As you hold Hansi mudra, take several natural breaths to attune to all the feelings and sensations awakened by this gesture.
- Notice how your breath is gently directed into your upper chest, neck and head, naturally instilling a sense of joy and happiness.
- As joy and happiness permeate your being, a soft smile spreads across your face naturally.
- Take several breaths to allow this smile to gradually infuse your entire being, from the crown of your head to your feet.
- As you sense your entire being smiling radiantly, all of your essential positive qualities are awakened naturally.
- Begin by awakening the quality of joyfulness, taking several breaths to sense uplifting energy spreading throughout your being, a feeling that every moment of life is worth living fully and completely.
- As joyfulness permeates your being, you naturally awaken the quality of appreciation of beauty, experiencing awe and wonder in everything you see, especially the small details of daily living.
- Living joyfully and with appreciation of beauty, you naturally awaken the quality of communion, a sense of oneness with all beings that allows you to live with inner and outer harmony.
- As you integrate joy, appreciation and communion, you naturally awaken to your inherent wholeness, a knowing that you are absolutely complete and nothing can be added or subtracted from your essential being.
- Aligned with your inherent wholeness, you turn inward naturally to rest in the silence of your true being, awakening the wisdom that guides you at each step of your journey.
- Within this space of sacred silence, you naturally experience your essential bliss, taking several breaths to bathe in your inherent radiance.
- Affirm your essential qualities, repeating the following three times, aloud or silently: **"My inner smile serves as a key for awakening all my inherent positive qualities."**
- Slowly release the gesture, taking several breaths to rest in your blissful essence.
- When you are ready, open your eyes, returning slowly and gently, more deeply aligned with the Anandamaya kosha, your bliss body.

Annamaya kosha (physical body)

• Directs breath and awareness to the area of the thymus gland.
• The enhanced positive mood supports the health of the immune system.
• Releases tension from the jaw, which may be helpful for TMJ dysfunction.
• The lightness cultivated by this gesture is generally helpful for Kapha imbalance.
• The joy cultivated is generally helpful for Pitta imbalance.

Pranamaya kosha (energy body)

• Activates Udana vayu, the uppermost current of energy.
• Opens and balances the fifth, sixth and seventh chakras, centers of spiritual purification, wisdom and unity.

Manomaya kosha (psycho-emotional body)

• Cultivates positive emotions, including contentment, lightness and joy.

Vijnanamaya kosha (wisdom body)

• As we become aware that positive qualities arise from within us, we naturally strengthen our connection to our true Self.

Anandamaya kosha (bliss body)

• As the inner smile is awakened, feelings of bliss and limitlessness naturally arise.

Chapter Six

Keys to Health and Healing

MUDRAS FOR HEALTH CHALLENGES

The word health is derived from the Old English *haelp*, meaning "whole," and is also related to the Old Norse *helge*, meaning "holy" or "sacred." [2] These root words convey the essence of health as wholeness at all levels of being, which occurs through reconnection with our spiritual essence. From this perspective, health and healing are a reflection of our journey toward wholeness and spiritual awakening. The five koshas are a model of the whole person that serve as a road map for this journey. Mudras are an important vehicle for supporting the journey of health, healing and awakening within all the dimensions of our being.

Physical Dimension - Annamaya Kosha

Mudras support health and healing within our physical being through their ability to direct breath, awareness and energy into specific areas of the body. As body awareness is increased, we are able to recognize and respond to the body's messages of balance or imbalance more easily. Directing the breath to particular areas of the body also creates a massaging effect that enhances circulation, supporting optimal nutrition and elimination. For example, Brahma mudra directs breath and awareness into the solar plexus, expanding the breath and creating a powerful massaging effect for the entire abdominal area, optimizing circulation to the digestive system.

The ability of mudras to direct the breath makes them an important support for cultivating optimal health. As we practice mudras, the gestures themselves take charge of the breath, changing the speed, focus, quality and location of our breathing almost instantly, allowing for beneficial changes to occur naturally within our physiology. For example, Adhi mudra slows the breath dramatically, thereby activating the relaxation response, reducing heart rate and blood pressure.

Another way that mudras support the health of the body is by balancing the five elements that make up our physical being. There are specific mudras for balancing each of the five elements, which can be used to restore equilibrium within the physical body. For example, Rupa mudra activates the earth element, with its qualities of strength and stability, making it useful for supporting the health of the skeletal system.

Mudra	Health Condition	Core Quality
20 Rupa	Osteoporosis & Health of the Skeletal System	Healthy Skeletal System
21 Anudandi	Back Pain & Health of the Spine	Back Pain Relief
22 Matsya	Osteoarthritis & Health of the Joints	Healthy Joints
23 Apanayana	IBS & Health of the Elimi-natory System	Balanced Elimination
24 Varuna	Cystitis & Health of the Urinary System	Healthy Urinary System
25 Yoni	PMS & Female Reproductive System	Female Reproduc-tive Health
26 Shankha	Prostate & Male Reproductive System	Male Reproductive Health
27 Trimurti	Menopause & Life Transi-tions	Harmonious Life Transitions
28 Pushan	Health of the Digestive System	Balanced Digestion
29 Brahma	Weight Management, Energy & Vitality	Awakening Energy and Vitality
30 Mira	Asthma & Health of the Respiratory System	Easeful Breathing
31 Vayan	Hypertension & Cardio-vascular Health	Optimal Circulation
32 Apana Vayu	Health of the Heart	Healthy Heart
33 Mahashirsha	Headache & Tension Relief	Headache Relief
34 Garuda	Thyroid & Health of the Endocrine System	Balanced Metabolism
35 Vajrapradama	Depression	Enthusiasm for Living
36 Pala	Anxiety	Anxiety Relief
37 Vyana Vayu	MS & Health of the Ner-vous System	Healthy Nervous System
38 Bhramara	Allergies & Health of the Immune System	Healthy Immunity
39 Mani Ratna	Integral Healing	Global Healing

Energy Dimension - Pranamaya Kosha

Within our energetic dimension, mudras deepen our sensitivity to the flow of energy throughout our subtle anatomy. Through this enhanced awareness, energy blockages can be sensed and released, thereby reestablishing the free flow of subtle energy. As energy flows more freely, the systems of our physical body are nourished more completely. There are specific mudras for balancing each component of our energetic anatomy, which includes the *chakras*, *prana vayus* and *nadis*. Through the use of mudras, we are able to channel energy to each component of our subtle anatomy, allowing us to reestablish energetic balance in the specific area where it is needed. For example, Svadhisthana mudra directs breath, awareness and energy to the pelvis, enhancing the flow of *Apana vayu* while balancing the second chakra. The reestablishment of energetic balance in the pelvis supports the health of the reproductive, urinary and eliminatory systems.

Psycho-Emotional Dimension - Manomaya Kosha

Mudras work with the mind and emotions in a number of important ways. Many of the gestures, such as Pala mudra, are calming and relaxing, thereby supporting stress reduction. Others, such as Rupa, instill a sense of stability and grounding that help relieve anxiety. Some gestures, such as Vajrapradama mudra, cultivate a sense of confidence and enthusiasm, which can support the treatment of depression. Gestures, such as Trimurti mudra, are centering, cultivating a sense of equanimity that helps us to move through life transitions more easily. Heart-opening gestures, such as Apana Vayu mudra, support us in welcoming and honoring our psycho-emotional being, which supports the release of tension and therefore contributes to overall health and healing.

Wisdom Dimension - Vijnanamaya Kosha

The wisdom body is the dimension of our being that allows us to grow and transform spiritually. Wisdom arises through awakening our inner witness, allowing us to perceive our limiting beliefs without identifying with them so completely. With the gradual release of these beliefs, we cultivate greater ease at the level of our thoughts and feelings, which subsequently allows energy to flow more freely within the subtle body. As energy flows more freely, our physical systems are nourished energetically, supporting their optimal functioning. Mudras play an important role in awakening the wisdom body. Gestures, such as Apana Vayu, cultivate sensitivity and inner listening to our own source of wisdom and guidance. Mudras, such as Garuda, open the throat chakra, creating space in which core beliefs can be seen and gradually released.

Bliss Dimension - Anandamaya Kosha

As limiting beliefs are released, space is created for revealing the inherent positive qualities that compose our body of bliss. Mudra practice supports us in awakening these qualities, including unconditional love, wholeness and limitlessness. Mudras, such as Mani Ratna, awaken us to our essential unity, which integrates all of these qualities, cultivating an experience of healing within all dimensions of our being.

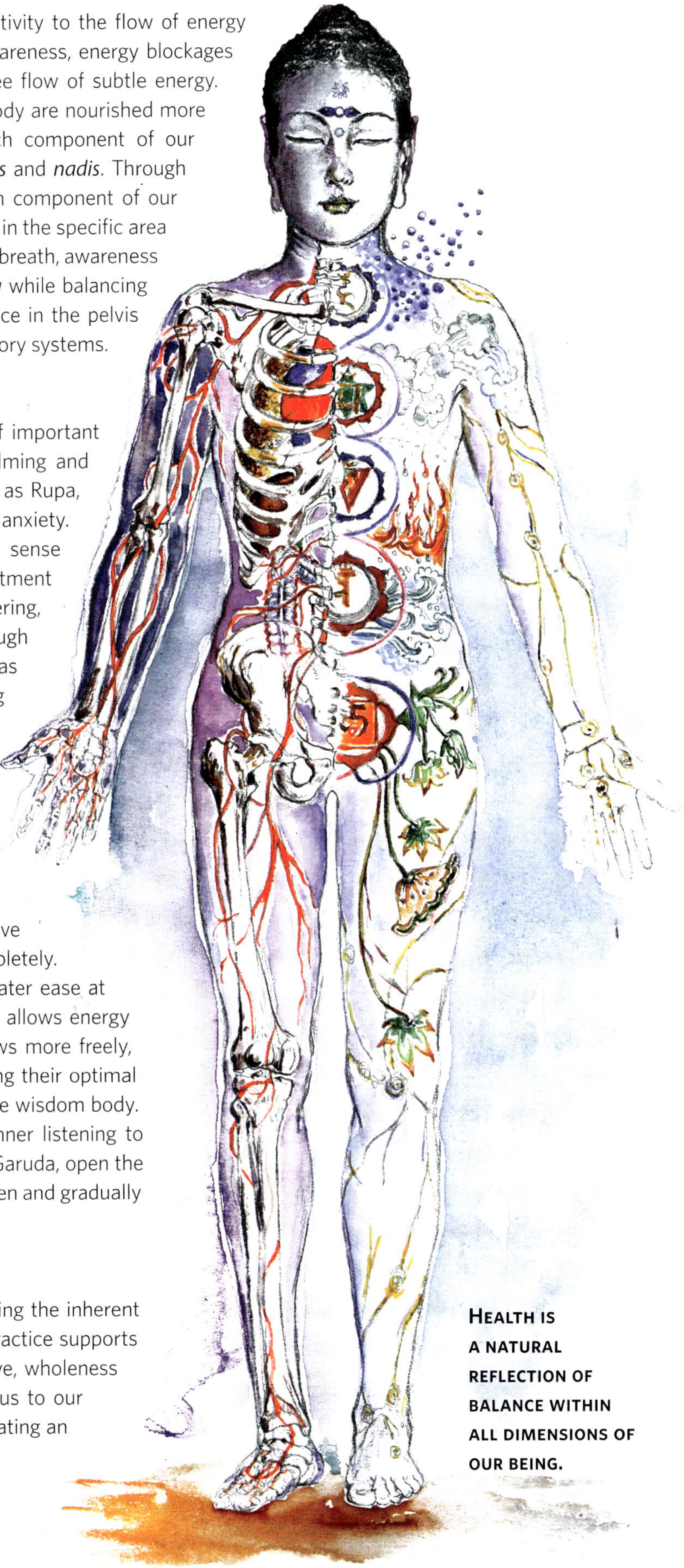

Health is a natural reflection of balance within all dimensions of our being.

20 RUPA MUDRA

Gesture of Form

For Osteoporosis & the Health of the Skeletal System

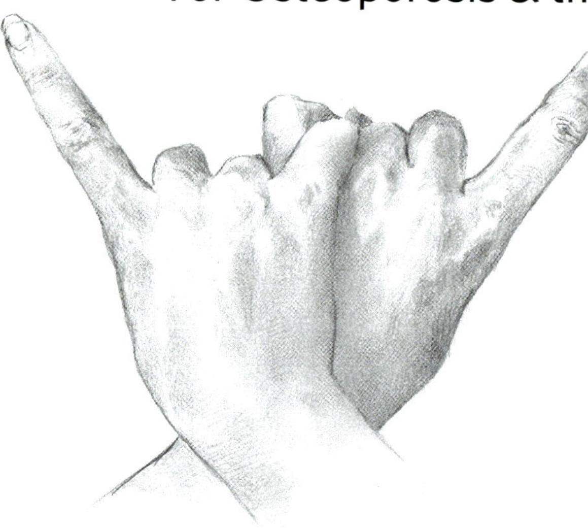

Nourished by the healing nectar of the earth,
I'm fully supported along my journey.

CORE QUALITY

Healthy Skeletal System

ESPECIALLY HELPFUL FOR

- Supporting bone strength and density.
- Instilling a sense of embodiment.
- Reducing stress.
- Enhancing a sense of support and safety.

MUDRAS WITH SIMILAR EFFECTS

Jalashaya, Adhi, Bhu, Apanayana

CAUTIONS

None

INSTRUCTIONS

1. Bend the thumbs into the palms of the hands and wrap the fingers over them.
2. Extend the little and index fingers straight out and turn the palms down.
3. Cross the right hand over the left so that the right wrist rests on the top of the left.
4. Interlace the little fingers, wrapping them gently around each other.
5. The index fingers are extended straight forward.
6. Hold the gesture below the navel or rest the hands on the lap.
7. Relax the shoulders back and down, with the spine naturally aligned.

Osteo means "bone," and *porosis* means "porous." Osteoporosis is a condition in which the bones become porous, and subsequently fragile, because the amount of new bone tissue being created is less than the amount being removed and recycled. Although some loss of bone density is a normal part of the aging process, the amount of bone loss in osteoporosis is such that the individual is subject to fractures. Osteoporosis is most common in postmenopausal women, due to the reduction of estrogen production. Estrogen stimulates osteoblasts (bone-building cells) and inhibits osteoclasts (cells that cause absorption of bone). In addition to the estimated 28 million Americans who have osteoporosis, many more, including those in a younger age group, have osteopenia, low bone density.[3]

Rupa means "form," "shape" or "structure," and Rupa mudra cultivates a feeling of support and stability throughout the entire body, especially within the musculo-skeletal system. This gesture directs breath, awareness and energy to the pelvis and the base of the body, deepening our connection with the earth and instilling a sense of stability and grounding. As stability and grounding increase, our sense of embodiment is enhanced naturally. Stress can be a factor in osteoporosis because during the stress response calcium and other minerals are taken from the bones.[3] Stress is also related to lifestyle habits, such as poor diet and sleep, as well as alcohol and tobacco use, which may be factors in osteoporosis. The stability, grounding and embodiment cultivated by Rupa mudra allow us to experience greater relaxation, reducing stress and thereby supporting the health of the musculo-skeletal system.

SYSTEMS BALANCED:

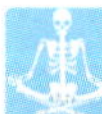

ELEMENTS ACTIVATED:

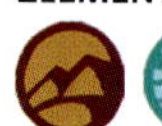
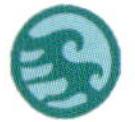

DOSHAS BALANCED:

PRANA VAYUS NOURISHED:

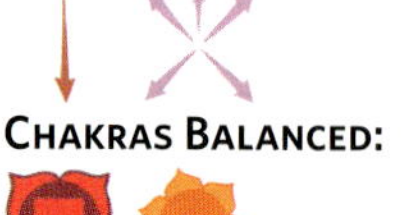

CHAKRAS BALANCED:

SCALE FROM CALMING TO ENERGIZING:

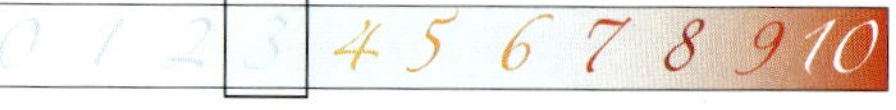

Guided Meditation: Nourishing Nectar of the Earth

- ॐ As you hold Rupa mudra, take several natural breaths to attune to all the feelings and sensations evoked by this gesture.
- ॐ Notice how your breath is gently directed down toward the base of your body, instilling a sense of support and grounding.
- ॐ Become aware of the points of contact between your body and the earth, as if you were growing roots down into its firm, but yielding surface.
- ॐ As you deepen your connection to the earth, visualize its essence as an amber colored nectar of healing, containing all the nutrients and minerals your body needs to nourish your skeletal system completely.
- ॐ With each inhalation, you draw this nectar up from the earth, and with each exhaling breath, this amber energy nourishes each part of your skeletal system with support, strength and stability.
- ॐ Begin by drawing the healing nectar of the earth into the bones of your legs and feet, taking several breaths to allow these areas to be nourished and strengthened optimally.
- ॐ Now, allow the amber nectar of the earth to be drawn up into your pelvis, sensing warmth and tingling as your hips are bathed with nourishing energy, cultivating optimal bone strength and density.
- ॐ For your next few breaths, sense the earth's nectar flowing smoothly up and down your spine, nourishing and strengthening each disc and vertebra.
- ॐ As your spine is fully nourished and aligned, amber nectar bathes your entire rib cage with healing energy, supporting your ability to breathe smoothly and freely.
- ॐ Now, the earth's healing essence bathes the bones of your shoulders, arms, elbows, forearms and wrists, all the way to your fingertips, infusing them with strength and nourishment.
- ॐ For your next few breaths, allow the healing nectar of the earth to gently flow up into your neck and head, fully nourishing these areas.
- ॐ As all the bones of your body are infused with the earth's nectar of healing, sense perfect harmony between bone cells being recycled and new cells coming into being.
- ॐ Deeply nourished by the earth's amber energy, its healing qualities permeate your entire being, providing you with the strength and stability to participate in all of your activities comfortably.
- ॐ Affirm balanced bone density, repeating the following three times, aloud or silently: **"Nourished by earth energy, my bones are infused with strength and stability."**
- ॐ Now, slowly release the gesture, taking several breaths to sense the earth's essential nourishment.
- ॐ When you are ready, open your eyes, returning slowly and gently, sensing your entire being nourished by the earth's amber, healing energy.

Annamaya kosha (physical body)

- **Directs breath and awareness to the base of the body and pelvis, creating a massaging effect that supports the release of muscular tension and promotes optimal circulation to these areas.**
- **Cultivates a feeling that the bones are strong and well nourished.**
- **Instills a sense of embodiment that supports balance and safe movement, which may help to prevent falls that could lead to injury.**
- **Slows the breath, which helps to reduce stress.**
- **The calming and grounding effects cultivated by this gesture are generally helpful for Vata imbalance.**

Pranamaya kosha (energy body)

- **Activates Apana vayu, the downward moving current of energy, as well as Vyana vayu, the all-pervading energy, moving from center to extremities.**
- **Opens and balances the first and second chakras, centers of safety and self-nourishment.**

Manomaya kosha (psycho-emotional body)

- **Instills a sense of stability and safety.**
- **Cultivates deep calm and serenity.**

Vijnanamaya kosha (wisdom body)

- **As we become grounded and serene, it is easier to attune to our inner being, whose very nature is support and safety.**

Anandamaya kosha (bliss body)

- **As we cultivate trust in the body, sensations of ease and well-being arise from within the skeletal system itself.**

21 Anudandi Mudra

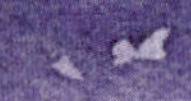

Gesture of the Backbone

For Back Pain & the Health of the Spine

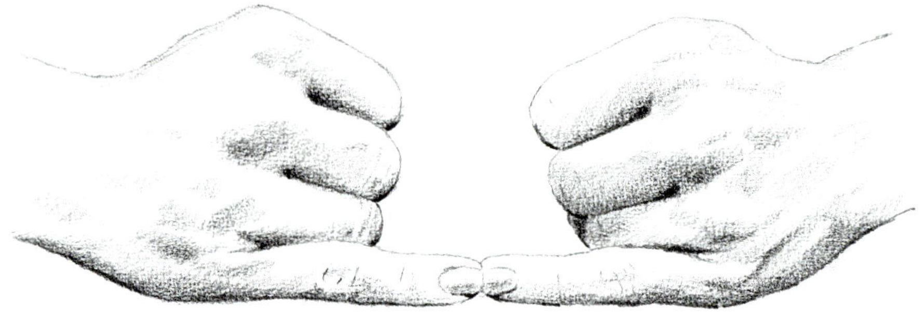

Waves of comfort flow through my back body,
Allowing me to experience greater harmony.

Core Quality

Back Pain Relief

Especially helpful for

- Releasing tension from the back.
- Supporting optimal posture.
- Providing a massaging effect for the area of the kidneys and adrenal glands.
- Reducing stress.

Mudras with similar effects

Dirgha Svara (upper back),
Vajra (mid back), Yoni (lumbar)

Cautions

None

Instructions

1. Make the hands into fists, with the thumbs inside and the palms facing the body.
2. Extend the little fingers and touch them firmly together at their tips.
3. Hold the gesture below the navel or rest the hands on the lap.
4. If there is discomfort in the seated position, use the restorative position, lying on your back.
5. Relax the shoulders back and down, with the elbows held slightly away from the body and the spine naturally aligned.

Back pain is a generic term for a wide range of conditions of the back and spine that share the common symptom of discomfort or pain. Back pain is a common complaint, especially in the lower back, with four out of five people in the United States experiencing lower back pain at least once during their lives. Acute back pain often comes on suddenly and usually lasts from a few days to a few weeks, while chronic back pain lasts for three months or more.[4] Stress reduction is an important part of back pain relief, because one aspect of the stress response is the contraction of the major skeletal muscles of the body as part of the fight, flight or freeze response. When the stress response becomes chronic, the muscles of the back tend to remain contracted, reducing circulation and leading to the accumulation of residues, resulting in inflammation and pain.

Anudandi means "spine," and Anudandi mudra directs breath, awareness and energy to the entire back of the body, releasing tension and instilling a sense of greater comfort. This gesture creates a rhythmic, wavelike movement of the breath, which flows up and down the back body, supporting the release of muscular contraction. As contraction is released, there is a growing sense of ease that helps to reduce stress, further supporting back pain relief. This combination of stress reduction and reduced muscular contraction can help to break the cycle of back pain. Anudandi mudra also supports awareness of optimal posture and alignment of the spinal column, which are important factors in the health of the back. Additionally, the enhanced breathing in the back creates a massaging effect for the kidneys and adrenal glands.

Systems Balanced:

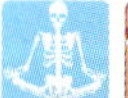
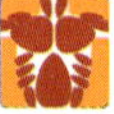

Elements Activated:

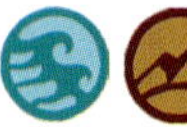
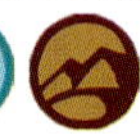

Doshas Balanced:

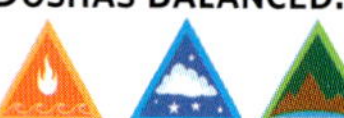

Prana Vayus Nourished:

Chakras Balanced:

Scale from Calming to Energizing:

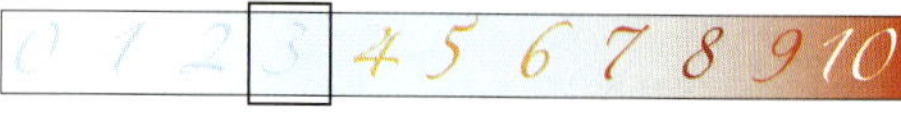

Guided Meditation: **Wave of Ease and Release**

- As you hold Anudandi mudra, take several natural breaths to attune to all the feelings and sensations evoked by this gesture.
- Sense your breath as a wave of relaxation and ease that flows freely throughout the entire back of your body.
- With each inhalation, this wave rises up from your lower back to the top of your neck, and with each exhaling breath, this gentle wave descends, releasing all tension.
- By directing this wave of breath to each area of your back individually, you will bring greater lightness and ease to the entire back of your body.
- Begin by directing your wave of breath into your lower back. With each inhalation, this area is bathed with relaxing energy, and with each exhalation, all tightness and discomfort are naturally released.
- For your next few breaths, sense your lower back nourished by waves of relaxation and ease, deepening your sense of comfort and well-being.
- Now, your wave of breath moves up into your mid back. With each inhalation, sense your lower ribs expanding gently, and as you exhale, allow softness and ease to bathe the entire middle region of your body.
- For your next few breaths, sense all tension being released, allowing your mid back to relax completely.
- Now, direct your wave of breath into your upper back. With each inhalation, sense space being created between your shoulder blades, and with each exhalation, allow them to release down toward the base of your body.
- Take several breaths to sense greater lightness and ease as all tension is released from your upper back and the area between your shoulder blades.
- Your next wave of breath flows all the way up to the top of your neck, lengthening your cervical spine with each inhalation, and with each exhaling breath, allows this area to completely relax.
- Now, take some time to sense your wave of breath flowing smoothly and freely, bringing greater comfort and ease to the entire back of your body.
- Affirm your growing ease as you repeat the following three times, aloud or silently: **"As my wave of breath flows freely, I sense greater ease in the back of my body."**
- Slowly release the gesture, taking several breaths to sense increased comfort throughout your back.
- When you are ready, open your eyes, returning slowly and gently, continuing your activities with greater comfort and ease.

Annamaya kosha (physical body)

• Directs breath and awareness into the entire back, releasing tension and increasing circulation to the muscles of the back.
• Lengthens the exhalation, helping to reduce stress.
• The enhanced awareness and increased movement of the breath in the back supports optimal alignment of the spine.
• The enhanced circulation to the mid back supports the health of the kidneys and adrenal glands.
• The relaxing effects of this gesture are generally helpful for Pitta imbalance.
• The grounding and stabilizing effects of this gesture are helpful for Vata imbalance.
• The expansion of the breath at the back of the lungs is generally helpful for Kapha imbalance.

Pranamaya kosha (energy body)

• Balances Prana and Apana vayus, the upward and downward moving currents of energy.
• Opens and balances the first five chakras.

Manomaya kosha (psycho-emotional body)

• Facilitates relaxation and a sense of release that is helpful for back pain.

Vijnanamaya kosha (wisdom body)

• As we develop greater trust in the healing that arises from our inner being, our connection to our true Self, our own inner healer, deepens naturally.

Anandamaya kosha (bliss body)

• Cultivates a sense of well-being, allowing us to see that the body can be a source of positive feelings.

22 MATSYA MUDRA

Gesture of the Fish

For Osteoarthritis & the Health of the Joints

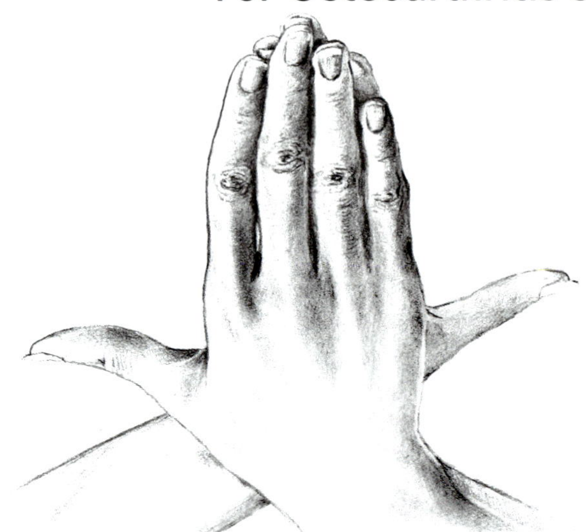

Bathed in waves of nourishing energy,
My body moves freely and comfortably.

CORE QUALITY

Healthy Joints

ESPECIALLY HELPFUL FOR

- Nourishing the joints.
- Releasing muscular contraction.
- Aligning the spine.
- Reducing stress.
- Instilling a sense of inner refreshment.
- Cultivating emotional fluidity.

MUDRAS WITH SIMILAR EFFECTS

Dvimukham, Mira, Svadhisthana, Vyana Vayu

CAUTIONS

None

INSTRUCTIONS

1. Hold the palms facing downward in front of the lower abdomen, with the fingers facing forward and no space between them.
2. Place the palm of the right hand onto the back of the left hand.
3. Extend the thumbs straight out like the fins of a fish.
4. Rest the forearms against the lower abdomen or rest the hands on the lap.
5. Relax the shoulders back and down, with the spine naturally aligned.

Osteoarthritis is the degeneration of the cartilage that protects the joints, resulting in inflammation, pain and movement restriction when the unprotected joint surfaces come into contact. Osteoarthritis most frequently occurs in joints that support weight, like the hip and knee; but it also occurs in the hands, feet, shoulders and spinal column. Almost everyone develops osteoarthritis to some degree with aging, which may or may not present symptoms. Women are twice as likely to suffer as men, partly because of the hormonal changes that occur with menopause. Those who tend to suffer joint trauma, such as athletes, are also more likely to develop osteoarthritis. Obesity, a diet lacking in calcium or high in acidity, a sedentary lifestyle and poor posture are also factors in osteoarthritis. Stress reduction is important in osteoarthritis management because the stress response increases chronic muscular contraction, reducing range of motion, which results in poor circulation and a buildup of toxins that can exacerbate osteoarthritis.[5]

Matsya means "fish," and refers to the fish-like shape of the hands in Matsya mudra. This gesture activates the water element, enhancing the qualities of fluidity, hydration and refreshment. This mudra directs breath and energy to the pelvis, cultivating soothing sensations that may provide relief from the discomfort experienced in osteoarthritis. The lengthening of the exhalation and the subsequent calming effects of this gesture help to reduce stress. This gesture further supports the treatment of osteoarthritis by cultivating optimal postural alignment, which helps to reduce pressure on the joints. At a psycho-emotional level, Matsya mudra instills a sense of fluidity and equanimity, supporting us in dealing with health challenges more easily.

SYSTEMS BALANCED:

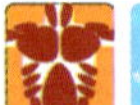
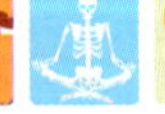
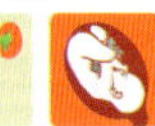
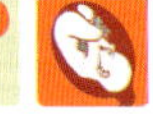
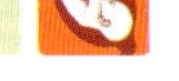
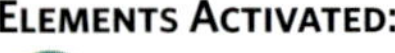

ELEMENTS ACTIVATED:

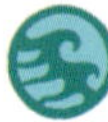

DOSHAS BALANCED:

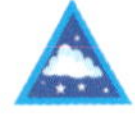

PRANA VAYUS NOURISHED:

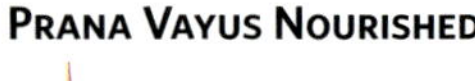

CHAKRAS BALANCED:

SCALE FROM CALMING TO ENERGIZING:

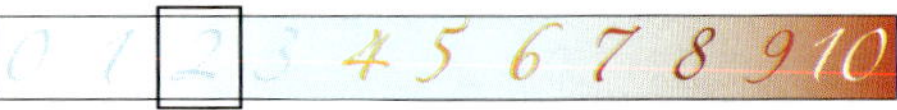

Guided Meditation: **Soothing Inner Tide Pool**

ॐ As you hold Matsya mudra, take several natural breaths to attune to all the feelings and sensations evoked by this gesture.

ॐ Notice how your breath is gently directed into your pelvis and lower abdomen, instilling a sense of ease and fluidity.

ॐ As your breath flows through your pelvic area more easily, visualize yourself floating in a crystal clear tide pool within a soothing tropical sea.

ॐ Your tide pool is shallow, calm and serene, allowing your soft rhythmic breathing to send gentle waves across its surface, caressing your entire body.

ॐ Take several breaths to attune to the rhythm of your soft breathing, naturally deepening your level of comfort and ease.

ॐ Now, allow gentle waves of ease to flow into each area of your body, bathing your joints in nourishing energy.

ॐ Begin by sensing soft waves of nourishment flowing through your ankles and feet, soothing and relaxing them completely.

ॐ Soft waves of healing circulate through your knees, cultivating relaxation and comfort throughout these areas of your being.

ॐ For your next few breaths, allow all the joints of your lower extremities to be bathed completely by gentle waves of healing energy.

ॐ Soft waves now flow through your hips, bathing them in comfort and nourishment while relaxing all the muscles that surround them.

ॐ Slow-motion waves of undulating energy now flow up and down your spine, creating space between each vertebra.

ॐ Soothing waves of healing now bathe your shoulders, elbows and wrists, instilling complete relaxation and a deep sense of nourishment.

ॐ Take several breaths to experience your arms soft and released, floating in a sea of ease, as all the small joints of your hands and fingers are bathed in healing energy.

ॐ Gentle undulating waves of healing now support the weight of your neck and head, allowing your senses to soften and completely rest.

ॐ Now, take several breaths to sense your entire being caressed by soft waves of nourishment and healing, allowing all the joints of your body to relax completely.

ॐ As your body floats comfortably, repeat the following three times, aloud or silently: **"Nourished by waves of healing, I experience comfort in all the joints of my body."**

ॐ Slowly release the gesture, taking several breaths to rest in your tide pool of inner nourishment.

ॐ When you are ready, open your eyes, returning slowly and gently, sensing greater ease within all the joints of your body.

Annamaya kosha (physical body)

• Directs breath and awareness to the pelvic area, enhancing circulation to the reproductive and urinary systems.
• Instills a sense of cooling, soothing energy that may provide relief from inflammation.
• Relaxes the muscles of the face and jaw, which may be helpful for TMJ dysfunction.
• The nourishing effects cultivated by this gesture are generally helpful for Vata imbalance.
• The calming effects are generally helpful for Pitta imbalance.

Pranamaya kosha (energy body)

• Activates Apana vayu, the downward moving current of energy.
• Opens and balances the second chakra, center of self-nourishment.

Manomaya kosha (psycho-emotional body)

• Cultivates relaxation and serenity.
• Instills a sense of fluidity.

Vijnanamaya kosha (wisdom body)

• As we relax and reduce stress, we are able to witness pain more easily without identifying with it so completely.

Anandamaya kosha (bliss body)

• The wavelike flow of the breath instills sensations of complete comfort and lightness.

23 Apanayana Mudra

Gesture of the Vehicle of Elimination

For IBS & the Health of the Eliminatory System

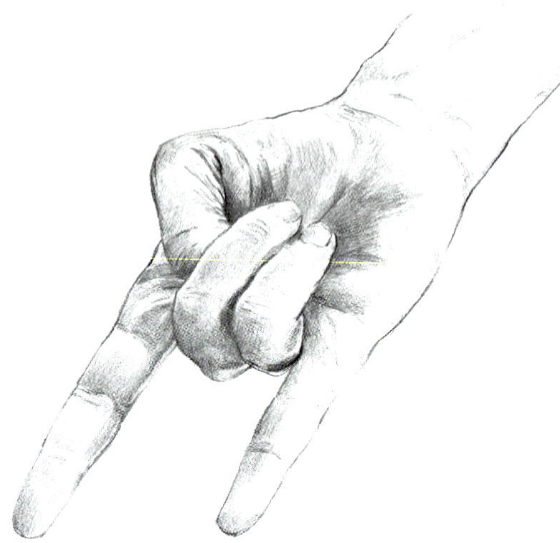

Balance in all of my activities
Supports my body in functioning optimally.

Core Quality
Balanced Elimination

Especially helpful for
- Supporting the treatment of IBS.
- Optimizing the health of the eliminatory, urinary and reproductive systems.
- Reducing stress.
- Instilling a sense of balance and conservation of energy.

Mudras with similar effects
Apana, Dvimukham, Pranidhana, Jalashaya

Cautions
None

Instructions
1. Make the hands into soft fists with the thumbs inside.
2. Extend the little and index fingers straight out.
3. Rest the backs of the hands on the thighs or knees.
4. Relax the shoulders back and down, with the spine naturally aligned.

Irritable Bowel Syndrome (IBS), also called spastic colitis, is characterized by cramping, abdominal pain, bloating, constipation and diarrhea. Up to twenty percent of the adult population in the United States have IBS symptoms. This condition is most common in women under the age of thirty-five. Symptoms vary from person to person, with some more prone to diarrhea and others to constipation while some alternate between the two. For some, symptoms can subside for a few months and return while others report a constant worsening over time.[6] There are several possible causes of IBS, including hyper-reactivity of the colon, food sensitivity, autoimmune dysfunction and bacterial infection. Chronic stress may be a factor in IBS. During the fight, flight or freeze response, blood is shunted away from the digestive system to meet the needs of the large working muscles. When the short-term source of stress has passed, digestive functions return to normal. When stress becomes chronic, however, the digestive system may lose its natural balance.[7]

Apanayana means "elimination" and also "healing," and Apanayana mudra directs breath, awareness and energy into the pelvis and lower abdomen, creating a massaging effect that enhances circulation to the entire eliminatory system. This gesture lengthens the exhaling breath as well as the pause at the end of the exhalation, instilling calm and relaxation, thereby reducing stress, which supports the optimal functioning of the eliminatory system. The lengthened exhalation is the vehicle of *Apana vayu*, the downward moving current, which is responsible for all processes of elimination. The massaging effect cultivated by this gesture together with the balanced flow of Apana vayu supports the health of the reproductive and urinary systems.

Systems Balanced:

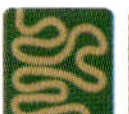 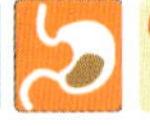 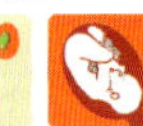 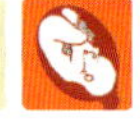 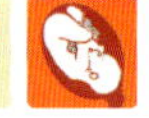

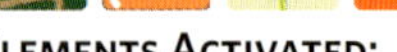

Prana Vayus Nourished:

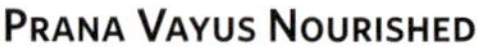

Elements Activated:

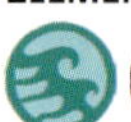 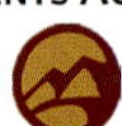

Chakras Balanced:

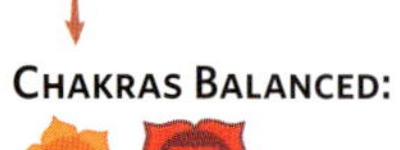

Doshas Balanced:

 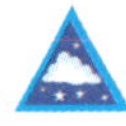

Scale from Calming to Energizing:

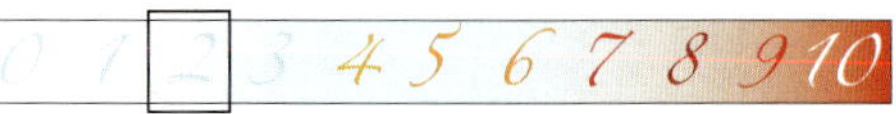

Guided Meditation: Balance in All of Your Activities

- As you hold Apanayana mudra, take several natural breaths to attune to all the feelings and sensations evoked by this gesture.
- With each inhalation, sense the slow, steady expansion of your lower abdomen, and with each exhaling breath, allow your entire abdominal area to soften and relax.
- Take several breaths to sense how your exhalation is lengthened naturally, cultivating a feeling of deep relaxation and release that supports your eliminatory system in functioning optimally.
- As you experience greater ease, envision the ways you can support the health of your eliminatory system by cultivating balance in all of your activities.
- Begin by seeing yourself waking up in the morning, relaxed and refreshed, starting your day in a calm and easeful way, with gentle exercise, a time of silence or prayer.
- Envision yourself eating nourishing food slowly and consciously, with a spirit of reverence and harmony, as an expression of gratitude for the gift of your body.
- After meals, see yourself taking a few slow, deep breaths or a time of rest, allowing your food to be fully digested, so that you receive optimal nourishment.
- Your more relaxed way of eating is reflected in your work and activities, allowing you to meet challenges from a place of greater calm and centering.
- Whenever you begin to feel anxious or stressed, you remember to take a few long, slow, deep breaths to regain your serenity, returning to your activities with greater equanimity.
- With your work day complete, you are ready to transition to a time of rest, which you appreciate more deeply, having cultivated balance in all of your activities.
- Now, as you prepare for sleep, take some time to reflect on all you've done and seen, naturally surrendering into deep sleep easily, allowing you to awake refreshed for another day of balanced living.
- Affirm your balance as you repeat the following three times, aloud or silently: **"With greater balance and ease, my eliminatory system functions optimally."**
- Slowly release the gesture, taking several breaths to experience greater balance.
- When you are ready, open your eyes, returning slowly and gently, with a greater sense of ease in all of your activities.

Annamaya kosha (physical body)

• Directs breath and awareness into the pelvis and lower abdomen, creating a massaging effect that enhances circulation to the eliminatory, reproductive and urinary systems.
• Lengthens the exhalation and the pause at the end of the exhalation, supporting relaxation and stress reduction, thereby cultivating balance in the digestive and eliminatory systems.
• The centering effects of this gesture are generally helpful for Vata imbalance.
• The calming effects of this gesture are generally helpful for Pitta imbalance.

Pranamaya kosha (energy body)

• Gently activates the flow of Apana vayu, the downward moving current of energy.
• Opens and balances the first and second chakras, centers of safety and self-nourishment.

Manomaya kosha (psycho-emotional body)

• Cultivates tranquility and stability in the mind, alleviating the worry and anxiety that can be factors in IBS.
• Supports the optimal digestion of thoughts, emotions and experiences.
• Helps to release resentment and anger.

Vijnanamaya kosha (wisdom body)

• As we experience greater balance in all activities, we attune more easily to our true being, whose very nature is equanimity.

Anandamaya kosha (bliss body)

• With greater relaxation, sensations of deep comfort and well-being arise from within the abdomen.

24 Varuna Mudra

Gesture of the God of Water

For Cystitis & the Health of the Urinary System

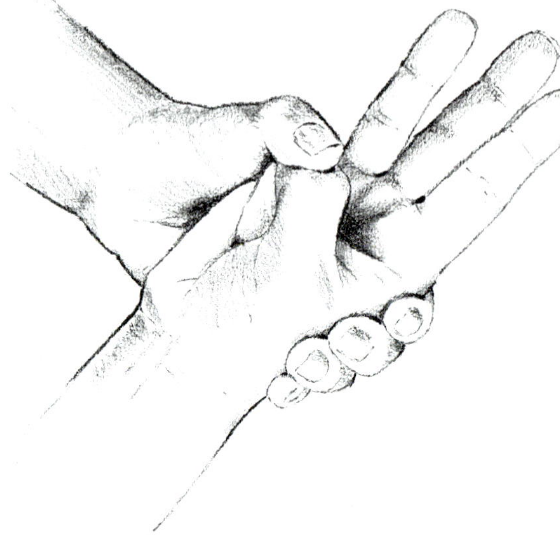

Moving through life with greater fluidity,
My liquid systems function harmoniously.

Core Quality

Healthy Urinary System

Especially helpful for

- Supporting the optimal functioning of the urinary and reproductive systems.
- Releasing muscular contraction from the pelvic floor, pelvis, and mid back.

Mudras with similar effects

Jala, Dvimukham, Matsya, Mira

Cautions

Contraindicated for those with an overactive bladder.

Instructions

1. Bend the little finger of the right hand to the base of the right thumb, securing the finger with the right thumb.
2. Extend the middle, ring, and index fingers of the right hand straight out.
3. Rest the back of the right hand onto the palm of the left hand so that the fingers of the left hand wrap around the outer border of the right hand.
4. Place the left thumb over the right thumb and right little finger.
5. Hold the gesture below the navel or on the lap.
6. Relax the shoulders back and down, with the spine naturally aligned.

Cystitis is an inflammation of the lining of the urinary bladder, whose symptoms include frequent urination, burning during urination and a feeling of fullness in the bladder even after urinating. Cystitis affects over six million adults in the United States, while over twenty percent of women experience urinary tract infections at some point in their lives. There are several causes of cystitis, the most common being a bacterial infection. Interstitial cystitis (IC), also known as bladder pain syndrome (BPS), is a chronic, often severely debilitating disease of the bladder, characterized by pain in the bladder and pelvic region along with urinary frequency. Theories as to the cause of IC/BPS are inflammation and heredity. Stress is thought to aggravate the symptoms of IC/BPS. [8]

Varuna is the "god of water," and Varuna mudra is the gesture traditionally recommended for urinary problems. This gesture directs breath, awareness and energy to the entire front of the pelvis and to the area of the bladder in particular, releasing tension and enhancing circulation. Varuna mudra also directs breath, awareness and energy to the area of the kidneys, supporting their optimal functioning. This mudra cultivates a cooling and refreshing sensation, which increases the level of comfort within the urinary tract, especially when inflammation is present. This gesture also creates a massaging effect within the pelvic floor, releasing tension and enhancing circulation, which supports the health of the urinary and reproductive systems, especially the prostate gland.

Systems Balanced:

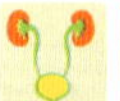 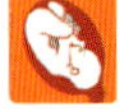

Elements Activated:

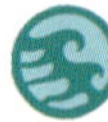

Doshas Balanced:

 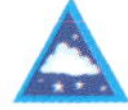

Prana Vayus Nourished:

Chakras Balanced:

Scale from Calming to Energizing:

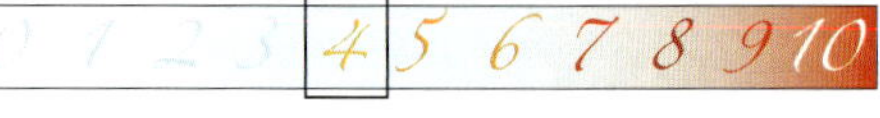

Guided Meditation: Refreshing Inner Stream

ॐ As you hold Varuna mudra, take several natural breaths to attune to all the feelings and sensations evoked by this gesture.

ॐ Notice how your breath is gently directed into your pelvis, instilling a sense of inner refreshment and ease that supports your urinary system in functioning optimally.

ॐ To deepen your sense of refreshment and ease, visualize a soothing stream that bathes each part of your urinary system in refreshing energy.

ॐ Begin by bringing your awareness to your kidneys, one on each side of your mid back, sensing how they filter your blood and remove excess liquid.

ॐ Take several breaths to sense your soothing inner stream flowing through your kidneys, nourishing them to support their optimal functioning.

ॐ Your stream of nourishment and healing now bathes your ureters, the long muscular tubes that transfer liquid smoothly downward.

ॐ Take some time to sense your ureters expanding and releasing in synchrony with your smooth, rhythmic breathing, allowing stress and tension to be released, ensuring their optimal functioning.

ॐ Your healing stream now flows into your bladder, where liquid is stored for release, massaging your pelvis internally, allowing the muscles in this area to relax completely.

ॐ Take several breaths to sense the walls of your bladder expanding and releasing, nourished with your rhythmic breathing, completely healing this area of your being.

ॐ Now, visualize your healing stream flowing through your entire urinary system, nourishing it completely, supporting its optimal functioning.

ॐ Affirm your urinary health, repeating the following three times, aloud or silently: **"Bathed in nourishing, refreshing energy, my urinary system functions optimally."**

ॐ Slowly release the gesture, taking several breaths to rest in the complete ease that allows your urinary system to function perfectly.

ॐ When you are ready, open your eyes, returning slowly and gently with a greater sense of ease and fluidity.

Annamaya kosha (physical body)

• Directs breath and awareness to the pelvis and mid back, releasing tension and enhancing circulation to the urinary system.
• Lengthens the exhalation and creates a longer pause at the end of the exhaling breath, instilling a sense of calm and serenity, reducing stress.
• The feeling of enhanced hydration cultivated by this gesture is generally helpful for Vata imbalance.
• The calming and refreshing qualities of this gesture are generally helpful for Pitta imbalance.

Pranamaya kosha (energy body)

• Activates Apana vayu, the downward moving current of energy.
• Opens and balances the second chakra, center of self-nourishment.

Manomaya kosha (psycho-emotional body)

• Cultivates calm and a sense of emotional well-being.
• Instills a sense of inner refreshment.

Vijnanamaya kosha (wisdom body)

• The lengthened pause at the end of the exhalation instills a sense of serenity, which serves as a portal to our true being.

Anandamaya kosha (bliss body)

• As tension from the pelvis is released, sensations of pleasure and comfort arise naturally.

25 YONI MUDRA

Gesture of the Womb

For PMS & Female Reproductive Health

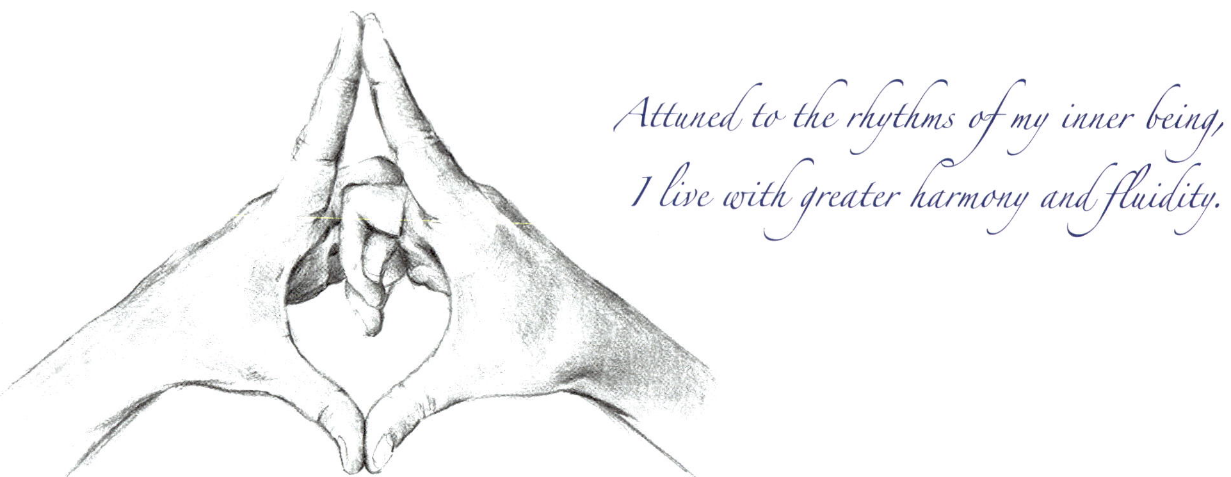

*Attuned to the rhythms of my inner being,
I live with greater harmony and fluidity.*

CORE QUALITY

Female Reproductive Health

ESPECIALLY HELPFUL FOR

- PMS and reproductive health, including menstrual imbalances, infertility and menopausal symptoms.
- Supporting the health of the urinary system.
- Attuning to the feminine, intuitive aspect of our being.

MUDRAS WITH SIMILAR EFFECTS

Trimurti, Mira, Matsya, Svadhisthana

CAUTIONS

This gesture should be used cautiously during pregnancy and should not be held for extended periods.

INSTRUCTIONS

1. Interlace the fingers inward with the left little finger on the bottom.
2. Join the pads of the index fingers and extend them forward.
3. Join the pads of the thumbs and extend them back toward the body.
4. Rest the hands below the navel or on the lap.
5. Relax the shoulders back and down, with the elbows held slightly away from the body and the spine naturally aligned.

Premenstrual syndrome (PMS) is a collection of symptoms that appear during the two weeks preceding menstruation. PMS symptoms include feelings of bloating, mood swings, anxiety and tiredness. These symptoms affect up to seventy-five percent of women at some point in their childbearing years, being moderate to severe in approximately five percent of the female population. Lifestyle modifications, such as diet, exercise and adequate rest can be helpful in reducing symptoms of PMS. Stressful experiences, especially during the two weeks prior to menstruation, can make PMS worse.[9] PMS is associated with reduced levels of serotonin, and meditation has been shown to raise serotonin levels.[10] Mudra practice, especially when accompanied by a guided meditation, may produce similar effects, thereby supporting the treatment of PMS.

Yoni refers to the "female reproductive system" at the physical level and also at a symbolic level as the "womb of creation." Yoni mudra directs breath, awareness and energy to the pelvic area, creating a massaging effect that enhances circulation to the reproductive organs while cultivating sensations of inner nourishment. This gesture slows the breath rate and lengthens the exhalation, which reduces stress, thereby helping to alleviate symptoms of PMS. The lengthened pause at the end of the exhalation cultivates a space of inner silence that allows us to turn inward and attune to our own natural rhythms and cycles. Yoni mudra instills a sense of comfort and ease, which may be helpful in reducing the irritability associated with PMS. The overall health of the reproductive and urinary systems are benefited by the increased sense of comfort and ease cultivated by this gesture.

SYSTEMS BALANCED:

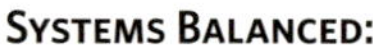
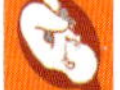
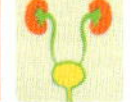

ELEMENTS ACTIVATED:

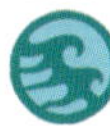

DOSHAS BALANCED:

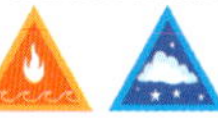

PRANA VAYUS NOURISHED:

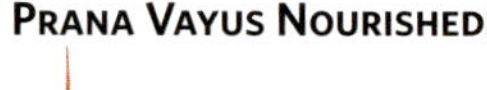

CHAKRAS BALANCED:

SCALE FROM CALMING TO ENERGIZING:

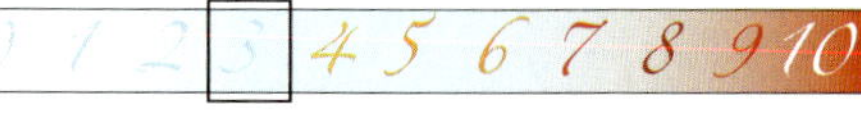

Guided Meditation: **Attuning to Your Inner Rhythms**

ॐ As you hold Yoni mudra, take several natural breaths to attune to all the feelings and sensations evoked by this gesture.

ॐ Notice how your breath is gently directed down into your pelvis, creating a massaging effect that cultivates a sense of deep inner nourishment.

ॐ Each inhalation bathes your pelvis in soft waves of comfort and ease, and each exhalation allows your pelvic area to relax completely.

ॐ As your breath flows through your pelvis more freely, sense gentle undulations nourishing this area of your being with soft waves of healing energy.

ॐ Experience these waves as a reflection of nature's rhythms, guiding the seasons, the tides of the sea, the phases of the moon and the natural cycles within your own being.

ॐ Sense your waves of inner healing nourishing you with the essential qualities that help to reestablish balance in all of your inner cycles and rhythms.

ॐ As you inhale, attune to your inner sea, sensing the quality of fluidity arising naturally. As you exhale, allow gentle waves of fluidity to bathe your reproductive organs completely.

ॐ Take several breaths to sense this area of your being nourished with soft waves of healing.

ॐ With your next inhalation, return to the inner sea at the center of your being, opening to receive the quality of release. As you exhale, sense yourself letting go of all you no longer need, dissolving stress and tension naturally.

ॐ As you sense greater release, you are able to move through your day, from the time you wake until you sleep, more attuned to the rhythms and cycles of your inner being.

ॐ With your next inhalation, return to the calm depths of your inner sea, allowing a sense of equanimity to arise naturally.

ॐ As you exhale, sense yourself opening to all life brings, allowing your relationships and interactions to flow more harmoniously.

ॐ With greater equanimity, you naturally develop sensitivity to your true needs, naturally finding a balance between rest and activity.

ॐ Now, return to the calm sea at the center of your being, integrating the qualities of fluidity, release and equanimity, naturally reestablishing balance within all of your inner cycles and rhythms.

ॐ Affirm your inner equilibrium, repeating the following three times aloud or silently: **"Attuned to my calm inner sea, my cycles and rhythms are balanced naturally."**

ॐ Now, slowly release the gesture, taking several breaths to experience your essential balance.

ॐ When you are ready, open your eyes, returning slowly and gently, bringing greater harmony to all of your activities.

Annamaya kosha (physical body)

• Directs breath and awareness into the pelvis, creating a massaging effect that enhances circulation to the reproductive and urinary systems.
• The lengthened exhalation reduces stress, which supports the release of the muscular tension from the pelvic area that may be helpful in reducing cramping.
• The calming and cooling effects cultivated by this gesture are generally helpful for Pitta imbalance.
• The centering effects of this gesture are generally helpful for Vata imbalance.

Pranamaya kosha (energy body)

• Activates the flow of Apana vayu, the downward moving current of energy.
• Opens and balances the second chakra, center of self-nourishment.

Manomaya kosha (psycho-emotional body)

• Cultivates a sense of serenity.
• Instills a sense of fluidity and inner nourishment.
• Cultivates emotional balance and the ability to deal with challenges more easily.

Vijnanamaya kosha (wisdom body)

• Instills a feeling of going back to the womb, creating a sense of comfort and security that are reflections of our true being.

Anandamaya kosha (bliss body)

• As we attune to our inner rhythms, a feeling of deep comfort and inner peace arises from within the pelvis.

26 SHANKHA MUDRA

Gesture of the Conch

For the Prostate & Male Reproductive Health

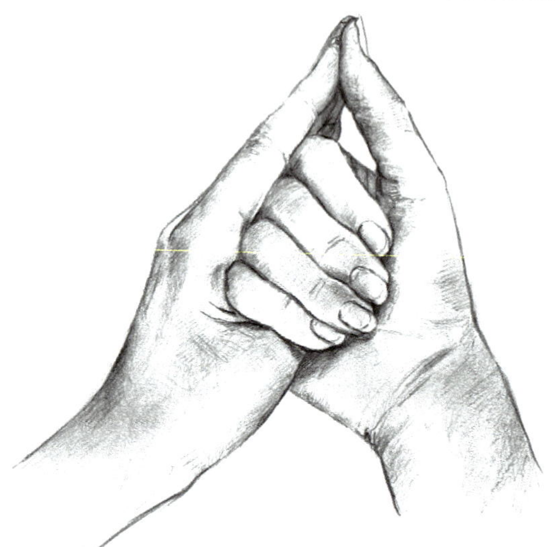

Resting in the comfort of my inner spring,
I experience healing in all dimensions of being.

CORE QUALITY

Male Reproductive Health

ESPECIALLY HELPFUL FOR

- Reproductive issues, including prostate problems.
- Releasing tension from the pelvis.
- Instilling a sense of grounding, safety and inner nourishment.

MUDRAS WITH SIMILAR EFFECTS

Prajna Prana Kriya, Adho Merudanda, Svadhisthana

CAUTIONS

None

INSTRUCTIONS

1. Secure the left thumb with all four fingers of the right hand and rest the back of the right hand onto the left palm.
2. Touch the tip of the right thumb to the tip of the left index finger.
3. Wrap the fingers of the left hand around the edge of the right hand.
4. Place the wrists below the navel or rest the gesture on your lap.
5. Relax the shoulders back and down, with the elbows held slightly away from the body and the spine naturally aligned.

Benign prostate hypertrophy (BPH) is an increase in the size of the prostate gland, a walnut-sized gland found in men, located beneath the bladder and surrounding the urethra. Its glandular part secretes fluid into semen, and its smooth muscular part assists in ejaculation. The majority of men over fifty experience some degree of BPH, and with age, about ninety percent of men will have some enlargement. A small increase in the size of the prostate is normal after middle age, but becomes a problem when the gland compresses the urethra, causing difficulty in urination and a sensation that the bladder is never completely evacuated.[11] Another prostate issue is prostatitis, an acute inflammation in the prostate that sometimes becomes chronic, causing pain. Prostatitis is often caused by a bacterial infection.[12] Prostate issues may be affected by stress, as blood is shunted away from the reproductive organs during the fight, flight or freeze response.

Shankha means "shell," and Shankha mudra directs breath, awareness and energy into the pelvis and base of the body, promoting relaxation of the musculature and improving circulation in this area. This increased awareness and circulation to the pelvic floor is especially important in prostate issues, because the prostate lies in an area prone to poor circulation.[11] As this gesture directs breath into the pelvis, it creates a sense of inner nourishment and contentment that helps to reduce tension and stress, which may be factors in prostate problems. Shankha mudra also instills a sense of safety and security that may assist in reducing the anxiety that can accompany prostate issues.

SYSTEMS BALANCED:

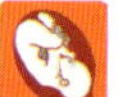 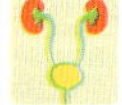

ELEMENTS ACTIVATED:

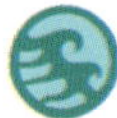

DOSHAS BALANCED:

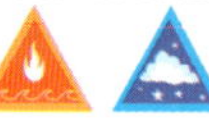

PRANA VAYUS NOURISHED:

CHAKRAS BALANCED:

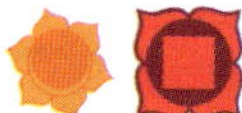

SCALE FROM CALMING TO ENERGIZING:

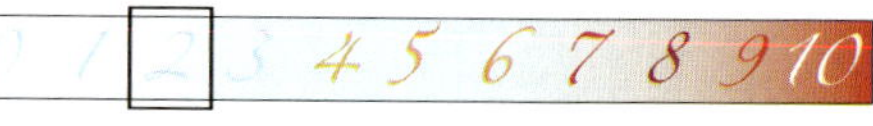

Guided Meditation: **Spring of Well-Being**

- As you hold Shankha mudra, take several natural breaths to attune to all the feelings and sensations evoked by this gesture.
- Notice how your breath is gently directed into your pelvis and the base of your body, instilling a sense of ease and well-being that allows these areas to relax completely.
- To deepen your sense of well-being, visualize yourself seated in a natural warm water spring, allowing its currents to bathe your pelvic area with nourishing energy.
- As the waters of your spring flow through the base of your body, the muscles of your pelvic floor soften naturally, increasing the flow of vital energy.
- As these muscles release, the waters of your inner spring bathe your reproductive system with healing energy, allowing circulation to flow through this area more freely.
- As you sense greater ease within your pelvis and the base of your body, the healing waters of your spring gradually flow out to nourish your entire being.
- Take several breaths to sense the waters of your healing spring bathing your legs and feet, allowing them to soften and relax completely.
- Warmth and inner nourishment now flow up into your abdomen and low back, allowing these areas to soften and fully relax.
- Now, sense the waters of your spring nourishing your solar plexus, chest and upper back, allowing your breath to flow smoothly and freely as all tension is released.
- The warmth of your inner spring now flows through your shoulders, arms and hands, all the way to your fingertips, bathing these areas with nourishment.
- Your soothing waters now flow up into your neck and head, gently dissolving all tension, allowing your senses to fully rest.
- Finally, take several breaths to allow the healing waters of your spring to flow serenely throughout your entire being as a source of nourishment and healing.
- Affirm your complete well-being, repeating the following three times, aloud or silently: **"In the healing waters of my inner spring, I experience complete well-being."**
- Now, slowly release the gesture, taking several breaths to sense complete inner nourishment.
- When you are ready, open your eyes, returning slowly and gently, with a greater sense of well-being.

Annamaya kosha (physical body)

• Directs breath and awareness to the pelvis and pelvic floor, creating a massaging effect that relaxes the musculature of this area, enhancing circulation to the reproductive and urinary systems.
• Slows the breath, reducing stress, which helps to reestablish the healthy flow of circulation to the pelvis.
• The centering effects cultivated by this gesture are generally helpful for Vata imbalance.
• The calming effects of this gesture are generally helpful for Pitta imbalance.

Pranamaya kosha (energy body)

• Activates the flow of Apana vayu, the downward moving current of energy.
• Opens and balances the first and second chakras, centers of safety and self-nourishment.

Manomaya kosha (psycho-emotional body)

• Cultivates a sense of safety as if moving into a shell of protective energy.
• Instills a sense of calm and serenity.

Vijnanamaya kosha (wisdom body)

• As comfort and safety increase, we are able to glimpse our true being, whose very nature is absolute serenity.

Anandamaya kosha (bliss body)

• As we relax the pelvic area, feelings of nourishment and well-being arise naturally.

27 Trimurti Mudra

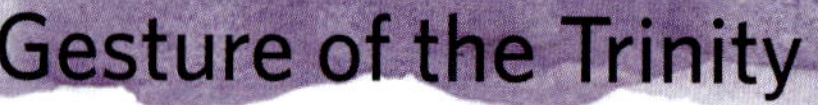

Gesture of the Trinity

For Menopause & All Life Transitions

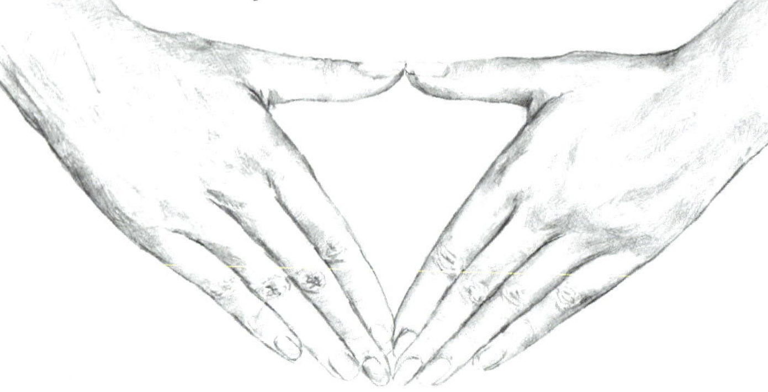

Balanced at the center of my being,
I embrace life's transitions as opportunities.

Core Quality

Harmonious Life Transitions

Especially Helpful For

- Menopause and other reproductive issues, including infertility.
- Reducing stress.
- Supporting all life transitions.
- Instilling equanimity and a sense of centering.

Mudras with Similar Effects

Dharma Chakra, Mira, Abhaya Varada

Cautions

None

Instructions

1. Hold the hands in front of the pelvis with the palms facing the body and the fingers together and pointing downward.
2. Extend the thumbs out to touch at their tips and join the index fingers to form a downward facing triangle.
3. Rest the hands onto the pelvis below the navel.
4. Relax the shoulders back and down, with the elbows held away from the body and the spine naturally aligned.

Menopause is a natural stage in a woman's life when the female reproductive cycle comes to completion. In many societies menopause is perceived positively, especially in those that revere aging. For many women, however, menopause may be accompanied by symptoms of discomfort, including hot flashes, mood swings, difficulty concentrating, depression, anxiety and decreased libido. Loss of bone tissue and a possible increased risk for hypertension and heart disease may also occur. Menopause may have a cultural factor, with symptoms being more pronounced in developed societies.[13] Stress may aggravate the symptoms of menopause because it affects the body's ability to produce estrogen and progesterone, the primary hormones of the female reproductive system. From a wider perspective, menopause is one of many transitions that are a natural part of the life journey. To the extent that change is embraced with balance and harmony, these transitions occur more smoothly.

Trimurti means "three deities," and refers to the three male deities and their female consorts who embody the three facets of existence: *Brahma* and *Sarasvati*, creation; *Vishnu* and *Lakshmi*, sustenance; and *Shiva* and *Parvati*, transformation. Trimurti mudra directs breath, awareness and energy to the center of the pelvis, instilling a sense of balance and harmony that supports us in embracing transitions more easily as a natural part of the life journey. This gesture is a symbol of sacred femininity, and as it directs breath, awareness and energy into the pelvis, it creates a massaging effect that enhances circulation to the reproductive system. The triangular shape of this gesture symbolizes the balance of body, mind and spirit, whose integration supports us in remaining centered within our being, allowing us to embrace transitions as opportunities.

Systems Balanced:

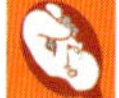 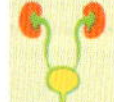

Elements Activated:

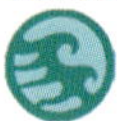

Doshas Balanced:

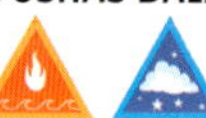

Prana Vayus Nourished:

Chakras Balanced:

Scale from Calming to Energizing:

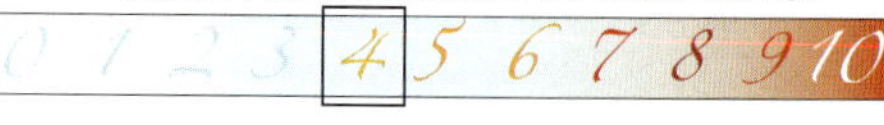

Guided Meditation: Triangle of Inner Balance

- As you hold Trimurti mudra, take several natural breaths to attune to all the feelings and sensations evoked by this gesture.
- Notice how your breath is naturally directed into the triangle formed by your hands, instilling a sense of harmony that arises from the very center of your being.
- The three sides of your triangle represent body, mind and spirit, symbolizing the balance that allows you to make life transitions with greater equanimity.
- With greater equanimity, you embrace transitions as opportunities for growth and learning, transforming uncertainty into enthusiasm for new possibilities.
- In order to envision these new possibilities more clearly, take some time to bring to mind a transition that you are currently experiencing.
- Begin by sensing how this transition is reflected in your physical body, honoring the changes that are occurring by embracing them as a natural part of your life journey.
- Notice any areas of tension related to this transition. As you inhale, focus on your triangle of equanimity, and as you exhale, all tension is released from your physical being, allowing you to relax completely.
- Next, take some time to sense how this transition is reflected in your psycho-emotional being, honoring the thoughts and feelings that arise as a natural part of the transformation you are experiencing.
- Sense any stress, worry or anxiety that are arising at this moment in your journey. As you inhale, focus on your triangle of equanimity, and as you exhale, all stress is naturally released, allowing you to experience greater lightness and ease.
- Finally, sense how this transition serves as an opportunity to bring your deepest core beliefs into the light of clear seeing, honoring them as a field of learning while recognizing that they no longer support your journey.
- Take some time to explore the limiting beliefs that keep you from making this life transition harmoniously.
- As you inhale, focus on your triangle of equanimity, and as you exhale, your identification with these beliefs dissolves gradually as they lose their power to color your way of seeing and being.
- Now, return to your triangle of equanimity, sensing the comfort and clarity that allow you to step forward into the next chapter of your life smoothly and easily.
- Affirm your equanimity as you repeat the following three times, aloud or silently: **"Centered in my triangle of equanimity, I embrace life transitions smoothly and easily."**
- Now, slowly release the gesture, taking several breaths to sense complete balance.
- When you are ready, open your eyes, returning slowly and gently, with an enhanced ability to embrace life transitions harmoniously.

Annamaya kosha (physical body)

• Directs breath and awareness into the pelvis, creating a massaging effect that enhances circulation to the reproductive system.
• This massaging effect may be helpful for PMS discomfort and menstrual cramps.
• The centering effects cultivated by this gesture are generally helpful for Vata imbalance.
• The equanimity cultivated by this gesture is generally helpful for Pitta imbalance.

Pranamaya kosha (energy body)

• Activates the flow of Apana vayu, the downward moving current of energy.
• Opens and balances the second chakra, center of self-nourishment.

Manomaya kosha (psycho-emotional body)

• Instills a sense of serenity that allows us to embrace life transitions more easily.
• Cultivates integration of body, mind and spirit.

Vijnanamaya kosha (wisdom body)

• Cultivates the ability to see all of life's transitions as part of a larger journey in which each chapter has its own lessons and opportunities.

Anandamaya kosha (bliss body)

• As tension is released from the pelvic area, a greater sense of well-being and equanimity arise naturally.

28

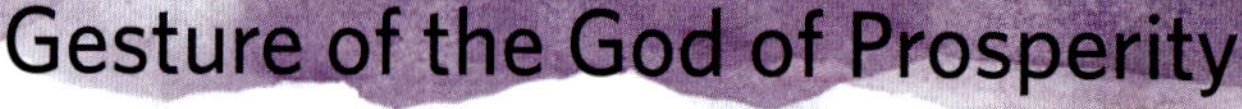

Pushan Mudra

Gesture of the God of Prosperity

For the Health of the Digestive System

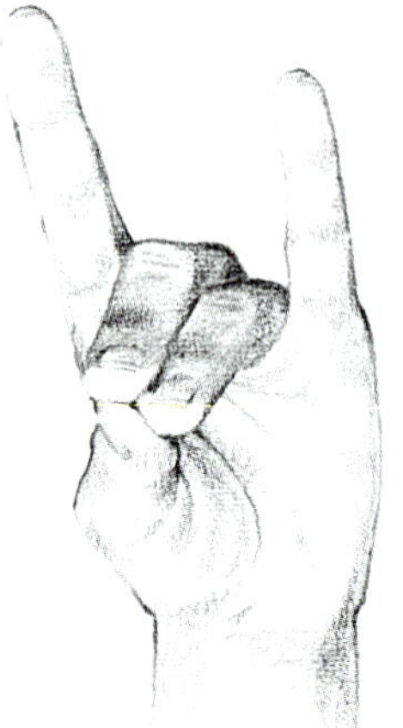

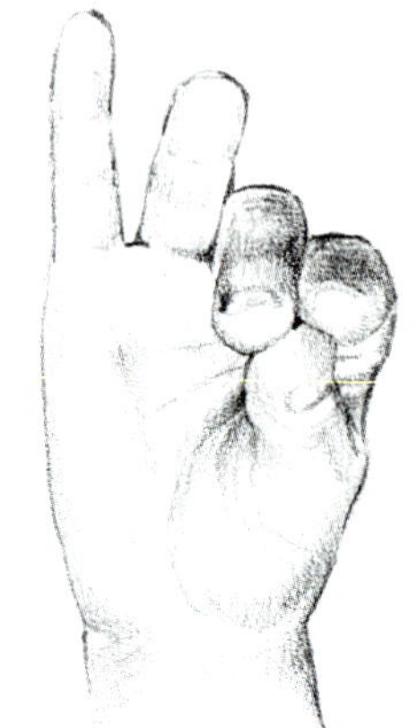

As my entire being is nourished completely, I experience optimal health and vitality.

Core Quality

Balanced Digestion

Especially helpful for

- Supporting optimal digestion, assimilation and elimination.
- Facilitating digestion of life experiences.

Mudras with similar effects

Kubera, Achala Agni, Surya, Vajra

Cautions

None

Instructions

1. Left hand: Touch the tip of the thumb to the tips of the middle and ring fingers while extending the little and index fingers straight out.
2. Right hand: Touch the tip of the thumb to the tips of the index and middle fingers while extending the little and ring fingers straight out.
3. Rest the backs of the hands onto the thighs or knees.
4. Relax the shoulders back and down, with the spine naturally aligned.

From the perspective of Ayurveda, the ancient healing science of India, optimal digestion is key to health because it provides the body with essential nourishment and vitality. Additionally, optimal digestion supports the removal of waste products, whose accumulation is a main factor in disease.[14] Optimal digestion requires healthy eating habits as well as a balanced lifestyle, which includes eating consciously in a stress free environment. Stress management is essential for healthy digestion because the stress response shunts blood away from the digestive system to the large working muscles of the body. This serves to conserve energy during periods of stressful activity, but when stress becomes chronic, the entire digestive system tips toward imbalance.[15]

Pushan is the "solar deity of sustenance and prosperity." Pushan mudra directs breath, awareness and energy to the solar plexus and abdomen, creating a massaging effect that increases circulation to the digestive system. This gesture further optimizes digestion by deepening our awareness of the process of digestion, allowing us to perceive the first signs of imbalance before they evolve into more serious digestive conditions. This heightened sensitivity also makes us more conscious of how and what we eat, and the subsequent effects on our body. Pushan mudra enhances *agni,* the subtle digestive fire, which is essential for optimal digestion, nutrition and elimination. Balanced agni also improves the subtle digestion of life experiences, which further helps to reduce stress, thereby improving physical digestion.

Systems Balanced:

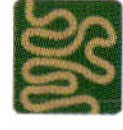

Elements Activated:

Doshas Balanced:

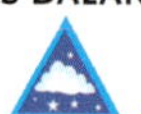
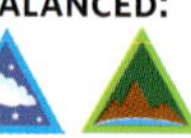

Prana Vayus Nourished:

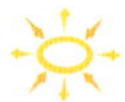

Chakras Balanced:

Scale from Calming to Energizing:

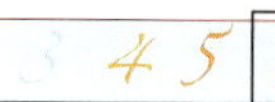
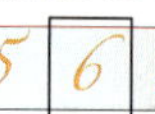

Guided Meditation: Cultivating Optimal Digestion

- As you hold Pushan mudra, take several natural breaths to attune to all the feelings and sensations evoked by this gesture.
- Notice how your breath is gently directed into your solar plexus, instilling a sense of gentle warmth and nourishment.
- With each inhalation, your solar plexus expands outward naturally, and with each exhaling breath, it softens inward, and relaxes completely.
- Take several breaths to sense how this rhythmic movement of expansion and relaxation deeply massages this area of your being, supporting your digestive system in functioning optimally.
- Visualize your power of digestion as a golden glow that radiates out from the center of your solar plexus, bathing each of your digestive organs with vital energy.
- Begin by taking several breaths to sense your golden glow bathing your stomach with nourishing energy, enhancing its ability to break down food more efficiently.
- Your golden glow is now gently directed into your pancreas, assisting it in completing the process of breaking down food completely.
- Now, visualize your small intestine filled with golden energy, sensing the rhythmic movement that allows nutrients to be absorbed into your bloodstream optimally.
- Next, your golden glow bathes your liver in nourishing vitality, allowing it to store nutrients and energy more efficiently while removing toxins from your bloodstream.
- With digestion and absorption of nutrients functioning harmoniously, your golden glow now flows through your large intestine, completing the process of healthy digestion by eliminating waste products efficiently.
- With your entire digestive system functioning smoothly, take several breaths to sense your golden glow radiating throughout your entire being, providing you with the vitality to live fully and vibrantly.
- Affirm your optimal digestion, repeating the following three times, aloud or silently: **"With my digestion functioning optimally, I am fully nourished with vital energy."**
- Slowly release the gesture, taking several breaths to sense complete nourishment.
- When you are ready, open your eyes, returning slowly and gently, continuing your journey with abundant vital energy.

Annamaya kosha (physical body)

• Directs breath and awareness into the solar plexus and abdomen, cultivating a massaging effect that enhances circulation to the digestive system.
• Lengthens the inhalation and the exhalation evenly, facilitating deeper, fuller breathing.
• Generally helpful for digestive imbalances in all three doshas.

Pranamaya kosha (energy body)

• Balances the flow of Samana vayu, the horizontal current of energy.
• Opens and balances the third chakra, center of personal power.

Manomaya kosha (psycho-emotional body)

• Cultivates calm and steadiness in the mind and breath.
• Instills a sense of emotional balance that helps digest and assimilate life experiences.

Vijnanamaya kosha (wisdom body)

• With enhanced ability to digest and assimilate life experiences, we use our life energy wisely, learning from experiences and then releasing what we no longer need to continue our journey with greater lightness and ease.

Anandamaya kosha (bliss body)

• Cultivates sensations of fullness and contentment within the solar plexus and abdomen.

29

Brahma Mudra

Gesture of Creative Energy

For Weight Management

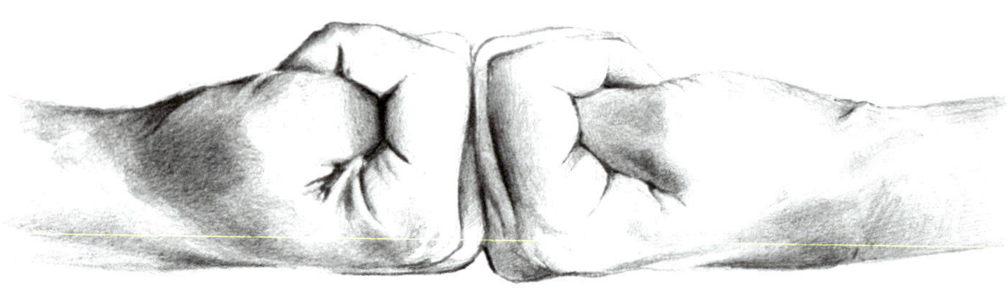

With radiant vitality at all levels of being,
I manifest my life purpose completely.

Core Quality

Awakening Energy and Vitality

Especially helpful for

- Supporting weight management.
- Optimizing digestion and elimination.
- Instilling energy and vitality.
- Building self-esteem and determination.
- Realizing our full potential.
- Developing self-mastery.

Mudras with similar effects

Matangi, Mushtikam, Merudanda

Cautions

Those with hypertension should begin with Pushan mudra, then continue with Surya, advancing to Vajra, and finally experimenting with Brahma, while monitoring the effects.

Instructions

1. Make the hands into fists with the thumbs inside.
2. Turn the palms upward and place the backs of the fists together, pressing them gently against each other.
3. Rest the gesture against the solar plexus.
4. Relax the shoulders back and down, with the elbows held away from the body and the spine naturally aligned.

At least twenty-five percent of adults in the United States are obese and an additional thirty-five percent are overweight. Genetics play a role, but lifestyle issues, including lack of exercise, overeating and unhealthy diets, are primary factors.[16] Stress is also a factor, contributing to weight gain in several ways. The pace of modern life tends to increase feelings of anxiety and eating is often used to provide temporary relief. Chronic stress also elevates cortisol levels, which increase abdominal fat storage. Advances in technology have created a virtual world leading to isolation and reduced physical activity, which are important factors in obesity, especially in childhood. The values of modern society also play a role in obesity. Consumerism encourages us to fill ourselves up from the outside, as opposed to finding nourishment and contentment through exploring our life's deeper values and meaning.

Brahma is the "deity of creation," and Brahma mudra directs breath, awareness and energy into the solar plexus, our center of personal power. This gesture is stimulating, enhancing the power of digestion as well as elimination, leading to increased vitality. This mudra cultivates enthusiasm and builds self-esteem, providing the determination that allows us to move toward our goals more easily, including those related to weight loss and dieting. Brahma mudra also instills a sense that we are inherently whole and complete, reducing the need to fill ourselves up from the outside by eating unconsciously. At the deepest level, Brahma mudra cultivates the clarity that allows us to see that we have the power to transform our lifestyle and habits to become the creators of our own destiny.

Systems Balanced:

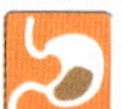 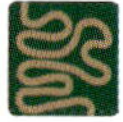

Elements Activated:

Doshas Balanced:

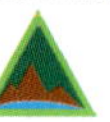

Prana Vayus Nourished:

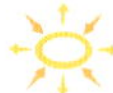

Chakras Balanced:

Scale from Calming to Energizing:

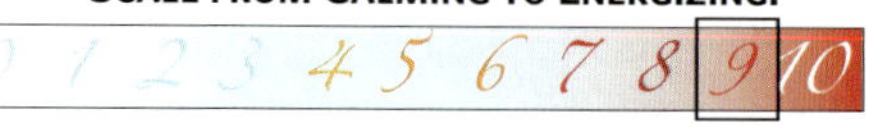

Guided Meditation: Radiant Inner Sun

- As you hold Brahma mudra, take several natural breaths to attune to all the feelings and sensations awakened by this gesture.
- Notice how your breath is naturally directed into your solar plexus, your center of empowerment, awakening the energy that allows you to live with greater vitality.
- In order to connect more deeply with your source of vital energy, visualize a golden sun at the center of your solar plexus shining brightly.
- With each inhalation, energy is concentrated at the center of your being, and with each exhalation, it radiates outward, filling you with the golden sunlight of vitality.
- Begin by sensing this radiant golden sunlight bathing your digestive system in vital energy, supporting it in functioning optimally.
- Take some time to sense radiant energy enhancing your body's ability to transform food into nutrients efficiently, assimilating them, and eliminating all waste products completely.
- With your physical digestion more complete, your golden sun enhances your ability to digest life experiences more easily, assimilating the learning you need while releasing all that no longer serves your journey.
- With enhanced ability to digest food and experiences easily, your inner sun now infuses your thoughts and feelings, cultivating the enthusiasm and vitality to live life more vibrantly.
- Living with greater enthusiasm and vitality, you are able to release habits and limiting beliefs that keep you from unfolding all of your talents and possibilities.
- As you release limiting beliefs, the rays of your inner sun fill you with the clarity and energy to define your life goals clearly and manifest them completely.
- With greater clarity and energy, you naturally adopt a lifestyle that supports your journey, including a balanced diet that provides optimal nutrition for all of your activities.
- Now, sense your golden sun illuminating all the dimensions of your being, providing you with the determination to overcome all obstacles along your journey, allowing you to live with radiant vitality.
- Affirm your radiant energy as you repeat the following three times, aloud or silently: **"As I awaken the sun of my inner being, I live with optimal energy and vitality."**
- Slowly release the gesture, taking several breaths to sense your inner radiance.
- When you are ready, open your eyes, returning slowly and gently, integrating greater energy and vitality into all of your activities.

Annamaya kosha (physical body)

- **Directs breath and awareness to the area of the solar plexus, cultivating a massaging effect that enhances circulation to the digestive system.**
- **Strengthens the diaphragm, enhancing respiration.**
- **Creates a massaging effect in the mid back that enhances circulation to the area of the kidneys and adrenal glands.**
- **Cultivates energy and vitality that supports weight loss.**
- **The stimulating effects cultivated by this gesture are generally helpful for Kapha imbalance.**

Pranamaya kosha (energy body)

- **Activates the flow of Samana vayu, the horizontal current of energy.**
- **Opens and balances the third chakra, center of personal power.**

Manomaya kosha (psycho-emotional body)

- **Builds self-esteem.**
- **Instills confidence and determination for achieving goals, including weight loss.**
- **Cultivates a sense of contentment and satisfaction, reducing the need to eat as a substitute for unfulfilled emotional needs.**

Vijnanamaya kosha (wisdom body)

- **Awakening our inner sun gives us the clarity to discern between the compulsions of the personality and the essential wholeness of our true being.**

Anandamaya kosha (bliss body)

- **The rays of our inner sun fill us with luminosity and radiant vitality.**

30 Mira Mudra

Gesture of the Ocean

For Asthma & Easeful Breathing

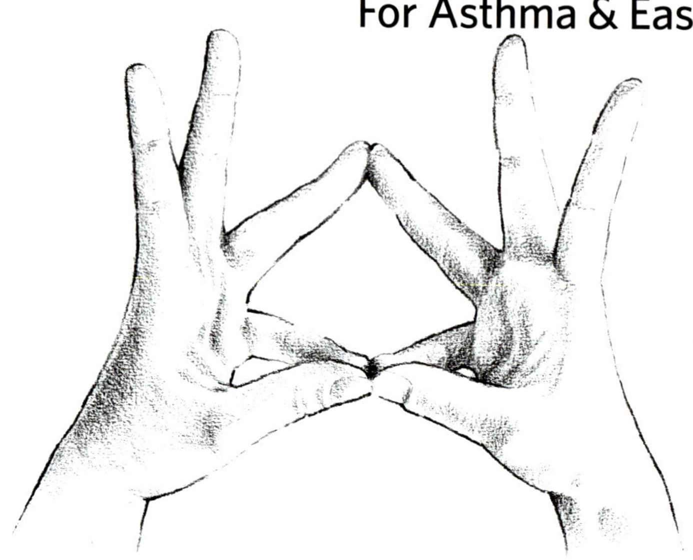

Greater harmony in all my activities
Supports me in breathing freely and easily.

Core Quality
Easeful Breathing

Especially helpful for
- Asthma and other respiratory issues.
- Supporting the health of the sacrum, pelvis and hip joints.
- Supporting the reproductive, urinary and eliminatory systems.
- Enhancing abdominal breathing, reducing stress and relieving anxiety.

Mudras with similar effects
Svadhisthana, Prajna Prana Kriya, Dvimukham, Pranidhana, Dirgha Svara

Cautions
Dirgha Svara should be used only when out of crisis and when you feel comfortable with all the other mudras above.

Instructions
1. Join the tips of the thumbs to the tips of the little fingers of the same hand.
2. Bring the joined fingers and thumbs of each hand together.
3. Touch the tips of the ring fingers together.
4. Extend the index and middle fingers.
5. Rest the hands below the navel.
6. Relax the shoulders back and down, with the spine naturally aligned.

Asthma is a respiratory condition whose main symptom is difficulty in breathing, accompanied by wheezing and tightness in the chest. This condition is caused by hypersensitivity of the bronchial tree, which activates an immune reaction, narrowing the breathing passages as a defense against irritants. Asthma may be accompanied by a persistent dry cough, sensations of tightness in the chest, shortness of breath and difficulty exhaling. Asthma can also be accompanied by a sense of panic, exhaustion and a state of confusion. Any number of factors such as pollen, dust, animal hair, certain food substances or physical exercise can bring on an asthma attack. Stress can be a factor both in the onset of an asthma attack and in the duration and intensity of symptoms.[17]

Mira means "ocean," and Mira mudra cultivates a feeling of fluidity and serenity, thereby reducing stress and allowing freer breathing. This gesture directs breath, awareness and energy into the pelvis and low abdomen. It calms the breath and also lengthens the exhalation, which is especially important for those who suffer from asthma. As Mira mudra cultivates calm and serenity, it helps to relieve the fear and anxiety that often accompany asthma. This gesture balances the first and second *chakras*, cultivating grounding and security while instilling a sense of nourishment and fluidity. This combination of grounding and fluidity supports the release of tightness and constriction, both at the physical and psychological levels, enhancing our ability to flow with life more easily.

Systems Balanced:

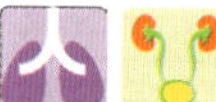

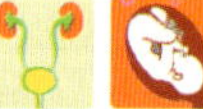

Elements Activated:

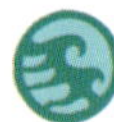

Doshas Balanced:

Prana Vayus Nourished:

Chakras Balanced:

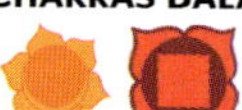

Scale from Calming to Energizing:

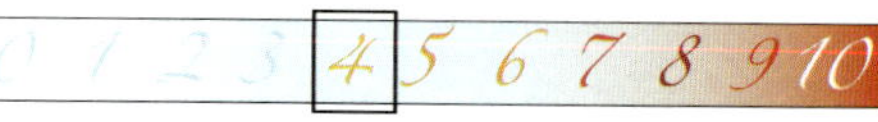

Guided Meditation: Wave of Easeful Breathing

- As you hold Mira mudra, take several natural breaths to attune to all the feelings and sensations evoked by this gesture.
- Notice how your breath is gently directed down into your pelvis and lower abdomen, instilling a sense of comfort and ease that allows your breath to flow smoothly and freely.
- Experience your breathing as soft waves rolling slowly up onto the shore and then gently returning to the sea.
- Take some time to ride your wave of breath as it comes and goes smoothly, allowing you to become more comfortable with the natural flow of your breathing.
- Sense your breathing as a natural giving and receiving between the atmosphere, your source of vital energy, and your lungs, where air is transformed to nourish your entire body.
- Take several breaths to attune to this natural giving and receiving, cultivating a growing friendship between your surroundings and your inner being.
- As you become more comfortable with giving and receiving within your breathing, allow this natural reciprocity to infuse all the dimensions of your being.
- Begin by envisioning a natural balance of giving and receiving within your relationships.
- As you inhale, sense yourself opening to receive love, support and caring, and as you exhale, sense your deepening ability to nourish others emotionally.
- Take several breaths to sense this natural giving and receiving within your emotional being, noticing how it naturally supports the free flow of your breathing.
- With greater emotional fluidity, you expand your balance of giving and receiving to encompass your career and role in the community.
- As you inhale, open to receive recognition for all of your talents and abilities, and as you exhale, see yourself sharing your gifts generously for the benefit of all beings.
- Take several breaths to sense this natural giving and receiving within your community, noticing how it naturally supports the free flow of your breathing.
- As the wave of giving and receiving touches all dimensions of your being, the frontiers of your heart expand naturally, allowing you to continue your journey joyfully and confidently.
- Affirm your easeful breathing, repeating the following three times, aloud or silently: **"The natural balance of giving and receiving is reflected in my easeful breathing."**
- Now, slowly release the gesture, taking several breaths to sense the complete harmony that allows you to live and breathe more easily.
- When you are ready, open your eyes, returning slowly and gently with deeper, freer breathing.

Annamaya kosha (Physical body)

• Directs breath and awareness to the pelvis, creating a massaging effect that enhances circulation to the reproductive and urinary systems.
• Cultivates a rhythmic abdominal breath and a lengthened exhalation, which are helpful for asthma.
• The calming effects cultivated by this gesture are generally helpful for Pitta imbalance.
• The centering effects of this gesture are generally helpful for Vata imbalance.

Pranamaya kosha (Energy body)

• Activates Apana vayu, the downward moving current of energy.
• Opens and balances the first and second chakras, centers of safety and self-nourishment.

Manomaya kosha (Psycho-emotional body)

• Instills a sense of fluidity.
• Cultivates a sense of trust and emotional balance.

Vijnanamaya kosha (Wisdom body)

• As we experience easeful breathing, we naturally release excessive fear and anxiety, recognizing the essential safety of our true being.

Anandamaya kosha (Bliss body)

• With greater fluidity in our breathing and a balance of giving and receiving, a deep sense of serenity arises naturally.

31 Vayan Mudra

Gesture of the Vehicle of the Air Element

For Hypertension & the Health of the Cardiovascular System

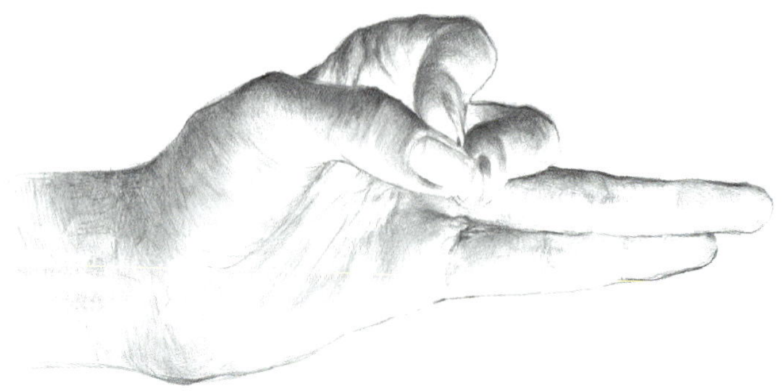

Releasing into the stream of serenity,
I experience complete inner nourishment and healing.

Core Quality
Optimal Circulation

Especially helpful for

- Hypertension and the health of the cardiovascular system.
- Releasing muscular tension from the entire body, especially the chest.
- Instilling fluidity and a sense of refreshment in the breath.
- Helping to reduce stress and anxiety, instilling a sense of serenity.

Mudras with similar effects
Chinmaya, Dvimukham, Pranidhana, Svadhisthana

Cautions
None

Instructions

1. Touch the tips of the thumbs to the tips of the index and middle fingers of each hand.
2. Extend the ring and little fingers straight out.
3. Rest the backs of the hands on the thighs or knees.
4. Relax the shoulders back and down, with the spine naturally aligned.

Hypertension is the chronic elevation of blood pressure in the arteries. When the circulatory system is functioning normally, blood pressure rises and falls dynamically, depending on our perceived needs for energy. In hypertension, this flexibility is lost, and the pressure within the arteries remains elevated. Factors in hypertension include genetics, diet, lifestyle, lack of exercise and especially stress. When we face stressful situations, blood pressure is elevated to provide energy to meet a perceived need, and when the stressor has passed, it then normalizes. In the case of chronic stress, however, this demand for energy is ongoing and the body adapts by maintaining elevated blood pressure, leading to hypertension. Hypertension is often asymptomatic and is discovered by blood pressure monitoring. Long-term hypertension increases the risk of atherosclerosis, heart disease and stroke.

Vayan means "vehicle of the air element," and Vayan mudra is the gesture traditionally recommended for hypertension. This gesture gently expands the chest, instilling a sense of ease and openness. It cultivates an optimal ratio within the breath, with the exhalation slightly longer than the inhalation, ideal for relaxation. This gesture instills a sense of fluidity in our breathing, along with a feeling that the entire circulatory system is flowing smoothly and easily. At the energetic level, this gesture gently activates *Prana vayu*, the upward moving current of energy, instilling a refreshing quality, like a soothing stream flowing throughout the chest. Vayan mudra also activates *Apana vayu*, the downward moving current, releasing tension from the chest, while enhancing relaxation. This gesture opens *Anahata chakra*, cultivating positive emotions, which help to reduce stress and blood pressure.

Systems Balanced:

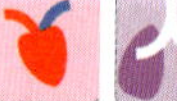
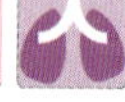

Elements Activated:

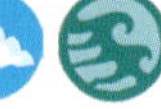

Doshas Balanced:

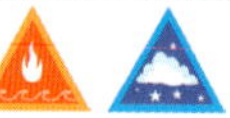
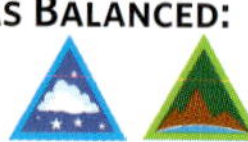

Prana Vayus Nourished:

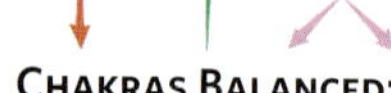

Chakras Balanced:

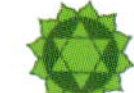

Scale from Calming to Energizing:

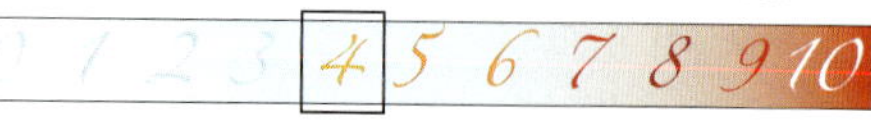

Guided Meditation: **Stream of Serenity**

- As you hold Vayan mudra, take several natural breaths to attune to all the feelings and sensations awakened by this gesture.
- Notice how your breath flows smoothly along the entire front of your body, instilling a sense of comfort and ease, as if bathing in a soothing stream of serenity.
- Take several breaths to allow your stream of serenity to nourish your heart completely, allowing it to beat calmly and easily.
- As your heart beats more easily, a sense of relaxation and ease flows outward through your bloodstream to relax and heal each part of your body.
- Begin by sensing your inner stream flowing down into your legs and feet, bathing these areas with nourishment and healing, allowing them to soften and relax completely.
- Now, for your next few breaths, sense your pelvis and hips infused with healing and nourishment, allowing these areas to become absolutely soft and serene, as you relax more deeply.
- With circulation flowing smoothly throughout your lower body, your inner stream of serenity continues its journey, nourishing your abdomen and low back, allowing these areas to soften and completely relax.
- Your soft, slow, soothing stream now flows into your solar plexus and mid back, allowing the entire middle region of your body to be infused with absolute serenity.
- Now, your stream of serenity flows gently into your upper back and chest, taking several breaths to allow your heart and lungs to be fully nourished and deeply rest.
- As your torso and lower extremities relax completely, your shoulders, arms and hands, all the way to your fingertips, are filled with healing and nourishment.
- Your stream of serenity now flows gently up into your neck and head, relaxing your jaw, eyes and forehead, taking several breaths to sense a soft smile naturally spreading across your face, as all tension is soothed away.
- Now, as your soothing stream flows softly throughout your entire being, you sense your heart becoming even more calm and serene, allowing you to relax deeply and completely.
- Affirm your complete ease as you repeat the following three times, aloud or silently: **"As my stream of serenity flows smoothly through my being, I relax completely."**
- Slowly release the gesture, taking several breaths to rest in absolute serenity.
- When you are ready, open your eyes, returning slowly and gently, integrating greater serenity in all of your activities.

Annamaya kosha (physical body)

• Gently directs breath and energy into the chest, instilling a sensation of coolness and relaxation.
• Lengthens the exhalation, cultivating relaxation and reducing blood pressure.
• Cultivates a fluid, rhythmic breath that helps regulate the cardiovascular system.
• The balancing effects cultivated by this gesture are generally helpful for Vata, Pitta and Kapha imbalances.

Pranamaya kosha (energy body)

• Gently activates Prana vayu, the upward moving current of energy.
• Activates Apana vayu, the downward moving current of energy, as well as Vyana vayu, the all-pervading energy, moving from center to extremities.
• Opens and balances the fourth chakra, center of unconditional love.

Manomaya kosha (psycho-emotional body)

• Cultivates an overall feeling of contentment and serenity that reduces stress and anxiety.
• Instills a sense of fluidity and ease.

Vijnanamaya kosha (wisdom body)

• As we develop greater fluidity and ease in the body, breath and mind, we are able to witness stressful situations with greater equanimity.

Anandamaya kosha (bliss body)

• As we become one with the stream of serenity, a sense of deep contentment flows through our entire body.

32 Apana Vayu Mudra

Gesture of the Downward Current of Energy

For the Health of the Heart

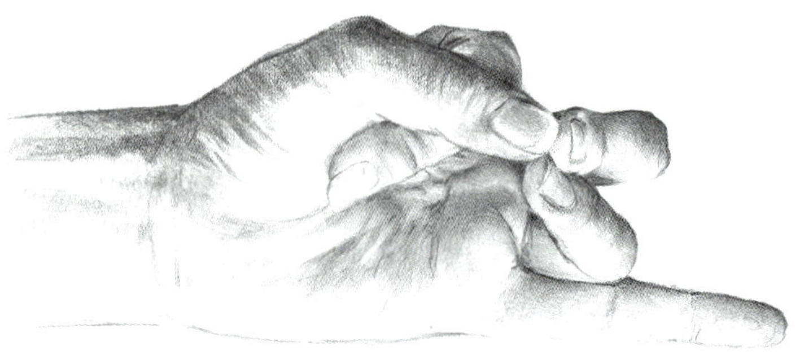

Listening to my heart sensitively
Naturally supports its health and vitality.

Core Quality

Healthy Heart

Especially helpful for

- Supporting optimal health of the heart and circulatory system.
- Releasing constriction from the chest.
- Reducing stress.
- Instilling calm and confidence.
- Cultivating intuition.

Mudras with similar effects

Padma, Purna Hridaya, Kapota, Karuna

Cautions

Discontinue if chest or upper body discomfort, fatigue or shortness of breath occur.

Instructions

1. Bend the index fingers down to touch the base of the thumbs.
2. Touch the tips of the thumbs to the tips of the middle and ring fingers.
3. Extend the little fingers straight out.
4. Rest the backs of the hands on the thighs or knees.
5. Relax the shoulders back and down, with the spine naturally aligned.

The human heart is an engineering miracle. It pumps 2,000 gallons of blood per day and fifty-five million gallons in a lifetime. With an average of eighty beats per minute, the heart beats 2.5 billion times in seventy years. Resting, the heart pumps about twelve pints each minute, but exercise can increase heart rate to 200 beats, pumping nearly 100 pints per minute. Incredibly, two heart cells from different beings, when placed together, begin to beat in synchrony. Exquisitely designed, the heart is prepared to survive almost anything, except the pace of modern life, where chronic stress and sedentary lifestyle have become the heart's worst enemy. The heart has one phase of contraction for each two phases of rest, and the heart's own physiology is an appropriate metaphor for what it needs to remain healthy. For most people, however, life is just the opposite - constant stress with very little time for complete rest. Because so few people listen to their own hearts, it's not surprising that heart disease is the leading cause of death in developed countries.

Apana vayu means "purifying current." Apana Vayu mudra is a composite of Apana mudra and Vayu mudra. Vayu mudra lengthens the inhalation, gently expanding the chest while Apana mudra lengthens the exhalation, releasing tension and stress from the chest area. The combination of expansion of the chest and deep relaxation cultivated by Apana Vayu mudra supports the optimal health of the heart and the entire circulatory system. This gesture cultivates a long natural pause at the end of the exhalation, creating a space of silence and deep rest in which we can attune to the rhythm of our own heart and begin to listen to its messages. As we listen more deeply, the heart reveals what it needs for its optimal health and well-being.

Systems Balanced:

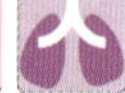

Elements Activated:

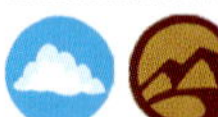
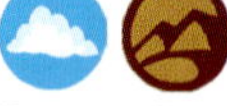

Doshas Balanced:

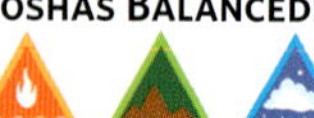

Prana Vayus Nourished:

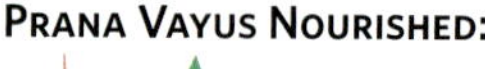

Chakras Balanced:

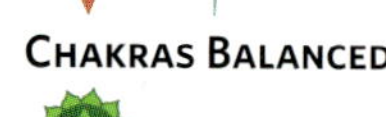

Scale from Calming to Energizing:

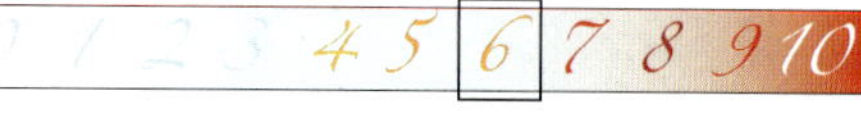

Guided Meditation: The Wisdom of the Heart

- As you hold Apana Vayu mudra, take several natural breaths to attune to all the feelings and sensations awakened by this gesture.
- Notice how your breath is gently directed into your chest, side ribs and upper back, cultivating a sense of lightness and openness.
- As your breath flows more freely, your rib cage expands and relaxes rhythmically, gently massaging your heart, supporting its optimal functioning.
- Take several breaths to listen to your heart more deeply, sensing how its every beat sends vitality to all the cells of your body while nourishing itself lovingly.
- As you attune to your heart with greater sensitivity, allow it to speak, opening to receive the guidance that would support its optimal health.
- Begin by listening to your heart with regard to changes you could make in your lifestyle, diet and daily activities.
- Take several breaths to reflect on which of your habits need to be gradually released, and what new activities would support your overall health and well-being.
- Listen to your heart's guidance sensitively, envisioning how its wisdom could be integrated into your daily routine.
- Now, attune to your heart and ask for guidance in relation to your thoughts and feelings, helping you to recognize the emotional patterns that cause stress and disharmony.
- Take several breaths to listen to your heart's guidance carefully, sensing the qualities you can cultivate, such as acceptance and empathy, that would lead to greater harmony in all of your interactions and activities.
- Now, attune to your heart even more sensitively, asking for guidance with regard to your life's purpose and deeper meaning.
- Take several breaths to reflect on your entire life journey, both the learnings and the blessings, embracing all you have done and been, while trusting your heart to guide you toward the manifestation of your true purpose and meaning.
- Listen to your heart's guidance lovingly, envisioning how its inherent wisdom can support your optimal health at all levels of being.
- Affirm the wisdom of your heart, repeating the following three times, aloud or silently: **"Listening to my heart with sensitivity, its wisdom guides my life journey."**
- Now, slowly release the gesture, taking several breaths to rest in your heart's inherent wisdom.
- When you are ready, open your eyes, returning slowly and gently, allowing your heart to guide your journey.

Annamaya kosha (physical body)

- **Gently directs breath and awareness into the chest, side ribs and upper back, releasing muscular contraction from these areas.**
- **Cultivates a healthy rhythm in the breath with the exhalation slightly longer than the inhalation, supporting the optimal functioning of the cardiovascular system.**
- **The expansion of the chest on the inhalation is generally helpful for Kapha imbalance.**
- **The calming effects together with enhanced sensitivity are generally helpful for Pitta imbalance.**
- **The rhythmic breathing and subsequent centering are generally helpful for Vata imbalance.**

Pranamaya kosha (energy body)

- **Gently activates the flow of Prana vayu, the upward moving current of energy.**
- **Activates Apana vayu, the downward moving current of energy.**
- **Opens and balances the fourth chakra, center of unconditional love.**

Manomaya kosha (psycho-emotional body)

- **Instills calm, confidence and open-heartedness.**
- **Releases psycho-emotional tension that constricts the subtle heart.**

Vijnanamaya kosha (wisdom body)

- **As tension is released, a space is created for listening to the heart's wisdom.**

Anandamaya kosha (bliss body)

- **As we listen to our hearts with sensitivity, openness, joy and love unfold naturally.**

33 MAHASHIRSHA MUDRA

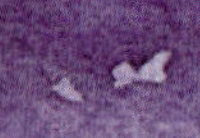

Gesture of the Great Head

For Headache & Tension Relief

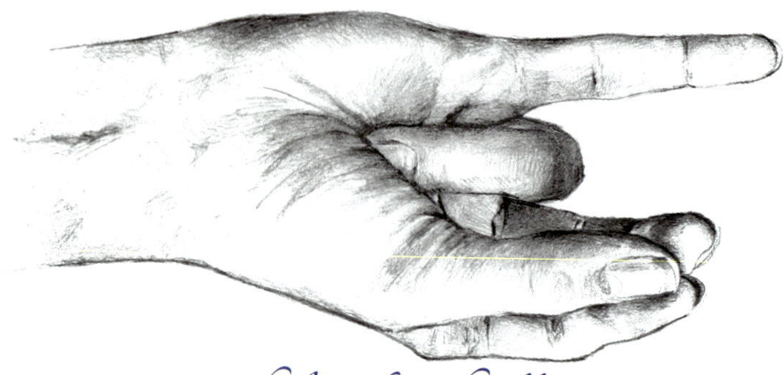

My exhaling breath allows me
To release stress and tension from my entire being.

CORE QUALITY

Headache Relief

ESPECIALLY HELPFUL FOR

- Relieving tension headache.
- Reducing muscular tension from the entire body, especially from the neck and head.
- Releasing tension from the jaw, which may be helpful for TMJ dysfunction.
- Reducing stress.

MUDRAS WITH SIMILAR EFFECTS

Pranidhana, Dvimukham, Apana, Apanayana

CAUTIONS

None

INSTRUCTIONS

1. Tuck the ring fingers into the palms.
2. Touch the tips of the thumbs to the tips of the index and middle fingers.
3. Extend the little fingers straight out as much as possible.
4. Rest the backs of the hands onto the thighs or knees with the palms facing upward.
5. Relax the shoulders back and down, with the spine naturally aligned.

About forty-five million Americans suffer from chronic headaches.[18] There are many types of headaches, with tension headache being among the most common. Factors in tension headache include poor posture, sleep deprivation, irregular meal times, eye strain and accumulated muscular tension. Stress is a factor in tension headaches, because during the stress response the breath moves to the upper chest, engaging the muscles of the shoulders and neck, increasing the breath rate to provide energy in preparation for the fight, flight or freeze response. When stress becomes chronic, these areas tend to remain contracted, creating the conditions in which a tension headache can occur. The stress response also increases circulation to the brain and head to enhance alertness, which is helpful for meeting a short-term challenge, but when stress becomes chronic, elevated blood pressure may become a factor in headaches.

Mahashirsha means "big head," referring to the sensation of lightness and comfort in the head cultivated by Mahashirsha mudra. This gesture releases muscular tension from the face, jaw and around the eyes, which may provide relief from tension headaches. As tension is released from the face and jaw, there is a natural softening around the area of the temporomandibular joint, which may be helpful for TMJ dysfunction. In this gesture, the inhalation instills a cooling effect, while the lengthened exhalation cultivates a sense of relief, a feeling that tension is being drained down and out of the head, shoulders and neck into the earth beneath. This gesture also instills a sense of letting go at the level of thoughts and emotions, which further supports headache relief.

SYSTEMS BALANCED:

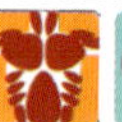
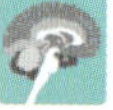
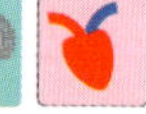

ELEMENTS ACTIVATED:

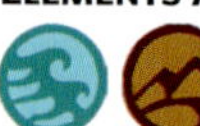
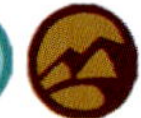

DOSHAS BALANCED:

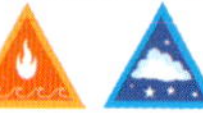

PRANA VAYUS NOURISHED:

CHAKRAS BALANCED:

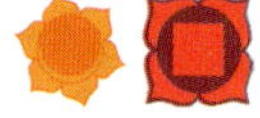

SCALE FROM CALMING TO ENERGIZING:

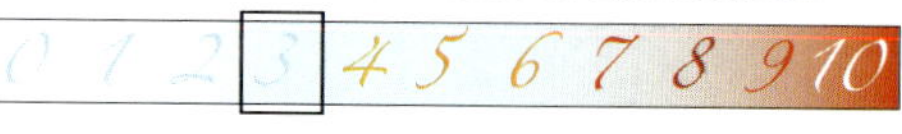

Guided Meditation: **Releasing Tension Downward**

ॐ As you hold Mahashirsha mudra, take several natural breaths to attune to all the feelings and sensations evoked by this gesture.

ॐ Sense how your exhalation is lengthened naturally, supporting the release of tension down and out into the earth beneath, allowing you to experience greater comfort and ease.

ॐ Begin by taking some time to sense your lengthened exhalation flowing down through your legs and feet, releasing tension from these areas into the earth beneath.

ॐ Now, your lengthened exhalation flows down into your abdomen, pelvis and hips, allowing all tension to naturally melt into the earth.

ॐ Your lengthened exhalation now dissolves all tension from your solar plexus and mid back, allowing these areas to completely soften and relax.

ॐ Now, sense all tension being released from your chest and upper back, down into the earth beneath, cultivating lightness and ease that allows you to breathe more freely.

ॐ Your lengthened exhaling breath now cascades down through your shoulders, arms and hands, releasing all tension.

ॐ Now, your exhalation flows gently down through your head, throat and neck, allowing all tension to be dissolved from these areas.

ॐ As tension from your head is released, sense your forehead, temples and eyes relax completely, allowing a serene smile to spread across your face and permeate your entire being.

ॐ Now, as your exhaling breath flows smoothly downward from the crown of your head to the soles of your feet, all remaining tension is naturally released into the earth beneath, allowing you to rest in absolute comfort and ease.

ॐ Affirm your complete relief as you repeat the following three times, aloud or silently: **"As tension is released into the earth beneath, I rest in absolute comfort and ease."**

ॐ Slowly release the gesture, taking several breaths to deeply rest.

ॐ When you are ready, open your eyes, returning slowly and gently, with a greater sense of comfort and ease throughout your entire being.

Annamaya kosha (physical body)

• Lengthens the exhaling breath, cultivating relaxation that reduces stress.
• Releases tension from the muscles of the shoulders, neck, jaw and head.
• The cooling effects cultivated by this gesture are generally helpful for Pitta imbalance.
• The calming effects of this gesture are generally helpful for Vata imbalance.

Pranamaya kosha (energy body)

• Activates Apana vayu, the downward moving current of energy.
• Opens and balances the first and second chakras, centers of safety and self-nourishment.

Manomaya kosha (psycho-emotional body)

• Instills a sense of release.
• Helps to let go of worry and anxiety.

Vijnanamaya kosha (wisdom body)

• The feeling of release allows us to surrender into the lightness and ease of our true inner being.

Anandamaya kosha (bliss body)

• As we learn to let go, we experience a sense of freedom and limitlessness.

34

Garuda Mudra

Gesture of the Eagle

For the Thyroid & the Health of the Endocrine System

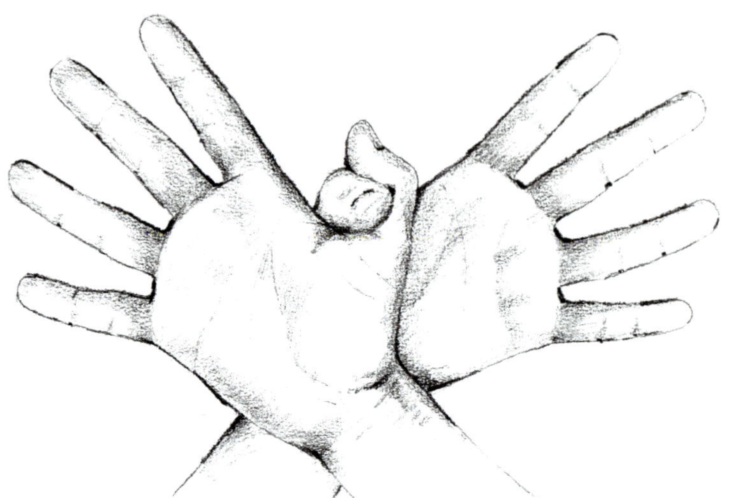

A balance of rest and activity
Supports all my body systems
In functioning optimally.

Core Quality

Balanced Metabolism

Especially helpful for

- Supporting the health of the thyroid.
- Aligning the cervical spine.
- Supporting the health of the throat and vocal cords.
- Releasing tension from the neck and jaw, which may be helpful for TMJ.
- Balancing rest and activity.

Mudras with similar effects

Kaleshvara, Vishuddha, Angushtha

Cautions

Those taking medications for the thyroid should monitor hormone levels regularly.

Instructions

1. Hold the right palm facing the chest.
2. Place the palm of the left hand onto the back of the right hand.
3. Slide the thumbs toward each other until they interlock.
4. The hands are angled diagonally, forming wings, with the fingers held together or slightly open.
5. Relax the shoulders back and down, with the elbows held slightly away from the body and the spine naturally aligned.

The thyroid gland is an organ of the endocrine system that regulates metabolism. In hypothyroidism, which affects ten percent of Americans, the thyroid produces insufficient quantities of its main hormones. Its most common symptoms include fatigue, weakness, weight gain, constipation, depression and irritability. Though far less common, the thyroid may also be overactive, as in Grave's Disease, whose symptoms include rapid heartbeat, increased bowel movements, nervousness and weight loss. Genetics, aging, diet and lifestyle are factors in thyroid conditions.[19] Stress is also a factor, because a higher rate of metabolism is essential for increasing energy and activity during the stress response. Like all other systems of our body, the thyroid functions optimally during periods of activity, followed by rest and regeneration. When stress becomes chronic, however, the thyroid is asked to function at a high level continuously, which may impair its functioning.

Garuda is a "mythical eagle," the vehicle for the god *Vishnu*, the deity who sustains creation. Garuda mudra directs breath, awareness and energy into the upper chest and neck with a special focus on the throat, where the thyroid is located. As breath and awareness are focused into the throat, circulation to this area is increased which supports the thyroid's functioning. This mudra enhances our awareness of the importance of balance in all of our activities that support the thyroid in functioning optimally. The position of the hands in this mudra, resembling two wings, is similar to the shape of the two lobes of the thyroid gland. These two wings symbolize the balance of rest and activity needed for the optimal functioning of the thyroid gland and the entire endocrine system.

Systems Balanced:

 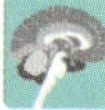 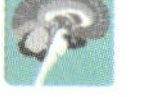

Elements Activated:

Doshas Balanced:

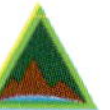

Prana Vayus Nourished:

Chakras Balanced:

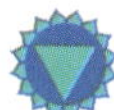

Scale from Calming to Energizing:

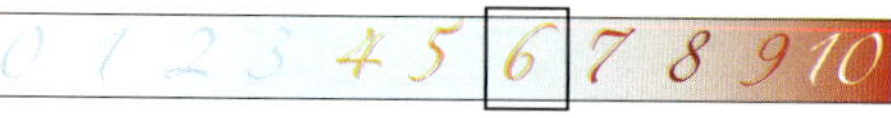

Guided Meditation: Wings of Balance

- As you hold Garuda mudra, take several natural breaths to attune to all the feelings and sensations awakened by this gesture.
- Notice how your breath is gently directed into your upper chest, throat and neck, naturally releasing tension from these areas.
- As tension is released, you experience greater balance and harmony throughout your entire being.
- To deepen your sense of balance and harmony, you will explore some of your body's polarities, naturally leading to an overall feeling of integration and unity.
- Begin by taking some time to sense your breath flowing through your left nostril and the left side of your body, experiencing the cooling and refreshing qualities that arise naturally.
- Now, bring your awareness to your right nostril and right side of your body, taking several breaths to sense the warming and energizing qualities that arise.
- Next, allow your breath to flow through both nostrils and both sides of your body evenly, experiencing an enhanced sense of integration and harmony.
- Continue your journey by taking several breaths to bring awareness to the right hemisphere of your brain: the intuitive, receptive aspect of your being.
- Next, take several breaths to bring awareness into the left hemisphere of your brain: the dynamic, cognitive aspect of your being.
- Now, allow your awareness to rest in both hemispheres evenly, taking several breaths to experience the integration and harmony that arise naturally, balancing your receptive and dynamic polarities.
- Continue your journey of balance and harmony by bringing breath and awareness to your thyroid gland, at the center of your throat, an essential organ for regulating metabolism.
- This gland has two lobes, shaped like wings, serving as a symbol for the balance of rest and activity that allows you to live with inner and outer harmony.
- Begin by bringing breath and awareness to your thyroid's left wing as a symbol for restoration and recovery, the time your body needs for complete healing.
- Next, bring breath and awareness to your thyroid's right wing, and sense its symbolic meaning: providing abundant vitality and energy for all of your activities.
- Now, bring breath and awareness into both sides of your thyroid evenly, sensing the perfect balance of rest and activity that supports the health of your endocrine system, allowing your whole body to function optimally.
- As all the polarities of your body are balanced naturally, sense your entire being resting in perfect harmony.
- Affirm your harmony as you repeat the following three times, aloud or silently: **"With all of my polarities balanced naturally, I experience perfect harmony."**
- Slowly release the gesture, taking several breaths to experience complete balance.
- When you are ready, open your eyes, returning slowly and gently, with a greater sense of the harmony of your essential being.

Annamaya kosha (physical body)

• Directs breath and awareness to the upper chest, neck and throat, enhancing circulation to the area of the thyroid gland.
• Releases tension from the throat and vocal cords, which may be helpful for those who sing or speak professionally.
• Releases tension from the jaw, which may be helpful for TMJ dysfunction.
• Supports alignment of the cervical spine.
• The mildly energizing effects cultivated by this gesture are generally helpful for Kapha imbalance.

Pranamaya kosha (energy body)

• Activates Udana vayu, the uppermost current of energy.
• Opens and balances the fifth chakra, center of spiritual purification.
• Balances Ida and Pingala nadis.

Manomaya kosha (psycho-emotional body)

• Cultivates a sense of balance in the mind and emotions.
• Supports clear communication.

Vijnanamaya kosha (wisdom body)

• Cultivates integration, harmony and equanimity as reflections of our true being.

Anandamaya kosha (bliss body)

• As balance is increased, we sense greater lightness and freedom, like a bird in flight.

35

Vajrapradama Mudra

Gesture of Unshakable Trust

For Depression

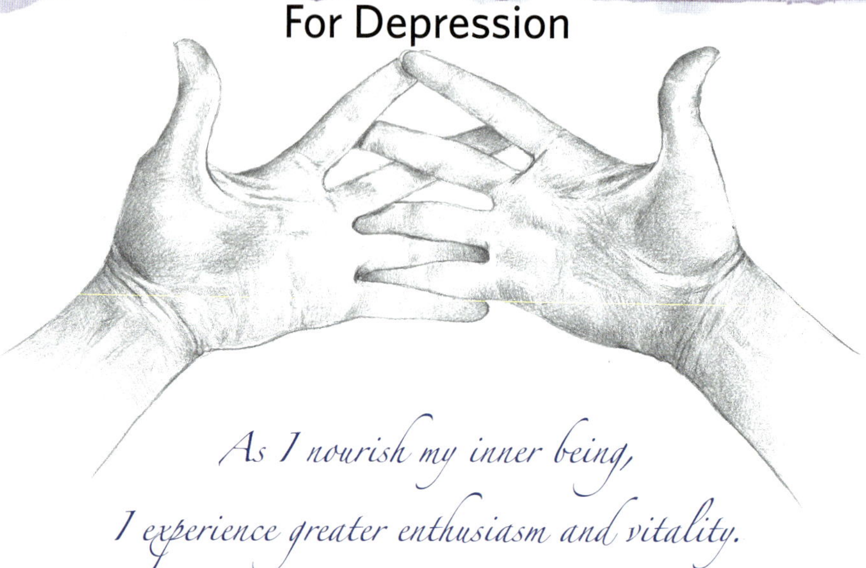

As I nourish my inner being,
I experience greater enthusiasm and vitality.

Core Quality

Enthusiasm for Living

Especially Helpful For

- Supporting treatment of depression.
- Releasing constriction from the chest, ribs and upper back.
- Enhancing self-trust and confidence.
- Increasing energy and enthusiasm.
- Enhancing sensitivity to the qualities of the subtle heart.

Mudras with Similar Effects

Padma, Purna Hridaya, Dirgha Svara, Kaleshvara

Cautions

None

Instructions

1. Hold the palms one hand's width away from the chest facing the body.
2. Open the fingers and interlace them at the middle digits, with the left little finger on the bottom while extending the thumbs upward.
3. Angle the fingers slightly upward, creating a small space between the webbing of the fingers.
4. Relax the shoulders back and down, with the elbows slightly away from the body and the spine naturally aligned.

Depression is a psychological condition whose symptoms include sadness, melancholy, pessimism, hopelessness and low self-esteem. Physical symptoms include lethargy, sleep disturbances and reduced sexual activity. Mild, short-term depression is experienced by almost everyone at some time in life as we face challenges and crises. In major, or clinical depression, which affects approximately 20 million Americans, there tends to be a pattern of helplessness in which the individual generalizes negative experiences to all of life.[20] Depression may be precipitated by life events and changes, including financial difficulties, job problems, relationship troubles, separation, bereavement and health challenges. In addition to the psychological factors, depression may have biological and genetic influences. Psychological stress is a factor, both in the onset of depression and in its continuing presence.

Vajrapradama means "unshakable trust and confidence." Vajrapradama mudra directs breath, awareness and energy into the chest, side ribs and upper back, cultivating a sense of openness and trust in ourselves and in life. The expanded thoracic breathing releases muscular tension from the chest and rib cage, cultivating a sense of relaxation and ease. The gentle lengthening of the inhalation instills a feeling of uplifting energy and vitality, which is helpful in improving mood and motivation. Vajrapradama mudra also directs breath, awareness and energy to the area of the thymus gland, supporting healthy immunity, which may be reduced during episodes of depression. This gesture opens *Anahata chakra*, at the center of the chest, increasing sensitivity to the heart's subtle qualities, which when nurtured carefully, reawaken enthusiasm and the joy of living.

Systems Balanced:

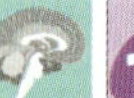 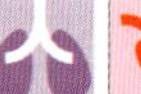 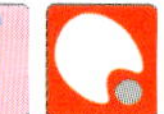

Prana Vayus Nourished:

Elements Activated:

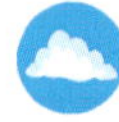

Chakras Balanced:

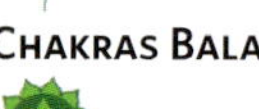

Doshas Balanced:

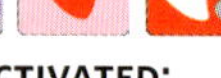 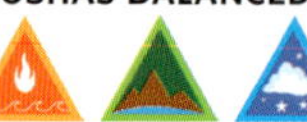

Scale from Calming to Energizing:

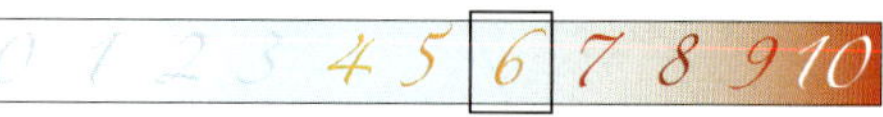

Guided Meditation: Nurturing your Heart's Essential Qualities

ॐ As you hold Vajrapradama mudra, take several natural breaths to attune to all the feelings and sensations awakened by this gesture.

ॐ Notice how your breath gently expands your chest, side ribs and upper back, allowing you to breathe more freely throughout your entire upper body.

ॐ With each inhaling breath, sense your lungs filled with uplifting energy and with each exhalation, sense all tension being released, allowing you to relax completely.

ॐ Take several breaths to sense how this harmony between vitality and release cultivates openness within your heart center that allows all of its essential qualities to unfold naturally.

ॐ Visualize these qualities as seeds, which blossom gradually when nurtured carefully within the garden of your heart.

ॐ Begin by taking several breaths to envision yourself planting the seed of self-nourishment.

ॐ As you nurture this seed lovingly, create an intention to honor and care for yourself by listening to your body's messages with sensitivity.

ॐ As self-nourishment blossoms within your heart, you plant the seed of self-esteem, recognizing that you are worthy to receive all of life's gifts and blessings.

ॐ Take several breaths to nurture the seed of self-esteem, envisioning its blossoming as your growing ability to honor and unfold all of your unique talents and possibilities.

ॐ Now, visualize yourself planting the seed of trust within the garden of your heart, allowing you to perceive that life's deepest intention is always to support your journey.

ॐ Take some time to envision yourself nurturing the seed of trust, sensing its blossoming as your ability to move forward in life confidently.

ॐ With self-nourishment, self-esteem and trust blossoming more fully, you now plant the seed of enthusiasm.

ॐ Take several breaths to see yourself nourishing this seed carefully, allowing you to reach out to life by embracing new projects and possibilities with energy and vitality.

ॐ Now, see all of your heart's essential qualities, nurtured tenderly, blossoming within the garden of your heart as full and joyful living.

ॐ Affirm your growing openness, repeating the following three times, aloud or silently: **"Nurturing my heart's essential qualities, I reawaken the joy of living."**

ॐ Now, slowly release the gesture, taking several breaths to sense the natural blossoming of your heart's essential qualities.

ॐ When you are ready, open your eyes, returning slowly and gently, with a greater sense of enthusiasm and vitality for living.

Annamaya kosha (physical body)

- **Directs breath and awareness into the chest, side ribs and upper back, enhancing breath capacity.**
- **Gently lengthens the inhalation, increasing metabolism and energy.**
- **Creates space between the shoulder blades, while lengthening and aligning the thoracic spine.**
- **The vitality cultivated by this gesture is generally helpful for Kapha imbalance.**
- **The heart-opening cultivated by this gesture is generally helpful for Pitta imbalance.**
- **The enhanced confidence and self-trust are generally helpful for Vata imbalance.**

Pranamaya kosha (energy body)

- **Gently activates Prana vayu, the upward moving current of energy.**
- **Opens and balances the fourth chakra, center of unconditional love.**

Manomaya kosha (psycho-emotional body)

- **Cultivates self-esteem and self-trust.**
- **Cultivates energy, enthusiasm and optimism.**

Vijnanamaya kosha (wisdom body)

- **Gradually opens the subtle heart, releasing negativity and awakening the heart's inherent positive qualities.**

Anandamaya kosha (bliss body)

- **As the subtle heart opens, enthusiasm and joy unfold naturally.**

36

Pala Mudra

Gesture of the Alms Bowl

For Anxiety

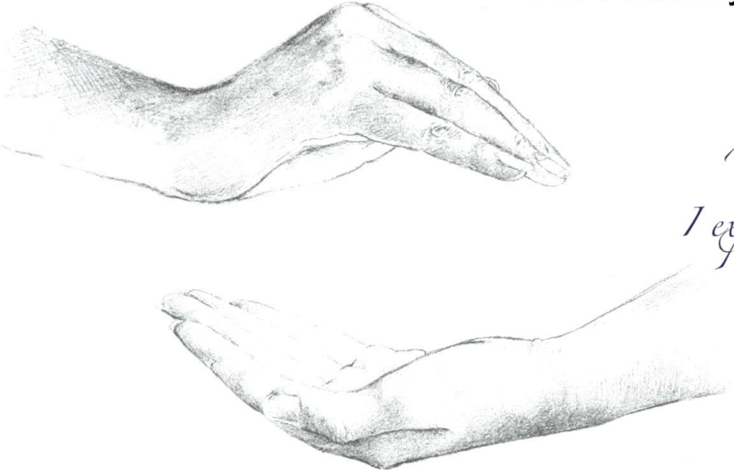

At peace within my inner being,
I experience a greater sense of security.

Core Quality

Anxiety Relief

Especially helpful for

- Supporting the treatment of anxiety.
- Releasing stress and muscular tension.
- Reducing blood pressure.
- Supporting the health of the reproductive, digestive and eliminatory systems.
- Instilling a sense of trust and non-attachment.
- Cultivating a sense of wholeness.

Mudras with similar effects

Chinmaya, Dvimukham, Svadhisthana

Cautions

None

Instructions

1. Cup the hands and place the left hand with the palm upward four finger-widths below the navel.
2. Place the right hand with the palm downward at the level of the navel, just above the left hand, with the hands gently touching the abdomen.
3. Relax the shoulders back and down, with the elbows held slightly away from the body and the spine naturally aligned.

Fear and worry are natural responses to life challenges, but when they become chronic, impairing our ability to live and work, they are classified as anxiety disorders. Anxiety disorders include generalized anxiety disorder (GAD), post-traumatic stress disorder (PTSD), phobias, panic disorder, social anxiety and obsessive-compulsive disorder (OCD). Generalized anxiety disorder affects over six million Americans, with women twice as likely to be affected.[21] Individuals with GAD experience chronic excessive worry and feelings of apprehension that disrupt social activities and can interfere with work, school or family. Physical symptoms include restlessness, insomnia, irritability, muscular tension, fatigue, gastrointestinal discomfort, heart palpitations and difficulty concentrating.

Pala is a "monk's begging bowl" used in the practice of receiving alms, called *bhiksha*. Cultivating non-attachment is a main facet of this practice; the monks receive only that which is freely given, without expectation and with a sense of tranquility, trusting that the universe always provides for their needs. Pala mudra instills this same sense of trust and tranquility. It slows the breath, directing awareness and energy into the abdomen, whose steady rise and fall relaxes the body while calming the mind and emotions. The cupped shape of the hands in this gesture, together with the abdominal breathing, instills a sense of entering a sanctuary where we can rest in complete tranquility. This gesture also supports us in reconnecting with our inherent wholeness, which gradually decreases our level of worry and anxiety. The calming effects of Pala mudra support the health of the reproductive, eliminatory and digestive systems.

Systems Balanced:

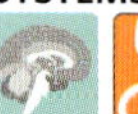
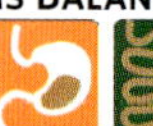
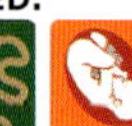
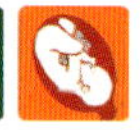

Elements Activated:

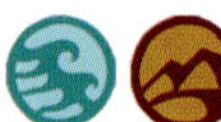

Doshas Balanced:

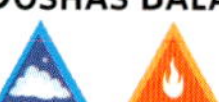

Prana Vayus Nourished:

Chakras Balanced:

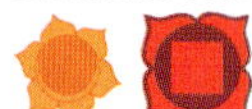

Scale from Calming to Energizing:

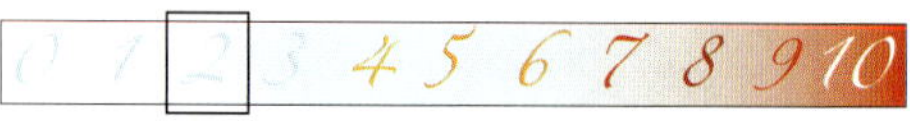

Guided Meditation: Sanctuary of Tranquility

ॐ As you hold Pala mudra, take several natural breaths to attune to all the feelings and sensations evoked by this gesture.

ॐ Notice how your breath is gently directed into your abdomen, instilling a sense of comfort and ease, as if entering your own inner sanctuary of tranquility.

ॐ Take some time to rest within this inner sanctuary, simply following the rhythmic rise and fall of your abdominal breathing, allowing you to relax completely.

ॐ To relax even more deeply, you will invite each area of your body into your inner sanctuary.

ॐ Begin by inviting your legs and feet into your sanctuary of tranquility, taking several breaths to allow these areas to relax completely.

ॐ Now, welcome your pelvis, abdomen and low back into your sanctuary, taking some time to sense these areas gently expanding and relaxing in synchrony with your soft, rhythmic breathing.

ॐ For the next few breaths, allow your chest and upper back to be bathed in absolute tranquility, naturally experiencing greater lightness and ease throughout these areas of your body.

ॐ Now, invite your shoulders, arms, hands and fingers into your sanctuary, allowing them to relax completely.

ॐ Your neck and head now enter and rest within your sanctuary of tranquility, allowing your eyes, ears, mouth and jaw to soften and relax completely.

ॐ Now, allow your entire being to rest within your inner sanctuary, taking several breaths to experience absolute tranquility.

ॐ Affirm your complete peace as you repeat the following three times, aloud or silently: **"Resting within my inner sanctuary, I experience absolute tranquility."**

ॐ Slowly release the gesture, taking several breaths to experience complete rest.

ॐ When you are ready, open your eyes, returning slowly and gently, bringing a deeper sense of tranquility into all of your activities.

Annamaya kosha (physical body)

• Directs breath and awareness into the abdomen, creating a gentle massaging effect that increases circulation to the reproductive, eliminatory and digestive systems.
• Lengthens the exhalation and slows the breath rate, helping to reduce anxiety.
• The stress reduction is helpful for hypertension.
• The calming effects cultivated by this gesture are helpful for Pitta imbalances.
• The centering effects are helpful for Vata imbalances.

Pranamaya kosha (energy body)

• Gently activates Apana vayu, the downward moving current of energy.
• Gently opens and balances the first and second chakras, centers of safety and self-nourishment.

Manomaya kosha (psycho-emotional body)

• Calms and relaxes the mind and creates space between thoughts.
• Cultivates a sense of safety and security.

Vijnanamaya kosha (wisdom body)

• With greater tranquility, we are able to witness fearful thoughts and feelings rather than identifying with them so completely.

Anandamaya kosha (bliss body)

• As the symptoms of anxiety decrease, we experience sensations of wholeness, well-being and ease.

37 Vyana Vayu Mudra

Gesture of All-Pervading Current of Energy

For MS & the Health of the Nervous System

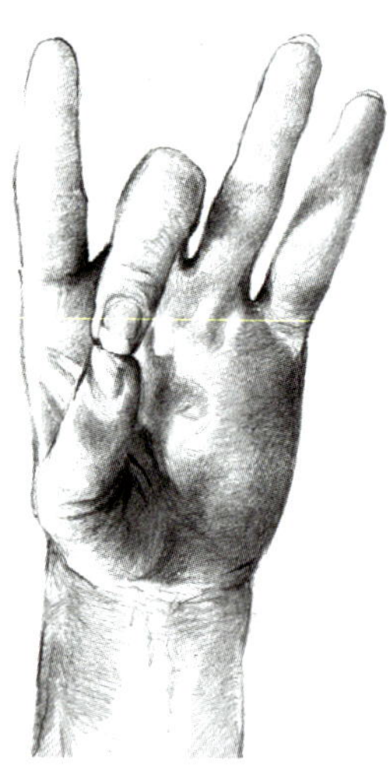

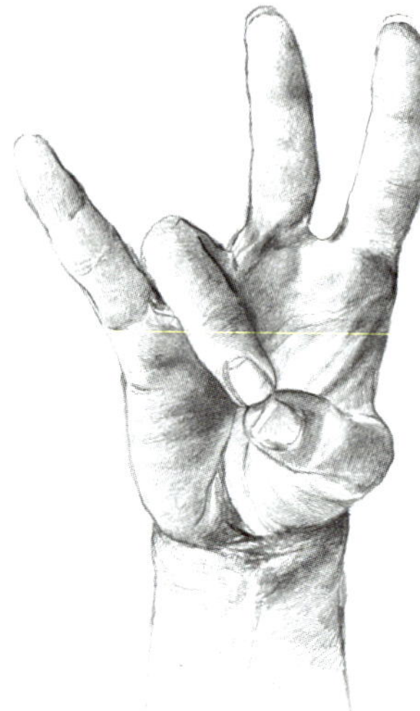

Nourishing all my energetic pathways
Supports my nervous system in
Functioning optimally.

Core Quality

Healthy Nervous System

Especially helpful for

- Supporting the health of the nervous system.
- Supporting the health of the joints.
- Improving circulation to the extremities.
- Enhancing body awareness.
- Promoting the free flow of energy within the subtle body.

Mudras with similar effects

Anushasana, Hakini, Dharma Chakra, Purna Jnanam

Cautions

For a more calming effect, those with MS should begin with the palms downward.

Instructions

1. Right hand: Touch the tip of the thumb to the tip of the ring finger. The other fingers are extended.
2. Left hand: Touch the tip of the thumb to the tip of the middle finger. The other fingers are extended.
3. Rest the hands onto the thighs or knees with the palms facing upward.
4. Release the shoulders back and down, with the spine naturally aligned.

Multiple Sclerosis (MS) is generally considered to be an autoimmune condition in which the immune system attacks and damages the myelin sheath that protects the nerves, thus impairing the transmission of nerve impulses from the brain to the body. Symptoms of MS vary widely, and in the earlier stages they may come and go, making diagnosis difficult. In its most severe form, individuals may lose their ability to walk and talk.[22] The exact causes of MS are unknown, but stress may be a factor. When the stress response becomes chronic, the sympathetic nervous system is activated continually to meet perceived needs. This is ideal for short-term challenges, because the brain, senses and nervous system are placed on high alert, increasing energy and concentration to deal with immediate threats. However, when the nervous system is activated constantly without sufficient time to recover, its functioning may become compromised.

Vyana vayu is the all-pervading current of energy that moves from the center of the body to the extremities. It supports the free flow of blood and nerve impulses at a subtle energetic level. Vyana Vayu mudra activates and balances the flow of Vyana vayu. This gesture directs breath and energy throughout the entire body, especially into the joints. It increases sensitivity within the extremities and is helpful for bringing warmth and energy to the hands and feet. Vyana Vayu mudra also nourishes the ayurvedic ***marmas***, the subtle energetic points located throughout the body. This gesture enhances body awareness both at the physical and subtle levels. The combination of enhanced body awareness, sensitivity and optimal flow of subtle energy cultivated by Vyana Vayu mudra may support the treatment of MS and other conditions of the nervous system.

Systems Balanced:

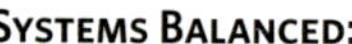
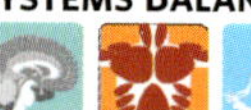
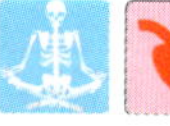
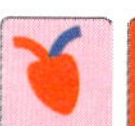
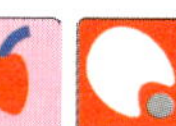

Elements Activated:

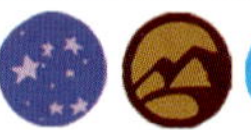

Doshas Balanced:

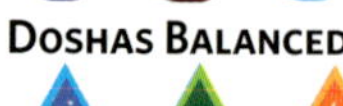

Prana Vayus Nourished:

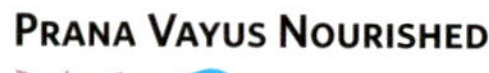
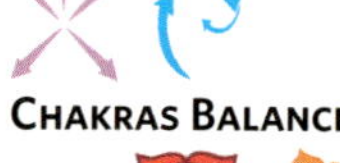

Chakras Balanced:

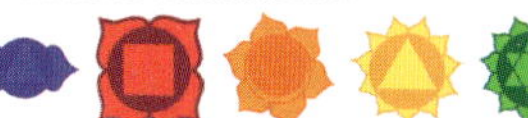

Scale from Calming to Energizing:

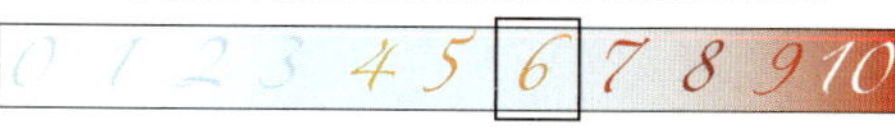

Guided Meditation: Restoring Clear Communication

ॐ As you hold Vyana Vayu mudra, take several natural breaths to attune to all the feelings and sensations awakened by this gesture.

ॐ Notice how your breath flows freely throughout your entire body, cultivating an overall feeling of integration and harmony.

ॐ Take some time to experience this harmony, noticing how it enhances your sensitivity to all of your body's subtle sensations and feelings.

ॐ With enhanced sensitivity, you are able to attune to the subtle energetic pathways from your brain to each area of your body, naturally nourishing them with vital energy.

ॐ Begin by bringing your awareness into your legs and feet. With each inhaling breath, trace the subtle pathways from these areas up to your brain, and with each exhaling breath, sense vital energy flowing back down to nourish them.

ॐ Take several breaths to attune to the free flow of energy from your brain to your lower extremities.

ॐ Next, bring your awareness to your pelvis, buttocks, abdomen and low back. With each inhalation, trace the pathways from these areas up to your brain, and with each exhaling breath, sense nourishing energy flowing back down again.

ॐ Take several breaths to sense these pathways more clearly, allowing vital energy to flow more freely throughout your pelvis, buttocks, abdomen and low back.

ॐ Next, bring awareness to your solar plexus, chest, mid and upper back. With each inhalation, trace the pathways from these areas up to your brain, and with each exhaling breath, sense these areas filled with vital nourishment.

ॐ As you attune to these pathways more completely, take several breaths to sense the free flow of vital energy bathing these areas of your being.

ॐ Now, your awareness rests in your shoulders, arms, hands and fingers. With each inhaling breath, trace the pathways from your fingertips, through your arms, all the way up to your brain, and with each exhaling breath, allow vital nourishment to flow back down into them.

ॐ Take several breaths to attune to the free flow of vital energy along these pathways, allowing greater feeling and sensitivity to infuse your upper extremities.

ॐ Now, bring your awareness into your neck and head. With each inhaling breath, trace the pathways from your neck and face into your brain, and with each exhaling breath, sense these areas fully nourished.

ॐ Take several breaths to attune to these pathways more clearly, allowing vital energy to flow through your neck, head and senses more freely.

ॐ Now, allow your awareness to encompass your entire body. With each inhalation, trace the energetic pathways from all areas of your body into your brain. With each exhalation, sense optimal communication and harmony throughout your entire being.

ॐ Affirm your enhanced sensitivity, repeating the following three times, aloud or silently: **"Attuned to my body's subtle pathways, clear communication is reestablished."**

ॐ Slowly release the gesture, taking several breaths to sense clear communication throughout all of your subtle pathways.

ॐ When you are ready, open your eyes, returning slowly and gently, with a greater sense of integration and harmony.

Annamaya kosha (physical body)

• Enhances body awareness, especially in the extremities, which may support improved balance and coordination.
• Creates a sense of enhanced communication between the central nervous system and the rest of the body.
• Enhanced body awareness, supports the functioning of the cardiovascular and immune systems.
• The centering effects are generally helpful for Vata imbalance.
• The increased sensitivity is generally helpful for Kapha imbalance.
• The awareness of the subtle body is generally helpful for Pitta imbalance.

Pranamaya kosha (energy body)

• Activates Vyana vayu, the all-pervading energy, moving from center to extremities.
• Gently activates Udana vayu, the uppermost current of energy.
• Opens and balances the first six chakras, with a special focus on the first and sixth.

Manomaya kosha (psycho-emotional body)

• Instills mental clarity.
• Instills a sense of trust in the self-healing process, thereby reducing stress and anxiety.

Vijnanamaya kosha (wisdom body)

• Cultivates integration of mind and body that serves as a doorway to self-healing.

Anandamaya kosha (bliss body)

• As we enhance our sensitivity to our subtle body, sensations of bliss arise naturally.

38 Bhramara Mudra

Gesture of the Bee

For Allergies & the Health of the Immune System

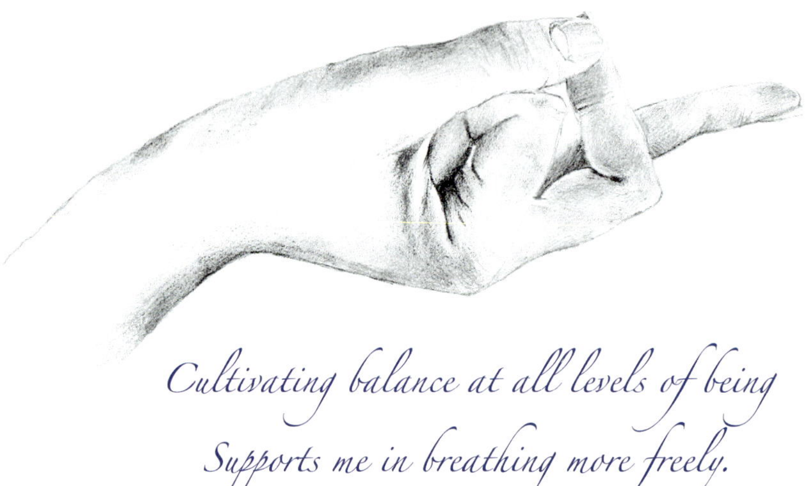

Cultivating balance at all levels of being
Supports me in breathing more freely.

Core Quality

Healthy Immunity

Especially helpful for

- Relieving allergies and nasal congestion.
- Balancing immune function.
- Establishing appropriate personal boundaries.
- Cultivating a positive attitude.

Mudras with similar effects

Chaturmukham, Kaleshvara, Dharma Chakra, Purna Jnanam

Cautions

None

Instructions

1. Press the tips of the index fingers into the crease of the lower joint of the thumbs, leaving a small open space.
2. Press the pads of the thumbs onto the outer borders of the upper digit of the middle fingers.
3. Extend the ring and little fingers.
4. Rest the hands onto the thighs or knees with the palms facing upward or hold the hands out to the side of the body facing upward.
5. Relax the shoulders back and down, with the spine naturally aligned.

Allergies are an excessive immune response to substances that are generally not harmful. Respiratory allergies, which affect one in five individuals in the United States, are the most common. Allergy symptoms include respiratory congestion, sinusitis and tearing or itchy eyes.[23] Allergies are just one of the many ways the immune system can over or under react. Autoimmune conditions are an example of an over reaction in which the immune system attacks healthy tissues. The immune system can also under react, as in the case of recurrent colds or flu, infection or the unchecked growth of cancer cells. The key to a healthy immune system is balance both at the physical level, in terms of diet and lifestyle, and at a psychological level. When our sense of boundaries is overly rigid, a message may be sent to the immune system to be hypervigilant, even against normally harmless substances. When we lack a clear sense of healthy boundaries, the immune system may lose its ability to maintain vigilance adequately.

Bhramara means "bee" and also "honey," and Bhramara mudra is the gesture traditionally recommended for allergies and the health of the immune system. This mudra directs breath, awareness and energy into the upper chest, throat, neck and head, including the area of the thymus gland, a maturation site for immune cells. Bhramara mudra instills a sense of opening within the sinuses and air passages. This gesture also instills a sense of clarity within the mind, supporting us in living more consciously through balanced diet and lifestyle, and appropriate personal boundaries. This enhanced equilibrium within all of our interactions and activities supports the optimal functioning of the immune system.

Systems Balanced:

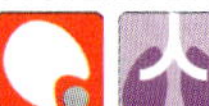

Elements Activated:

Doshas Balanced:

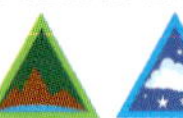

Prana Vayus Nourished:

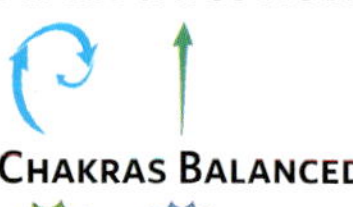

Chakras Balanced:

Scale from Calming to Energizing:

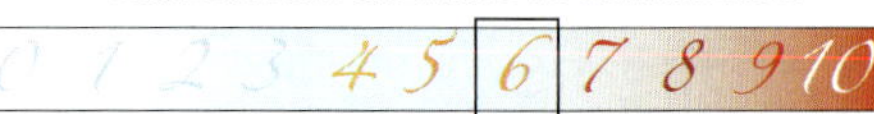

Guided Meditation: Establishing Healthy Boundaries

- As you hold Bhramara mudra, take several natural breaths to attune to all the feelings and sensations awakened by this gesture.
- Take some time to notice how your breath is gently directed into your upper chest, neck and head, instilling a sense of clearing throughout all of your breathing passages.
- As your air passages open, your breath flows through both nostrils more freely, cultivating greater comfort within your breathing.
- As you breathe more easily, you are able to sense the breath expanding beyond the frontiers of your physical body, allowing you to become more sensitive to your energetic being.
- Notice how the contours of your energy body naturally expand with each inhalation and soften with each exhaling breath, allowing you to sense more clearly your subtle energetic boundaries.
- Take several breaths to explore these boundaries, noticing the subtle field that surrounds your being, your aura of protective energy.
- Your experience of your energetic boundaries is a reflection of how you relate to the world and everyone around you. If your sense of boundaries is too rigid, you may overreact to life's challenges and, with the intention to protect, end up separating yourself from life's vital nourishment.
- If your boundaries are too porous, you lose the ability to distinguish "me" from "not me," allowing invaders to challenge your integrity.
- When your boundaries are balanced comfortably, you welcome all that is healthy and nurturing while maintaining an energetic shield that protects you adequately.
- Take several breaths to sense whether your energetic boundaries are too open, too rigid or balanced.
- Envision the changes you could make in your relationships and all your activities that would support greater balance in your energetic boundaries.
- With healthier boundaries, you perceive clearly the threats that compromise your body's integrity, without overreacting to your surroundings, thereby allowing your immune system to function optimally.
- With optimal immunity, you find a natural balance of giving and receiving, taking in vital nourishment while filtering out anything that could challenge your body's integrity.
- Affirm your healthy boundaries, repeating the following three times, aloud or silently: **"With clear and healthy boundaries, my immune system functions optimally."**
- Slowly release the gesture, taking several breaths to sense balanced protection.
- When you are ready, open your eyes, returning slowly and gently, with a greater sense of protection at all levels of your being.

Annamaya kosha (physical body)

• Directs breath and awareness to the upper chest, neck and head, enhancing circulation to the area of the thymus gland.
• Helps to open the sinuses and balance the breath evenly in both nostrils, which may provide relief from allergies.
• The mildly stimulating effects and the opening of the sinuses cultivated by this gesture are generally helpful for Kapha imbalance.
• The cultivation of healthy boundaries is generally helpful for Vata imbalance.
• The harmonizing effects are generally helpful for Pitta imbalance.

Pranamaya kosha (energy body)

• Activates Prana and Udana vayus, the upward moving and uppermost currents of energy.
• Opens and balances the fourth, fifth and sixth chakras, centers of unconditional love, spiritual purification and wisdom.

Manomaya kosha (psycho-emotional body)

• Cultivates a sense of contentment.
• Instills a sense of healthy boundaries.

Vijnanamaya kosha (wisdom body)

• Healthier boundaries support us in discerning between our personality and our true spiritual identity.

Anandamaya kosha (bliss body)

• As we become more balanced, feelings of integrity and equanimity unfold naturally.

39 Mani Ratna Mudra

Gesture of the Precious Jewel

For Healing the Whole Person

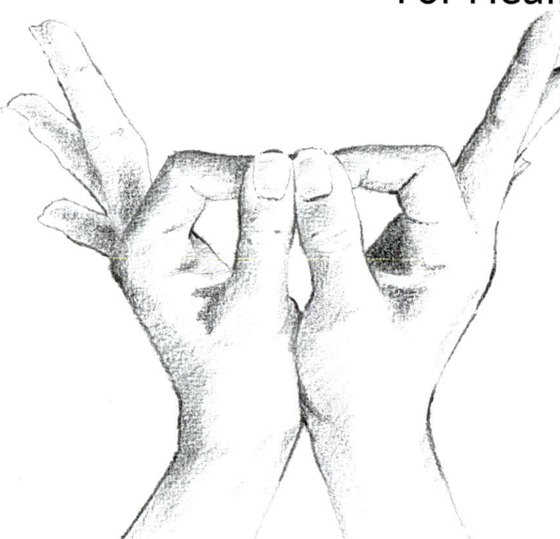

Bathed in the crystal light of healing,
I experience the sacred wholeness of my being.

Core Quality

Global Healing

Especially helpful for

- Integrating and balancing all the physical and subtle systems of the body.
- Relaxing the muscles of the face, neck and shoulders.
- Opening the crown chakra.

Mudras with similar effects

Hakini, Mandala, Dharma Chakra

Cautions

None

Instructions

1. Touch the tips of the index fingers to the thumbs of each hand.
2. Join the thumbs along their length and press the tips of the index fingers together, forming a straight line.
3. With the wrists together, spread the other fingers wide apart.
4. Relax the shoulders back and down, with the elbows slightly away from the body and the spine naturally aligned.

Health, in the ultimate sense, is an experience of radiant joyful living as a reflection of our growing connection to the wholeness of our true being. An essential part of the process of attuning to our inherent wholeness is the release of limiting beliefs, especially feelings of defectiveness, low self-esteem, resentment and inadequacy. As we bring light to these beliefs, the stress, worry and anxiety generated by them at the level of our thoughts and feelings are gradually released. As psycho-emotional tensions are released, so are the blockages in our subtle anatomy that obstruct the free flow of life force energy. As vital energy flows more freely, the physical systems are nourished energetically, allowing them to function optimally. Enhanced integration and optimal functioning within all dimensions of our being further supports our awareness of our essential wholeness and unity, thereby cultivating a cycle of optimal health as opposed to perpetuating a cycle of dis-ease.

Mani Ratna means "precious jewel," and Mani Ratna mudra awakens us to the inner jewel of our true being whose very essence is health and healing. This gesture directs breath, awareness and energy from the pelvic floor to the crown of the head, supporting the free flow of energy up and down the entire front of our body in synchrony with our rhythmic breathing. The free flow of energy cultivated by this gesture naturally reestablishes balance at all dimensions of our being, supporting our overall health and healing. Mani Ratna mudra supports the awakening of *Sahasrara chakra*, at the crown of the head, instilling a feeling of clarity in the form of crystal light that infuses our entire being with radiant healing energy.

Systems Balanced:

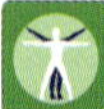

Elements Activated:

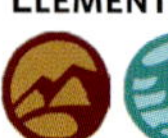

Doshas Balanced:

Prana Vayus Nourished:

Chakras Balanced:

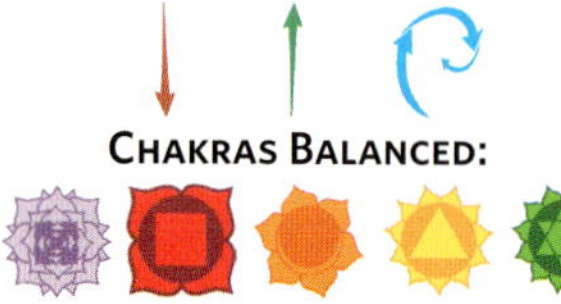

Scale from Calming to Energizing:

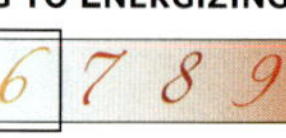

Guided Meditation: Healing all Dimensions of Being

- As you hold Mani Ratna mudra, take several natural breaths to attune to all the feelings and sensations awakened by this gesture.
- Notice how your breath flows smoothly and freely along the entire front of your body, cultivating greater openness and sensitivity.
- Take some time to attune to this flow of breath and energy, visualizing it as a crystal light that gently rises and falls in synchrony with your breathing.
- As you sense this crystal light more clearly, you are naturally guided to its source at the crown of your head, the seventh chakra, the center of pure Consciousness.
- Take some time to attune to your center of crystal light, recognizing it as the ultimate source of healing within all the dimensions of your being.
- Begin by taking several breaths to sense this light of healing reestablishing balance within every system, organ, tissue and cell of your physical body.
- As your physical body is infused with healing, allow crystal light to permeate your energy body, illuminating each of your chakras, restoring perfect balance within your subtle anatomy.
- Now, take some time to allow the light of healing to encompass your psycho-emotional being, permeating your thoughts and feelings with relaxation and ease, allowing you to rest in complete serenity.
- As the physical, energetic and psycho-emotional dimensions of your being are infused with healing energy, your crystal light illuminates all your limiting beliefs, allowing them to be gradually seen and released.
- Now, take several breaths to experience all the dimensions of your being infused with the light of healing.
- Affirm your complete healing as you repeat the following three times, aloud or silently: **"Filled with the light of healing, balance is reestablished at all levels of my being."**
- Slowly release the gesture, taking several breaths to rest in your healing essence.
- When you are ready, open your eyes, returning slowly and gently, nourished by the crystal light of healing.

Annamaya kosha (physical body)

- **Directs breath and awareness to the entire torso, neck and head, enhancing circulation to all the systems of the body.**
- **Softens and relaxes the muscles of the face, neck and shoulders.**
- **The overall balancing effects cultivated by this gesture are generally helpful for Vata, Pitta and Kapha imbalances.**

Pranamaya kosha (energy body)

- **Balances Prana and Apana vayus, the upward and downward moving currents of energy.**
- **Activates Udana vayu, the uppermost current of energy.**
- **Opens and balances all the chakras, with a special focus on the seventh chakra, center of unity.**

Manomaya kosha (psycho-emotional body)

- **Cultivates mental clarity.**
- **Instills a sense of self-trust in our powers of inner healing.**

Vijnanamaya kosha (wisdom body)

- **As the light of healing shines more clearly, we are able to perceive that it is actually a reflection of our own true being.**

Anandamaya kosha (bliss body)

- **The light of our inner jewel awakens an experience of radiance and unity.**

Chapter Seven

Finding Balance

MUDRAS FOR THE FIVE ELEMENTS

The model of the Five Elements, which forms the foundation of ayurvedic medicine, is one facet of an ancient Indian philosophy called *Samkhya.* This model describes all of creation as composed of five essential constituents or elements: earth, water, fire, air and space. Each of these elements embodies specific qualities. For example, the earth element embodies the physical qualities of density and stability, and the psychological qualities of grounding and security. Each individual is a unique combination of these five elements and their respective qualities. The balance of the elements within our being is an important foundation of health and healing.

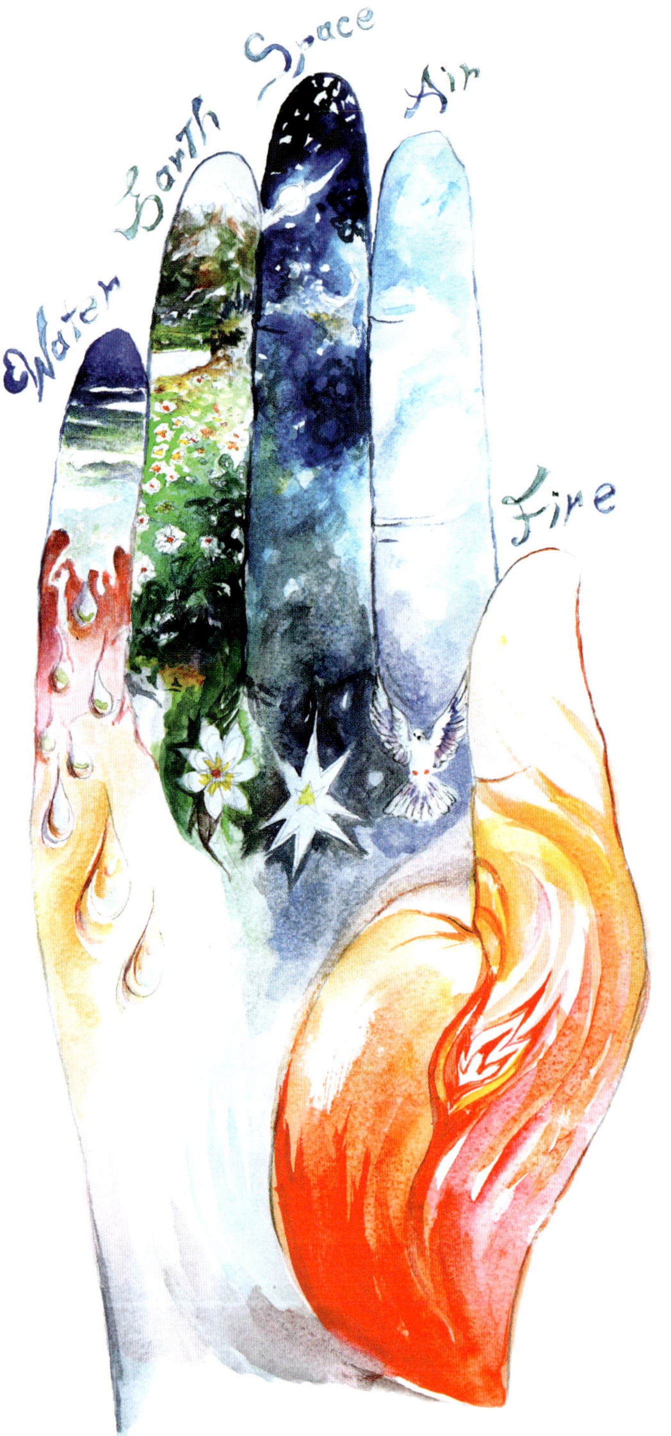

Mudras play an important role in activating the qualities of each of the elements and supporting the process of reestablishing balance. The wide variety of finger positions within the mudras allows us to rebalance the elements quickly and easily based on our individual needs. Within the mudra tradition, each finger is related to one of the five elements. In the system most commonly used, the relationship between the fingers and the elements is as follows:

- The fire element is associated with the thumb
- The air element is associated with the index finger
- The space element is associated with the middle finger
- The earth element is associated with the ring finger
- The water element is associated with the little finger

When the elements are balanced, we experience overall well-being both in the mind and in the body. When the elements are out of balance, we experience disharmony that can lead to illness. The first step in reestablishing balance within the five elements is becoming sensitive to the specific qualities that we need to cultivate harmony. As you practice each of the mudras in this family, along with their accompanying guided meditations, you will naturally begin to sense which gestures and which qualities are most helpful for you at this time. Among the different gestures for balancing the elements, one or two may resonate with you more strongly. These gestures can be practiced regularly, up to three times a day for at least one week, allowing you to experience the benefits and the growing sense of harmony as the elements come into balance.

Principal Mudra for each of the Five Elements	Name of Element, Sanskrit name & Symbol	Qualities related to each Element & Location in the Body	Color & Symbol Used for Meditation	Affirmations Used for Meditation
Bhu	Earth Prithivi	Solidity, density, immobility, grounding, security Base of the body, legs & feet	Red	"Embodying all of the earth's essential qualities, I experience complete stability."
Jala	Water Jala	Fluidity, flexibility, hydration, adaptability Pelvic bowl	Orange	"With greater fluidity at all levels of being, I move through life smoothly and easily."
Surya	Fire Tejas	Energy, luminosity, transformation, enthusiasm, determination Solar plexus	Gold	"Awakening my inner sun's radiant energy, I live with abundant vitality."
Vayu	Air Vayu	Mobility, lightness, sensitivity, openness, gracefulness Chest	Emerald green	"With greater lightness of being, I open my heart to embrace life completely."
Akasha	Space Akasha	Expansion, limitlessness, vastness, subtlety, all pervasiveness Throat	Sky-blue	"Attuned to the spaciousness of my true being, I open to my infinite possibilities."
Dharma Pravartana	All Elements Pancha Maha Bhuta	Integration Whole body	Violet	"With all five elements balanced completely, I experience perfect harmony."

40

Bhu Mudra

Gesture of the Earth

For Activating the Earth Element

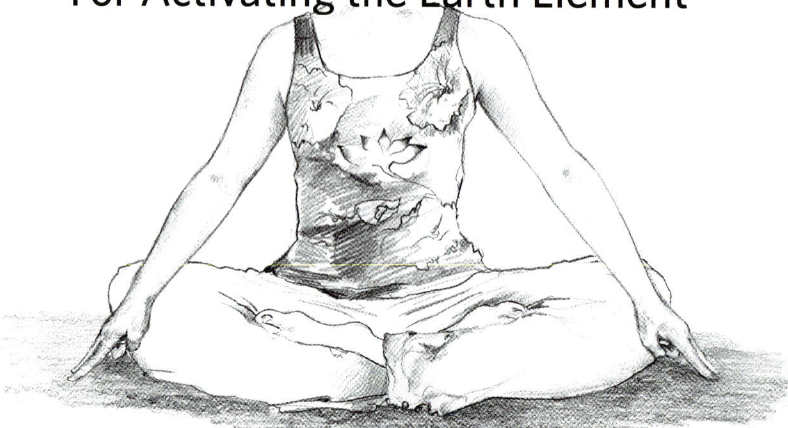

Attuned to the earth's stability, I move confidently along my life journey.

Core Quality

Stability of the Earth

Especially helpful for

- Cultivating a sense of stability both in the body and mind.
- Strengthening the bones.
- Facilitating optimal postural alignment.
- Reducing blood pressure.
- Cultivating grounding and embodiment.
- Supporting the treatment of anxiety.

Mudras with similar effects

Adhi, Prithivi, Rupa, Chinmaya, Murti

Cautions

None

Instructions

1. Curl the little and ring fingers comfortably toward the palms of the hands and place the thumbs on top of them.
2. Extend the middle and index fingers straight out in a "V" shape.
3. Touch the tips of the middle and index fingers firmly to the earth, out to the sides of the body so that the arms form a triangular mountain shape with the head as the summit.
4. Relax the shoulders back and down, with the spine naturally aligned.

Prithivi means "earth," and is the name of the earth element, whose qualities include solidity, firmness, immobility, security and stability. These qualities are experienced within the physical body as strength and structural support, especially in the bones and joints. The earth element is related to the sense of smell, and as we connect more deeply to the earth, we are able to appreciate all the fragrances of the natural world. As we attune to the qualities of the earth element within our being, we feel supported along our journey, with all our basic needs provided for naturally. At the psychological level, the earth element provides the emotional stability that allows us to move through life with a greater sense of trust and security, leading to enhanced serenity.

Bhu means "earth," and Bhu mudra activates the earth element, supporting us in integrating all of its essential qualities. In this gesture, the body forms a mountain shape, naturally cultivating a sense of stability and grounding. This sense of grounding is further enhanced by the activation of *Apana vayu,* the downward moving current of energy that naturally supports the eliminatory system in functioning optimally. As we develop greater stability and grounding, we naturally inhabit our bodies more completely, further enhancing our sense of security. This enhanced sense of embodiment facilitates optimal postural alignment. Bhu mudra opens and balances *Muladhara chakra*, further enhancing our sense of support and stability, allowing us to meet our survival needs more objectively, while releasing excessive fear and anxiety.

Systems Balanced:

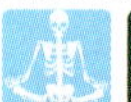
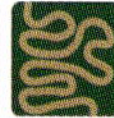

Prana Vayus Nourished:

Elements Activated:

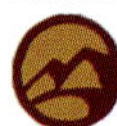

Chakras Balanced:

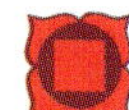

Doshas Balanced:

Scale from Calming to Energizing:

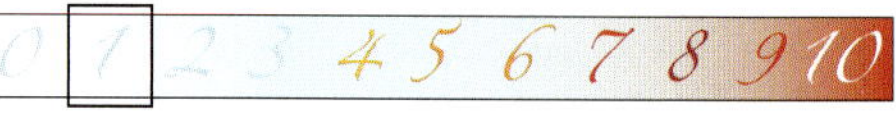

Guided Meditation: Stability of the Mountain

- ॐ As you hold Bhu mudra, take several natural breaths to attune to all the feelings and sensations evoked by this gesture.
- ॐ Visualize your body as a mountain with your legs as the base, your arms as the slopes stretching out to the sides, and the crown of your head as the mountain peak rising into the sky.
- ॐ With each inhalation, your spine lengthens naturally, and with each exhalation, the base of your body connects to the earth more firmly.
- ॐ Sense your breath flowing up and down your spine, creating space between each vertebra, cultivating a sense of alignment and stability throughout the entire structure of your body.
- ॐ Resting in your mountain's stability, take some time to notice how the pause at the end of your exhalation is lengthened naturally, allowing you to experience the earth's deep serenity.
- ॐ Attuned to the earth's stability and serenity, you naturally receive all of its healing qualities.
- ॐ Begin by taking several breaths to receive the earth's minerals in the exact quantities you need to support the structure of your body, cultivating optimal bone strength and density.
- ॐ With a greater sense of support, you naturally inhabit your body more completely, experiencing all areas of your being integrated as a seamless unity.
- ॐ As you inhabit your body more completely, the serenity of your mountain naturally permeates your thoughts and feelings, allowing you to experience absolute security at all times and places along your journey.
- ॐ With a deeper sense of security, a feeling of oneness with the natural world infuses your being, allowing you to feel completely at home within your surroundings.
- ॐ One with the earth and infused with its healing qualities, you rest within your mountain of stability, allowing its absolute stillness to permeate your entire being.
- ॐ Deeply attuned to the earth, repeat the following three times, aloud or silently: **"Embodying all of the earth's essential qualities, I experience complete stability."**
- ॐ Slowly release the gesture, taking several breaths to integrate all of the earth's healing qualities.
- ॐ When you are ready, open your eyes, returning slowly and gently, continuing your journey with a greater sense of support and stability.

Annamaya kosha (physical body)

- Directs breath and awareness to the base of the body, helping to release muscular tension, supporting the health of the eliminatory system.
- Cultivates a feeling of solidity and stability within the structure of the body that may facilitate healing in the musculo-skeletal system.
- Supports healthy embodiment and optimal postural alignment.
- The relaxing effects help reduce stress and blood pressure.
- The calming effects cultivated by this gesture are generally helpful for Pitta imbalance.
- The grounding effects are generally helpful for Vata imbalance.

Pranamaya kosha (energy body)

- Activates Apana vayu, the downward moving current of energy.
- Opens and balances the first chakra, center of safety.

Manomaya kosha (psycho-emotional body)

- Cultivates a feeling of grounding and stability, which may be helpful for anxiety.
- Instills the qualities of patience, security and consistency.

Vijnanamaya kosha (wisdom body)

- As we deepen our sense of grounding and stability, we recognize the essential security of our true being.

Anandamaya kosha (bliss body)

- As we connect deeply with the earth's essential qualities, a sense of oneness arises naturally.

41

Jala Mudra

Gesture of Water

For Activating the Water Element

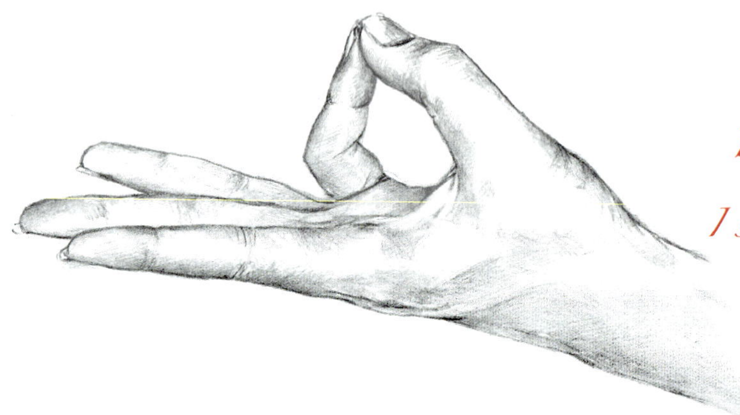

Bathed in water's soothing stream,
I savor life's sweetness more completely.

Core Quality
Fluidity of Water

Especially helpful for

- Instilling fluidity and flexibility in both the mind and body.
- Lubricating the joints.
- Supporting the health of the urinary, reproductive, digestive and eliminatory systems.

Mudras with similar effects
Mira, Yoni, Matsya, Svadhisthana

Cautions
None

Instructions

1. Touch the tips of the thumbs to the tips of the little fingers of the same hand and extend the other three fingers straight out.
2. Rest the backs of the hands on the thighs or knees.
3. Relax the shoulders back and down, with the spine naturally aligned.

Jala means "water," and is the name for the water element, whose qualities include fluidity, refreshment, hydration, lubrication, nourishment and purification. In the physical body, the water element, in the form of circulation, serves as a vehicle for nutrients, blood cells, hormones, oxygen and carbon dioxide. Water is associated with the sense of taste and is the essential vehicle for digestion, supporting the transformation of food and the absorption of nutrients. Water's qualities of hydration and flexibility are also essential for the healthy functioning of the muscles and joints, maintaining flexibility, which is especially important with aging. Water's subtle qualities, including fluidity and adaptability, are essential for the health of our psycho-emotional being, allowing us to flow with life's stream more easily.

Jala mudra directs breath, awareness and energy into the pelvis, the seat of the water element, enhancing the qualities of fluidity and flexibility in the physical body while cultivating greater ease and adaptability within our thoughts and feelings. This gesture creates a massaging effect within the pelvis and abdomen that supports the health of the reproductive and urinary systems. The enhanced abdominal breathing also supports the return of venous blood and lymphatic fluids from the lower body. As fluidity and flexibility are enhanced by this gesture, *Svadhisthana chakra* at the center of the pelvis opens naturally, supporting us in flowing with life changes more easily while developing relationships that are genuinely nourishing.

Systems Balanced:

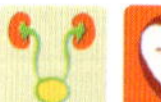  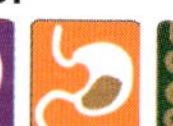 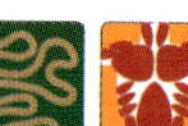 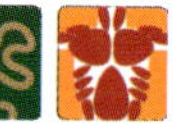

Prana Vayus Nourished:

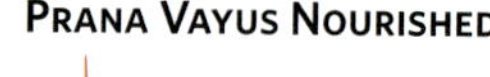

Elements Activated:

Chakras Balanced:

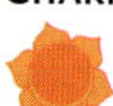

Doshas Balanced:

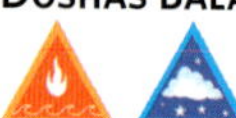 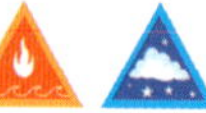

Scale from Calming to Energizing:

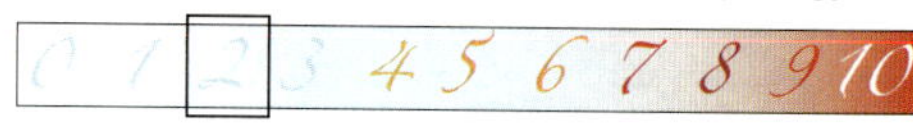

Guided Meditation: Flowing with the Stream of Life

- As you hold Jala mudra, take several natural breaths to attune to all the feelings and sensations evoked by this gesture.
- Notice how your breath flows gently down into your pelvic area, the home of the water element. Visualize all the expressions of water within your pelvis; the lakes and rivers, seas and streams infusing you with the quality of fluidity.
- Take several breaths to attune to your pelvis more deeply, sensing water's essential quality of fluidity bathing this area completely.
- As your pelvis is infused with fluidity, this stream of liquid energy flows outward to nourish your entire being.
- With your next inhaling breath, attune to your fluid essence within your pelvis, and as you exhale, sense your stream of liquid healing energy bathing your reproductive system completely, supporting its optimal functioning.
- With your next inhalation, return to the center of your being, and as you exhale, sense fluidity bathing your urinary system, from your kidneys down to your bladder, with soothing energy.
- With your next inhalation, attune to your center of fluidity, and as you exhale, sense how this quality supports your lymphatic system in removing residues from your body tissues efficiently.
- Take several breaths to sense your lymphatic system as a smoothly flowing stream whose purifying power allows all of your body's organs to function optimally.
- With your next inhaling breath, reconnect with the seat of the water element, and as you exhale, sense a stream of healing energy bathing all of your muscles, tendons and ligaments with suppleness and flexibility, allowing your joints to be lubricated naturally.
- As your body is infused with the quality of fluidity, you naturally experience greater ease within your psycho-emotional being, nourishing your relationships and allowing you to flow through life with greater equanimity.
- With greater equanimity, you naturally embrace transitions more easily, flowing with the stream of life at each moment of your journey.
- Affirm your essential fluidity as you repeat the following three times, aloud or silently: **"With greater fluidity at all levels of being, I move through life smoothly & easily."**
- Slowly release the gesture, taking several breaths to absorb water's healing essence.
- When you are ready, open your eyes, returning slowly and gently, experiencing greater fluidity within all dimensions of your being.

Annamaya kosha (physical body)

- **Directs breath and awareness into the pelvic area, which improves circulation to the urinary, reproductive, digestive and eliminatory systems.**
- **Facilitates deep abdominal breathing, which activates the relaxation response.**
- **Cultivates full movement of the diaphragm, helping to optimize lymphatic circulation.**
- **The nourishing effects cultivated by this gesture are generally helpful for Vata imbalance.**
- **The refreshing effects are generally helpful for Pitta imbalance.**

Pranamaya kosha (energy body)

- **Activates Apana vayu, the downward moving current of energy.**
- **Opens and balances the second chakra, center of self-nourishment.**

Manomaya kosha (psycho-emotional body)

- **Instills emotional fluidity.**
- **Cultivates the ability to flow with the seasons and cycles of life.**

Vijnanamaya kosha (wisdom body)

- **Developing greater flexibility supports us in releasing our rigid identification with the personality.**

Anandamaya kosha (bliss body)

- **The enhanced fluidity throughout the pelvic area allows us to sense inner comfort, ease, pleasure and well-being.**

42 Surya Mudra

Gesture of the Sun

For Activating the Fire Element

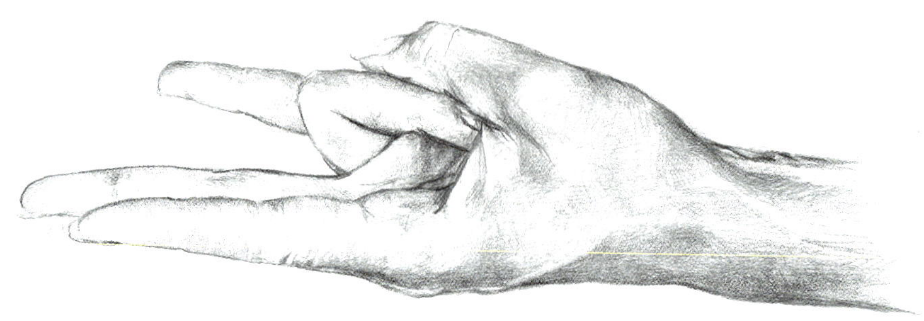

The radiant sun of my inner being
Fills me with abundant energy.

Core Quality
Radiant Energy of Fire

Especially helpful for

- Enhancing radiant energy in the mind and body.
- Supporting the health of the digestive system.
- Increasing metabolism, which may be helpful for weight loss.
- Building self-esteem.
- Allowing us to digest life experiences.
- Clarifying our life purpose.

Mudras with similar effects
Kubera, Vajra, Madhyama, Pushan

Cautions
Those with hyperacidity can use Pushan mudra as a substitute.

Instructions

1. Bend the ring fingers of each hand down to touch the rounded mounds just below the base of the thumbs.
2. Use the thumbs to gently secure the ring fingers in place.
3. Extend the little, middle, and index fingers straight out.
4. Rest the backs of the hands on the thighs or knees.
5. Relax the shoulders back and down, with the spine naturally aligned.

Tejas means "light" or "brilliance," and is the name for the fire element, whose qualities include energy, warmth, luminosity, radiance and the power of transformation. Within the physical body, the fire element provides the heat required for digestion and optimal assimilation of nutrients. At a subtle level, fire is the power of transformation that allows us to digest life experiences completely, absorbing the lessons we need while releasing accumulated emotions and memories. This optimal digestion in the body and mind allows us to live with radiant health and vitality. The fire element is related to the sense of sight, allowing us to see our life purpose more clearly while providing the energy and determination to manifest it completely. At the spiritual level, the fire element enhances discernment, the power to discriminate between the limited personality and our limitless true being.

Surya is one of the "solar deities," and Surya mudra activates the fire element and supports the integration of its qualities. This gesture directs breath, awareness and energy into the solar plexus, the seat of the fire element, instilling a sense of energy and vitality while removing lethargy. The enhanced breathing in the area of the diaphragm and solar plexus cultivated by this gesture increases circulation to the organs of digestion, supporting their optimal functioning. As Surya mudra enhances energy and vitality, *Manipura chakra*, located at the center of the solar plexus, opens naturally. This energetic opening cultivates personal power, determination and self-esteem, allowing us to clarify our life purpose and manifest it completely. This gesture supports the sense of sight and may be used together with exercises for the health of the eyes.

Systems Balanced:

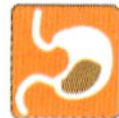

Elements Activated:

Doshas Balanced:

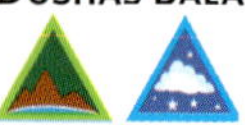

Prana Vayus Nourished:

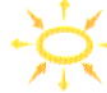

Chakras Balanced:

Scale from Calming to Energizing:

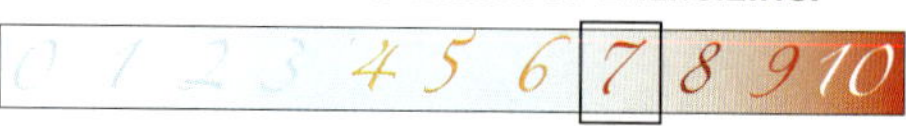

Guided Meditation: Sunlight of Transformation

- As you hold Surya mudra, take several natural breaths to attune to all the feelings and sensations awakened by this gesture.
- Notice how your breath is naturally directed into your solar plexus, the seat of the fire element, instilling a sense of energy and radiance.
- In order to enhance this experience of radiant energy, visualize a golden sun at the center of your being, infusing you with the fire element's essential qualities.
- Begin by sensing the light and warmth of the sun's golden rays bathing your digestive system, enhancing the power of transformation and assimilation of nutrients.
- Take several breaths to sense your inner sun illuminating all of your digestive organs, supporting them in functioning optimally, nourishing every cell of your body with vital energy.
- With your physical digestion more complete, the light of your inner sun now encompasses your thoughts and feelings, allowing you to digest life experiences more easily while releasing accumulated emotions and memories that drain your energy.
- With optimal digestion at all levels of your being, the light of your inner sun illuminates your vision, allowing you to perceive your life purpose more clearly.
- Take several breaths to envision the unfolding of all your possibilities while naturally receiving the determination to overcome any obstacles along your journey.
- As the rays of your inner sun grow in intensity, they naturally burn away any clouds of doubt and lethargy, allowing you to manifest your vision completely.
- Affirm your radiant energy as you repeat the following three times, aloud or silently: **"Awakening my inner sun's radiant energy, I live with abundant vitality."**
- Slowly release the gesture, taking several breaths to absorb the light of your inner sun.
- When you are ready, open your eyes, returning slowly and gently, infused with the fire element's radiant qualities.

Annamaya kosha (physical body)

• Directs breath and awareness into the solar plexus, creating a massaging effect that enhances circulation to the digestive system.
• Expands the lower ribs and diaphragm, facilitating fuller breathing, especially at the base of the lungs.
• Enhanced movement of the lower ribs supports optimal circulation to area of the kidneys and adrenal glands.
• Generates a sensation of gentle warmth throughout the body.
• The energizing effects cultivated by this gesture are generally helpful for Kapha imbalance.
• The gentle warmth and enhanced clarity are generally helpful for Vata imbalance.

Pranamaya kosha (energy body)

• Activates Samana vayu, the horizontal current of energy.
• Opens and balances the third chakra, center of personal power.

Manomaya kosha (psycho-emotional body)

• Illuminates our life purpose.
• Cultivates enthusiasm and vitality, which may be helpful for depression.

Vijnanamaya kosha (wisdom body)

• Enhanced digestion of life experiences promotes clarity, allowing us to see our life path and purpose more easily.

Anandamaya kosha (bliss body)

• The enhanced clarity allows us to experience the inner light that radiates throughout our being.

43

Vayu Mudra

Gesture of Wind

For Activating the Air Element

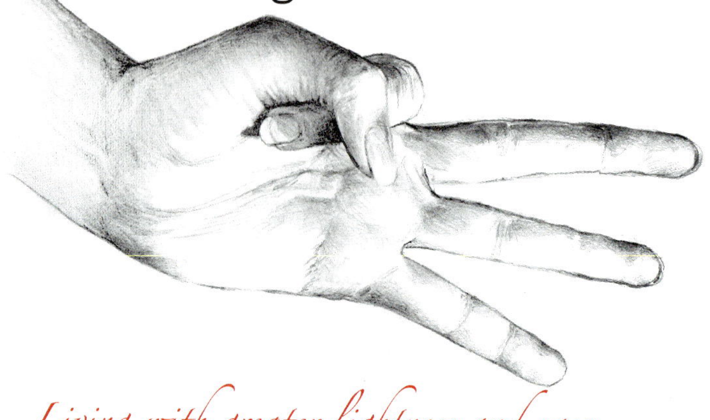

Living with greater lightness and ease,
I am naturally touched by all of life's beauty.

Core Quality

Lightness of Air

Especially helpful for

- Instilling a sense of lightness and ease in the body and mind.
- Supporting easeful breathing.
- Developing gracefulness and sensitivity.
- Cultivating appreciation of beauty.
- Opening the subtle heart.

Mudras with similar effects

Padma, Medha Prana Kriya, Purna Hridaya

Cautions

None

Instructions

1. Bend the index fingers of each hand down to touch the rounded mounds just below the base of the thumbs.
2. Use the thumbs to gently secure the index fingers in place.
3. Extend the little, ring and middle fingers straight out.
4. Rest the backs of the hands on the thighs or knees.
5. Relax the shoulders back and down, with the spine naturally aligned.

Vayu means "wind," and is the name for the air element, whose qualities include lightness, mobility, gracefulness and sensitivity. The essence of air is movement, reflected in the exchange of oxygen and carbon dioxide between the atmosphere and the lungs. The air element is also responsible for the movement of nerve impulses and the circulation of blood. At a subtle level, the air element supports psycho-emotional balance. When there is excessive movement within the mind, we may become unfocused and hyperactive. When air is deficient, the mind can become dull and lethargic. When air is balanced, thoughts and feelings arise and pass away easily, leaving the mind light and free. The air element is related to the sense of touch and naturally expands our sense of interconnectedness. This enhanced interconnectedness is experienced as a natural balance of giving and receiving in our rhythmic breathing and within all of our interactions and activities.

Vayu mudra activates the air element and supports the integration of its essential qualities. This gesture directs breath, awareness and energy to the chest, side ribs and upper back, gently lengthening the inhalation and optimizing respiration. This mudra activates *Prana vayu*, the upward moving current of energy, cultivating lightness and vitality. Vayu mudra naturally supports the opening of *Anahata chakra* at the center of the chest, the seat of universal love and compassion, allowing us to touch and be touched by life with greater sensitivity. As it awakens the air element, this gesture enhances enthusiasm, making it helpful in the treatment of depression. As the air element is integrated fully within our being, we experience greater lightness and ease, allowing us to journey forward in life gracefully.

Systems Balanced:

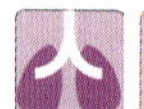 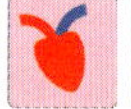 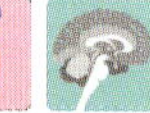

Elements Activated:

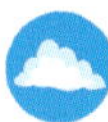

Doshas Balanced:

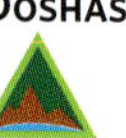

Prana Vayus Nourished:

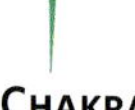

Chakras Balanced:

Scale from Calming to Energizing:

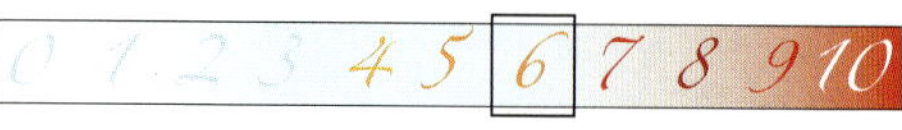

Guided Meditation: Lightness of Being

ॐ As you hold Vayu mudra, take several natural breaths to attune to all the feelings and sensations awakened by this gesture.

ॐ Sense each inhalation expanding your rib cage evenly while each exhaling breath allows your chest, side ribs and upper back to soften and relax completely.

ॐ Take several breaths to notice how this alternating expansion and release cultivates greater lightness and ease throughout your entire being.

ॐ To enhance your sense of lightness and ease, you will embark on a journey to an area of snow covered peaks.

ॐ As you begin your journey, your trail is naturally framed by wildflowers and tall trees, as your face is caressed by a gentle breeze.

ॐ The sky is bright blue and crystal clear, and in the distance, mountains stretch across the horizon endlessly, cultivating a sense of openness that allows you to breathe more freely.

ॐ As you breathe more freely, you become sensitive to the surrounding beauty: the wild flowers waving gracefully, the white clouds floating gently, and the sun's rays warming your entire being.

ॐ Touched by the beauty of your surroundings, your deepen your connection to the natural world, sensing your breath as a natural giving and receiving, an ongoing conversation with the entire web of creation.

ॐ As you journey higher, the air becomes light, fresh and clear, and you soon arrive at a meadow with butterflies gently floating in the mountain air.

ॐ A soft breeze invites you to sit and take in the scenery: a landscape of valleys, farms and fields, and in the distance, a panorama of snow covered peaks that evokes within you a sense of lightness of being .

ॐ Take several breaths to absorb this lightness within all dimensions of your being, within the cells of your body, in the flow of your breath, and within your thoughts and feelings.

ॐ As lightness permeates your being, your heart opens naturally, allowing you to embrace your life and all beings with an expanded sense of lightness and ease.

ॐ Affirm your lightness of being, repeating the following three times, aloud or silently: **"With greater lightness of being, I open my heart to embrace life completely."**

ॐ Slowly release the gesture, taking several breaths to rest in your essential lightness.

ॐ When you are ready, open your eyes, returning slowly and gently, integrating the essential lightness of the air element.

Annamaya kosha (physical body)

- **Directs breath and awareness into the entire rib cage, expanding breath capacity.**
- **Balance with the air element supports the health of the nervous and circulatory systems.**
- **The mildly energizing effects of this gesture are generally helpful for Kapha imbalance.**

Pranamaya kosha (energy body)

- **Activates Prana vayu, the upward moving current of energy.**
- **Softly opens and balances the fourth chakra, center of unconditional love.**

Manomaya kosha (psycho-emotional body)

- **Cultivates a healthy balance of giving and receiving.**
- **Supports the expansion of the frontiers of the heart, allowing us to embrace our own life journey.**

Vijnanamaya kosha (wisdom body)

- **Cultivates a lighter, more open attitude toward ourselves, others and life, reflecting the natural ease of our true being.**

Anandamaya kosha (bliss body)

- **As the heart opens, its inherent qualities of joy and delight arise naturally.**

44

Akasha Mudra

Gesture of Space

For Activating the Space Element

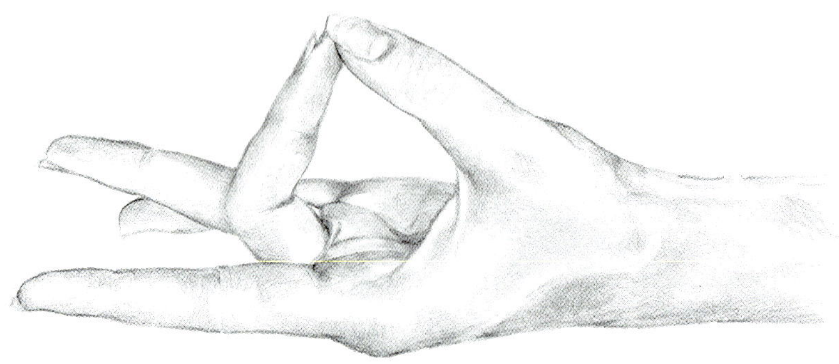

In a space of deep inner listening,
I receive guidance for my journey.

Core Quality

Vastness of Space

Especially helpful for

- Sensing the quality of spaciousness within our bodies and minds.
- Releasing muscular tension from the neck, shoulders and jaw.
- Supporting treatment of hypothyroid issues.
- Supporting treatment of hearing problems.
- Enhancing intuition.
- Opening to new possibilities.

Mudras with similar effects

Garuda, Shunya, Angushtha, Vishuddha

Cautions

Those with headaches, dizziness or light-headedness may choose to practice Garuda, which is less energizing.

Instructions

1. Touch the tips of the thumbs to the tips of the middle fingers.
2. Extend the little, ring and index fingers straight out.
3. Rest the backs of the hands on the thighs or knees.
4. Relax the shoulders back and down, with the spine naturally aligned.

Akasha means "space," and is the name for the space element, whose qualities include vastness, expansiveness, limitlessness and subtlety. The space element is the most subtle of the five elements and is the matrix that encompasses all of the other elements. At the physical level, space is an essential feature of our physiology, forming the body's hollow cavities, including the lungs, stomach, intestines and bladder. The quality of spaciousness is also important at the level of our psycho-emotional being. By creating space around heavy and dense thoughts and feelings, we gain the ability to not identify with them so completely. Spaciousness is also important for seeing beyond our limiting beliefs, thereby allowing us to unfold our infinite possibilities.

Akasha mudra activates the space element and supports the integration of its essential qualities. This gesture directs breath, awareness and energy into the throat and neck, the seat of the space element. The enhanced awareness and breath in this area increase circulation to the area of the thyroid gland, supporting its optimal health. The space element is related to the sense of hearing, and Akasha mudra cultivates a space of inner listening in which we receive guidance for our life journey. This gesture supports us in sensing the presence of space more palpably within our own bodies and surroundings. As we attune to the spaciousness within and around us, we naturally perceive the all-pervading intelligence and energy within all of creation.

Systems Balanced:

Elements Activated:

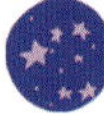

Doshas Balanced:

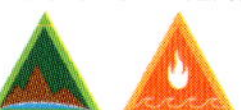

Prana Vayus Nourished:

Chakras Balanced:

Scale from Calming to Energizing:

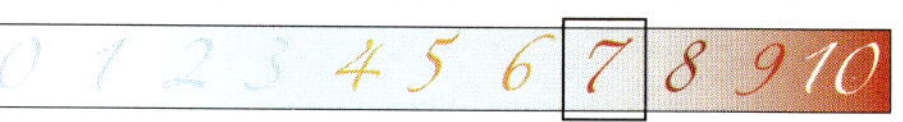

Guided Meditation: Cultivating Spaciousness

- As you hold Akasha mudra, take several natural breaths to attune to all the feelings and sensations awakened by this gesture.
- Notice how your breath is gently directed upward into your throat and neck, cultivating a greater sense of spaciousness.
- As you sense spaciousness more deeply, you naturally attune to the more subtle realms of your being, allowing you to see beyond your limitations and boundaries to glimpse your limitless possibilities.
- Begin by sensing the space around you, taking several breaths to notice how space forms the container in which you live, move and breathe, a matrix that allows everything to come into being.
- Now, sense the space occupied by your physical being, tracing your body's contours within the space around you.
- Take several breaths to notice how your body's contours expand and relax energetically with your breathing, allowing you to perceive that your physical boundaries are not as fixed as they initially appear to be.
- Now, explore the space within your body, taking some time to sense its hollow cavities, including your lungs, stomach, bladder and intestines, noting how spaciousness is essential for your body's functioning.=Next, choose any organ within your body, taking some time to notice its unique shape, volume and density.
- As you explore this organ more closely, you see that it is actually composed of individual cells forming an intelligent community, working in cooperation for your optimal health and well-being.
- Now, journey into one of these cells, noticing that it is made up of innumerable atoms. As you go inside one of these, you discover that it is mostly comprised of empty space.
- Within this vastness, subatomic particles appear and disappear within a field of infinite possibilities, reflecting the creative intelligence that is the matrix of everything.
- Take several breaths to sense yourself as one with the intelligence that is the essence of space, encompassing everyone and everything, including your own mind and body.
- As you sense the spaciousness of your essential being, take some time to open to perceive your own infinite possibilities.
- Affirm your spaciousness as you repeat the following three times, aloud or silently: **"Attuned to the spaciousness of my true being, I open to my infinite possibilities."**
- Now, slowly release the gesture, taking several breaths to rest in your inherent spaciousness.
- When you are ready, open your eyes, returning slowly and gently, sensing how the space element reveals your infinite possibilities.

Annamaya kosha (physical body)

• Directs breath and awareness to the throat and neck, enhancing circulation to this area.
• Gently increases circulation to the area of the thyroid gland.
• Helps to release chronic muscular contraction from the neck, shoulders and jaw, making it helpful for neck and shoulder pain, as well as TMJ .
• The spaciousness cultivated by this gesture is generally helpful for Kapha imbalance.
• The enhanced sensitivity to the subtle realms of our being is generally helpful for Pitta imbalance.

Pranamaya kosha (energy body)

• Activates Udana vayu, the uppermost current of energy.
• Opens and balances the fifth chakra, center of spiritual purification.

Manomaya kosha (psycho-emotional body)

• Creates space between thoughts.
• Promotes an openness to new ways of seeing.
• Supports us in releasing attachment to the past, opening us to new possibilities.

Vijnanamaya kosha (wisdom body)

• Cultivates inner listening, allowing us to release limiting beliefs and attune to the guidance of our inner being.

Anandamaya kosha (bliss body)

• The experience of spaciousness is accompanied by feelings of bliss, limitlessness and joy.

45 Dharma Pravartana Mudra

Gesture of Setting Dharma in Motion

For Balancing All Five Elements

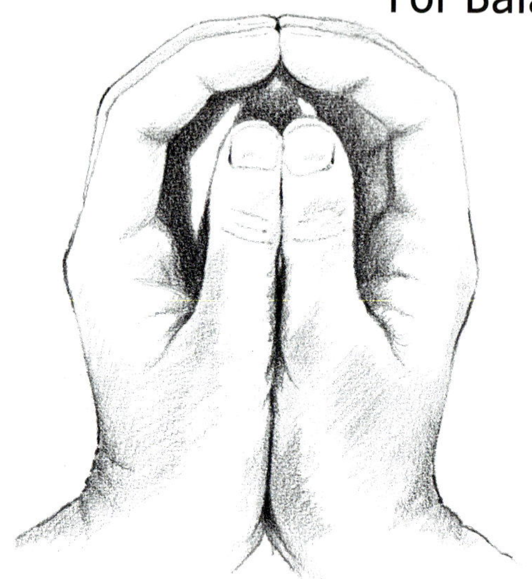

Attuned to all of the elements' essential qualities, I experience complete integration of mind and body.

Core Quality

Balancing all Five Elements

Especially helpful for

- Balancing the five elements.
- Instilling a sense of integration and harmony at all levels of being as the foundation of health and healing.

Mudras with similar effects

Hakini, Mandala, Dharma Chakra

Cautions

None

Instructions

1. Touch the fingertips of the right hand to the fingertips of the left hand.
2. Bring the outer edges of the thumbs together along their length.
3. The pads of the thumbs rest just below the index fingers without touching them.
4. Form a round space within the palms, as if holding a globe.
5. Place the hands facing forward in front of the solar plexus, with the forearms resting against the abdomen.
6. Relax the shoulders back and down, with the spine naturally aligned.

From the perspective of Yoga and Ayurveda, our physical body is composed of five elements and their balance is an essential foundation of health. When the elements are balanced, we experience integration and harmony at all levels of being. One of the most effective methods for integrating all of the elements is by combining mudra practice with a guided meditation called *Bhuta Shuddhi*, or "purification of the elements." In our adaptation of this meditation, which appears on the facing page, the symbols associated with each element are placed at that element's location in the body, awakening each element's essential qualities. The integration and harmony cultivated by this meditation supports healing within all dimensions of our being while naturally opening a doorway to spiritual awakening.

Dharma means "truth," and *Pravartana* means "to set in motion." Dharma Pravartana refers to the Buddha setting in motion the wheel of truth through his teachings. Dharma Pravartana mudra sets in motion the process of transformation leading toward health, healing and awakening through balancing the five elements. This gesture facilitates Full Yogic Breathing, optimizing the functioning of all systems of the body while cultivating an overall sense of integration and harmony at all levels of our being. This mudra opens and integrates the first six *chakras* and all five *prana vayus*, resulting in an overall sense of energetic well-being that supports the health of all the systems of the physical body, thereby establishing a firm foundation for the spiritual journey.

Systems Balanced:

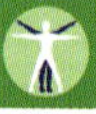

Elements Activated:

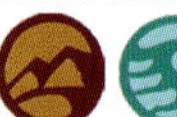
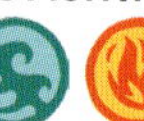

Doshas Balanced:

Prana Vayus Nourished:

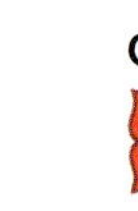

Chakras Balanced:

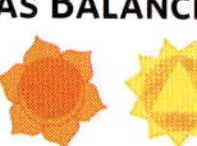
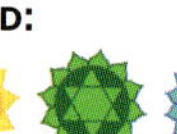
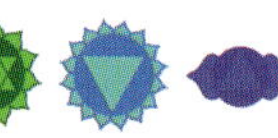

Scale from Calming to Energizing:

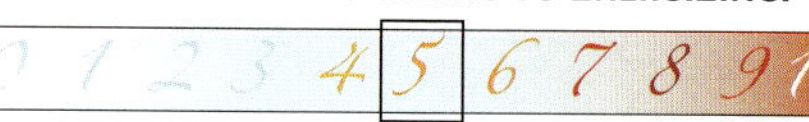

Guided Meditation: Balancing the Five Elements

- As you hold Dharma Pravartana mudra, take several natural breaths to attune to all the feelings and sensations awakened by this gesture.
- Notice how your breath flows freely throughout your entire torso, from your pelvic floor to the top of your chest and then back down again.
- As you follow the flow of your breathing, sense a growing equilibrium throughout your entire being as all of the elements come into balance naturally.
- By bringing awareness to each of the five elements individually, you will integrate all of their essential qualities, cultivating harmony within all dimensions of your being.
- Begin by visualizing a red square at the base of your body, the seat of the earth element. Envision a landscape spreading out from this square, encompassing all the features of the earth: mountains, plains, valleys and deserts.
- As you embody the earth element, take several breaths to smell its rich fragrance and absorb the quality of stability, allowing you to continue your journey in absolute safety.
- Now, visualize an orange circle within your pelvis, the home of the water element. Envision all the forms of water spreading out from this circle of life: the oceans and seas, rivers and lakes, clouds and rain that constantly renew life's ever flowing stream.
- As you embody the water element, take some time to savor its essential quality of fluidity, cultivating the ease that allows you to flow with all of life's changing seasons.
- Next, visualize an upward facing golden triangle at your solar plexus, the seat of the fire element. Envision the rays of an inner sun spreading out from this triangle, filling your entire being with light, warmth and energy.
- As golden rays fill your being, take some time to clarify your vision, seeing your life purpose clearly while receiving the energy and vitality to manifest it completely.
- Now, visualize an emerald six-pointed star at the center of your chest, the seat of the air element. Envision a meadow of green unfolding from your heart, with wildflowers swaying softly in the breeze.
- As the air element caresses your being, take all the time you need to sense lightness and ease permeating your thoughts and feelings, allowing you to embrace life completely with compassion and sensitivity.
- A silver crescent moon now arises within your throat center, the seat of the space element, opening a doorway through which you perceive the vastness of the universe with stars and galaxies unfolding and expanding infinitely.
- As you rest in the vastness of space, take several breaths to attune to the inherent spaciousness of your being, releasing all that limits your infinite possibilities.
- Now, direct your breath to your eyebrow center, visualizing there a luminous full moon, a symbol of the integration of all the elements.
- As you bathe in shimmering moonlight, sense all the elements aligned and balanced within your being, allowing you to experience perfect harmony.
- Affirm your integration as you repeat the following three times, aloud or silently: **"With all five elements balanced completely, I experience perfect harmony."**
- Slowly release the gesture, taking several breaths to sense the complete integration of the five elements.
- When you are ready, open your eyes, returning slowly and gently, sensing greater harmony throughout your entire being.

Annamaya kosha (physical body)

• Facilitates Full Yogic Breathing, which supports balance in all the systems of the body.
• Opens the breath in the front of the body, releasing muscular tension from the chest and sternum.
• Creates an ideal balance between rest and activity.
• The balancing effects of this gesture are generally helpful for Vata, Pitta and Kapha imbalances.

Pranamaya kosha (energy body)

• Activates and balances all prana vayus.
• Opens and balances the first six chakras.

Manomaya kosha (psycho-emotional body)

• Cultivates the essential qualities of each of the five elements in the proportion needed for optimal psychological health.

Vijnanamaya kosha (wisdom body)

• Instills an overall sense of integration and wholeness that allow us to align more easily with our true being.

Anandamaya kosha (bliss body)

• As the elements come into balance, we experience an overall feeling of harmony and unity.

Chapter Eight

Balancing the Three Doshas

MUDRAS FOR AYURVEDIC HEALING

Ayurveda, which means "knowledge of life," is the ancient healing art of India. From an ayurvedic perspective, health is a state of balance at all levels of being. When imbalance occurs, health is reestablished through a balancing diet, lifestyle, herbs, cleansing techniques and yogic practices based on an individual's unique ayurvedic constitution. There are three basic constitutional types or *doshas*: *Vata*, *Pitta* and *Kapha*. Each dosha is a combination of two of the five elements. Vata is a combination of air and space; Pitta is composed of fire and water; and Kapha is a combination of earth and water. Most individuals have a dominant dosha, and this is the one that tends to go out of balance most often.

Doshas are described as "out of balance" when their qualities become excessive, either at a physical or psychological level. For example, when the dry and rough qualities of Vata become excessive, dry skin problems can occur. At the psycho-emotional level, Vata's quality of movement, when excessive, can manifest as emotional instability, excessive fear or anxiety. There are a variety of mudras to balance each of the doshas, supporting optimal health and healing within each individual's unique constitution.

Vata

Vata is responsible for movement within all dimensions of our being. Individuals with a Vata-dominant constitution tend to be thin and slight in build. They are flexible and energetic when young, but with aging, tend toward stiffness and low energy. Vata imbalances include dry skin, coldness, poor digestion and elimination, and a tendency toward arthritis after age fifty. At the psychological level, individuals with a Vata-dominant constitution are creative and sensitive. When out of balance, Vata's tendency toward movement can manifest as hyperactivity, anxiety, fearfulness and instability. Abhaya Varada mudra, with its calming, grounding and centering qualities, is an excellent support for rebalancing Vata.

Pitta

Pitta is responsible for transformation at all levels of our being. Individuals with a Pitta-dominant constitution tend to be of medium build with good musculature, digestion, circulation and flexibility. When Pitta becomes excessive, inflammation, gastritis, heartburn or ulcers can occur. At the psychological level, Pitta dosha is characterized by determination, organization, rationality and the desire to succeed. Pittas are confident, courageous and enthusiastic. When out of balance, those with a Pitta-dominant constitution tend to become impatient and judgmental and can even become angry and aggressive. Imbalanced, Pitta's competitive tendencies can result in chronic stress, which may become a factor in high blood pressure or heart disease. Jalashaya mudra's soothing, cooling and relaxing effects are helpful for Pitta imbalance.

Kapha

Kapha is responsible for the physical structure of the body, providing protection and lubrication of the joints. Individuals with a Kapha-dominant body type are often short or medium in height, strong, round and full-bodied. They tend to have a slower metabolism and sluggish circulation. When individuals with a Kapha-dominant constitution are out of balance, their digestion and water metabolism tend to be slow and they may suffer from edema, excess mucus and high cholesterol. At the psychological level, Kaphas tend to be caring, compassionate and gentle. When out of balance, they can become depressed and stuck in the past. Kaphas may also become excessively attached to people and material possessions. Ratna Prabha mudra's vitalizing effects are helpful for rebalancing Kapha.

Mudras	Doshas	Qualities Cultivated
Achala Agni	**Tridosha**	Balances digestion, which is especially important for Kapha & Vata imbalances. Also supports Pitta's normally strong digestion.
Abhaya Varada	**Vata**	Cultivates a sense of centering, grounding & safety that counteract Vata's tendency toward excessive fear, instability & anxiety.
Jalashaya	**Pitta**	Cultivates coolness, calmness and serenity that counteract Pitta's tendency toward inflammation, competition & anger.
Ratna Prabha	**Kapha**	Cultivates warmth, energy & self-esteem that counteract Kapha's tendency toward lethargy & lack of enthusiasm.

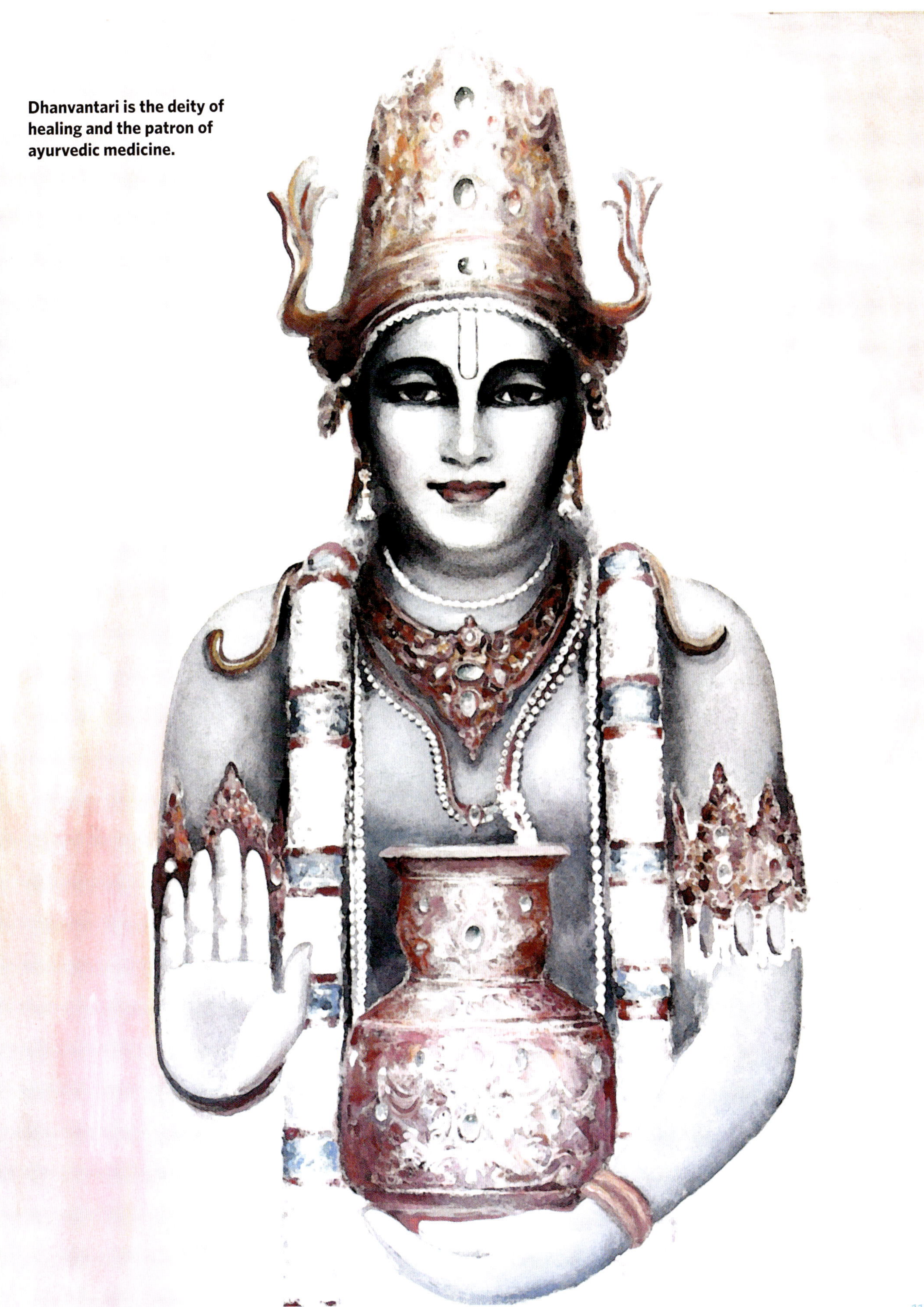

Dhanvantari is the deity of healing and the patron of ayurvedic medicine.

46 ACHALA AGNI MUDRA

Gesture of the Steady Fire

For Optimizing Digestion

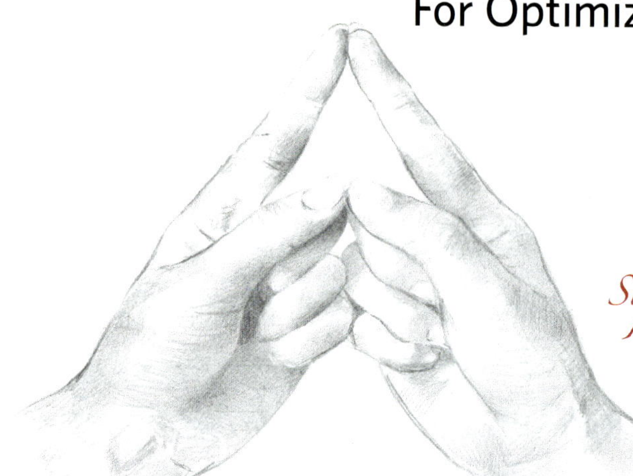

The light of agni purifies my being,
Supporting optimal digestion and balanced energy.

CORE QUALITY
Optimal Digestion

ESPECIALLY HELPFUL FOR
- Balancing physical digestion.
- Supporting digestion and assimilation of thoughts and feelings.
- Cultivating self-esteem.
- Instilling a sense of direction and clarity.

MUDRAS WITH SIMILAR EFFECTS
Pushan, Surya, Vajra, Kubera

CAUTIONS
None

INSTRUCTIONS
1. Make the hands into fists with the thumbs on the outside, resting on the second joint of the middle finger.
2. Extend the index fingers straight out.
3. Touch the inner borders of the tips of the index fingers together, as well as the knuckles of each hand.
4. The tips of the thumbs touch lightly with the palms facing upward.
5. Rest the forearms against the solar plexus with the index fingers forming an arrow that faces forward.
6. Relax the shoulders back and down, with the spine naturally aligned.

From the ayurvedic perspective, optimal digestion is essential for health and healing. Poor digestion and the subsequent accumulation of toxins, called *ama*, are main factors in disease. Optimal digestion is essential for the health of all three *doshas* and depends upon balanced *agni*, the subtle fire that supports all digestive processes. When agni is balanced, digestion is complete, providing optimal energy. When agni is imbalanced, digestion is compromised and toxins build up within the body. Ama is eliminated by improving the quality and quantity of what we ingest, digesting it fully, assimilating it thoroughly and eliminating waste products completely. Balanced agni within the physical body is supported by balanced agni at more subtle levels, especially the ability to digest sensory impressions. To the extent that these impressions, in the form of thoughts, feelings and memories, are digested fully, we receive the information we need while releasing residues held in the form of accumulated emotions, such as resentment or guilt.

Agni is the "subtle fire of digestion," and *achala* means "steady." *Achala agni* refers to steady, balanced digestion within the physical body and the mind. Achala Agni mudra directs breath, awareness and energy into the solar plexus, supporting all digestive processes. The regular practice of this gesture maintains a steady digestive fire that cultivates balanced energy while facilitating the release of toxins that could lead to dis-ease. At a psychological level, this gesture instills enthusiasm, vitality and a sense of clarity that supports the digestion of thoughts and feelings. The triangular shape formed by the index fingers symbolizes the flame of agni, which provides light and energy for all our activities while clarifying our life purpose.

SYSTEMS BALANCED:

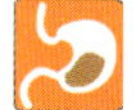
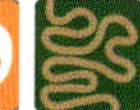

ELEMENTS ACTIVATED:

DOSHAS BALANCED:

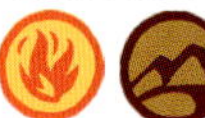
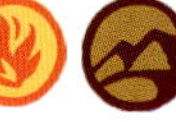
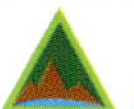

PRANA VAYUS NOURISHED:

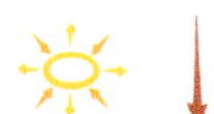

CHAKRAS BALANCED:

SCALE FROM CALMING TO ENERGIZING:

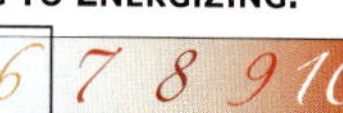

Guided Meditation: Cultivating Optimal Digestion

- As you hold Achala Agni mudra, take several natural breaths to attune to all the feelings and sensations awakened by this gesture.
- Notice how your breath is naturally directed into your solar plexus, instilling a sense of warmth and radiance.
- With each inhalation, your solar plexus expands outward horizontally, and with each exhalation, it softens inward completely.
- Sense how your rhythmic breathing gradually awakens vital energy, which you visualize as a flame at the center of your solar plexus.
- Take some time to kindle your inner flame with your breathing in exactly the right intensity to support optimal digestion at all levels of your being.
- Sense the steady flame of radiant energy infusing your stomach with warmth and vitality, allowing it to break down food more efficiently.
- Now, sense the light of your inner flame bathing your small intestine, balancing its rhythmic movement and optimizing the absorption of nutrients.
- As nutrients are assimilated more completely, take several breaths to sense optimal energy radiating out to nourish every cell of your body.
- As radiant energy flows throughout your being, the light of your inner flame naturally infuses your thoughts and feelings, allowing you to digest and assimilate life experiences more easily.
- Take several breaths to sense the release of any accumulated sensory impressions, thoughts, memories, feelings and beliefs, allowing you to move forward in life with radiant vitality.
- As you experience radiant vitality at all dimensions of your being, you naturally receive a clear vision for your life journey, along with the energy to manifest all of your possibilities.
- As energy and clarity infuse your entire being, you live each day vibrantly and joyfully.
- Affirm the light of vitality as you repeat the following three times, aloud or silently: **"Optimal digestion at all levels of being allows me to live with radiant vitality."**
- Slowly release the gesture, taking several breaths to experience the vitality that arises through balanced agni.
- When you are ready, open your eyes, returning slowly and gently, continuing your journey with perfect, balanced energy.

Annamaya kosha
(physical body)

• Directs breath and awareness to the solar plexus, enhancing movement of the abdomen and diaphragm that supports optimal digestion.
• Increases breathing in the mid back, creating a massaging effect that releases tension and increases circulation to the kidneys and adrenal glands.
• The mildly energizing effects of this gesture are generally helpful for Kapha imbalance.
• The enhanced clarity and sense of direction are generally helpful for Vata imbalance.
• The balancing effects support Pitta's generally strong digestion.

Pranamaya kosha
(energy body)

• Activates Samana and Apana vayus, the horizontal and downward moving currents of energy.
• Enhances the power of agni, the subtle digestive fire.
• Opens and balances the third chakra, center of personal power.

Manomaya kosha
(psycho-emotional body)

• Cultivates emotional balance.
• Assists in digesting sensory impressions and psycho-emotional experiences.

Vijnanamaya kosha
(wisdom body)

• Instills a sense of clarity, providing direction for our life journey.

Anandamaya kosha
(bliss body)

• As agni is balanced, our entire being is infused with light and radiance.

47 Abhaya Varada Mudra

Gesture of Fearlessness and Granting Wishes

For Balancing Vata Dosha

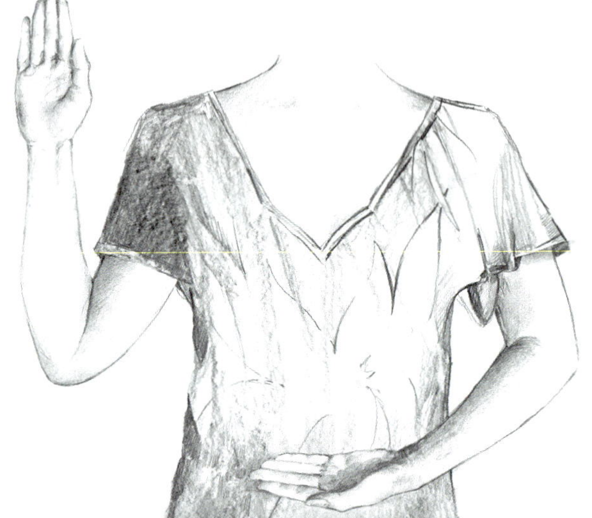

With a greater sense of grounding and centering, I move forward in life fearlessly.

Core Quality

Fearlessness

Especially helpful for

- Balancing Vata dosha by cultivating grounding and centering.
- Supporting the health of the eliminatory system.
- Reducing stress and anxiety.

Mudras with similar effects

Adho Merudanda, Chinmaya, Bhu, Adhi

Cautions

None

Instructions

1. Hold the left hand slightly cupped below the navel, gently touching the body, with the palm facing upward. The hand can also rest on the lap.
2. Hold the right hand slightly cupped at the level of the shoulder, with the palm facing forward.
3. The right elbow is held close to the waist with the forearm perpendicular to the earth.
4. Relax the shoulders back and down, with the spine naturally aligned.

The *Vata* constitution, composed of the air and space elements, is characterized by lightness and movement. Movement is essential for all our physiological functioning, including circulation, respiration, digestion, elimination and the transmission of nerve impulses. When movement becomes excessive, however, Vata imbalances, including dry skin, joint problems, poor digestion and elimination, gas and menstrual cramps can occur. At the level of the mind, individuals with a Vata-dominant constitution tend toward creativity and versatility. When imbalanced, however, Vatas can become unstable and ungrounded, resulting in excessive fear and anxiety.

Abhaya means "absence of fear," and *varada* means "granting wishes." Abhaya Varada mudra evokes the fearlessness that comes from being centered in our authentic being, whose essential nature is safety. This gesture directs breath, awareness and energy into the pelvis, the seat of Vata, enhancing abdominal breathing, which supports digestion and elimination. Abhaya Varada mudra lengthens the exhaling breath, which helps to reduce stress, release tension and improve elimination. This gesture also cultivates a sense of grounding and centering, which counteracts Vata's tendency toward insecurity. As grounding and centering increase, embodiment is enhanced along with the ability to live in the present moment more completely. Centered in the present moment and fully embodied, emotional stability is enhanced naturally, allowing Vatas to move forward in life more confidently. Finally, Abhaya Varada mudra cultivates a feeling of oneness and unity, further supporting imbalanced Vatas in releasing excessive fear and anxiety.

Systems Balanced:

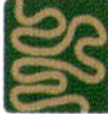

Elements Activated:

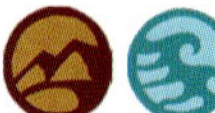
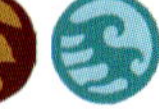

Doshas Balanced:

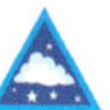

Prana Vayus Nourished:

Chakras Balanced:

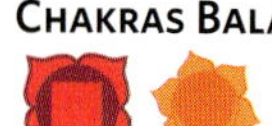

Scale from Calming to Energizing:

Guided Meditation: Centered Within Your Being

- As you hold Abhaya Varada mudra, take several natural breaths to attune to all the feelings and sensations evoked by this gesture.
- Notice how your breath is gently directed into your pelvis, instilling a sense of centering that allows you to journey forward confidently.
- You will deepen your sense of centering by visualizing yourself at the beginning of a trail in completely new surroundings.
- As you begin your journey, sense each of your steps firmly supported by the earth beneath, allowing you to move forward surely and steadily.
- Supported by the earth and centered within your being, you inhabit your physical body more completely, allowing you to be fully present at each step along your journey.
- As you move forward steadily, you attune to your rhythmic breathing, which naturally deepens your sense of centering.
- More attuned to your body and breath, your connection to the earth deepens naturally, cultivating a sense of oneness with your surroundings, allowing you to journey forward with greater security.
- As you continue along your way, you see in the distance an area of dense forest, a tunnel of trees, where almost no light is entering.
- You hesitate for a moment, but then reconnect with the steady flow of your breath, the support of the earth beneath and your sense of centering, allowing you to continue forward confidently.
- Once within the shade of these sheltering trees, your sense of oneness with the earth beneath allows all fear to be released, and you journey on with a renewed sense of safety.
- Soon, you come to a clearing with sunlight shimmering through the leaves and, at the very center, you are inspired by the sight of an ancient majestic tree.
- As you come nearer, you find a hollow within its huge trunk and roots, forming walls and a roof that invite you to sit within this natural room.
- As you sit, you sense your roots reaching deep into the earth, allowing you to become one with this ancient tree, naturally deepening your sense of centering.
- Fully centered within your being and deeply connected to the earth beneath, you rest in absolute tranquility, fully supported along your life journey.
- Affirm your centering as you repeat the following three times, aloud or silently: **"One with the earth and centered within my being, I journey in complete safety."**
- Slowly release the gesture, taking several breaths to rest in absolute tranquility.
- When you are ready, open your eyes, returning slowly and gently, integrating your enhanced sense of centering into all of your activities.

Annamaya kosha (physical body)

• Directs breath and awareness into the pelvis and pelvic floor, cultivating a massaging effect for the colon, the seat of Vata, supporting optimal elimination.
• Slows and stabilizes the breath while lengthening the exhalation, thereby helping to reduce stress and blood pressure.
• The grounding and centering effects of this gesture are generally helpful for Vata imbalance.

Pranamaya kosha (energy body)

• Activates Apana vayu, the downward moving current of energy.
• Opens and balances the first and second chakras, centers of safety and self-nourishment.

Manomaya kosha (psycho-emotional body)

• Cultivates a sense of inner safety that serves as an antidote for the excessive fear and anxiety that may accompany Vata imbalance.
• Cultivates grounding and centering, which are helpful antidotes for Vata instability.

Vijnanamaya kosha (wisdom body)

• As fear and insecurity are reduced, it becomes easier to align with our true being whose essential nature is safety.

Anandamaya kosha (bliss body)

• As grounding and centering increase, a sense of absolute safety arises naturally.

48

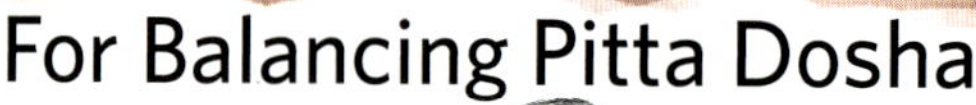

Jalashaya Mudra

Gesture of the Lake

For Balancing Pitta Dosha

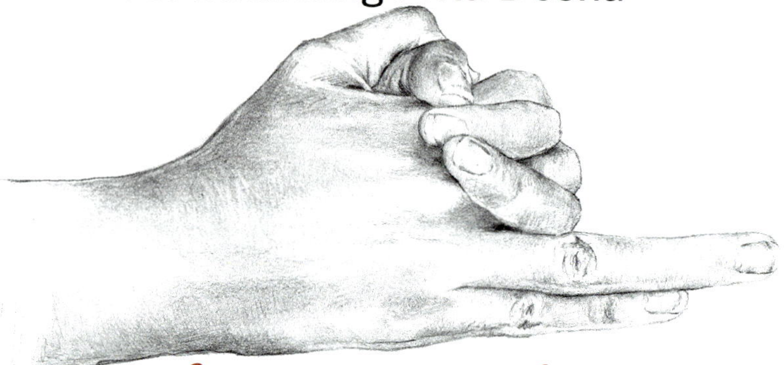

Bathing in my inner lake of serenity,
I experience complete peace and harmony.

Core Quality

Serenity

Especially helpful for

- Balancing Pitta dosha by soothing and calming the body and mind.
- Releasing tension from the lower back.
- Instilling a cooling effect that helps to relieve inflammation.
- Cultivating a sense of serenity that helps to release any tendency toward judgment, conflict or competition.

Mudras with similar effects

Jala, Dvimukham, Matsya, Pranidhana

Cautions

None

Instructions

1. Interlace all the fingers to the outside, with the right thumb on top.
2. Extend the ring and little fingers straight forward, joined along their length.
3. Rest the gesture below the navel with the forearms against the abdomen or on the lap.
4. Relax the shoulders back and down, with the elbows held slightly away from the body and the spine naturally aligned.

The *Pitta* constitution, composed of the fire and water elements, is characterized by heat and energy. When Pitta is balanced, optimal digestion and assimilation of nutrients occur naturally, providing a steady level of energy and vitality. When Pitta becomes excessive, however, symptoms of imbalance, including heartburn, hyperacidity, inflammation, gastritis and ulcers may occur. At the psycho-emotional level, the Pitta-dominant constitution is industrious, dynamic and extremely efficient at organizing and managing. When Pittas become imbalanced, they tend toward hyperperfectionism and criticism. Imbalanced Pittas may also become demanding, harsh and sharp, generating inner and outer conflict. Pitta's hypercompetitive behavior makes them more vulnerable to stress, and when stress becomes chronic, it may manifest as stress-related illness, including hypertension.

Jalashaya means "lake," and is formed from two Sanskrit words: *jala* meaning "water," and *shaya* meaning "calm," "peaceful," "nighttime" or "sleep." Jalashaya mudra cultivates the cooling, refreshing qualities of a peaceful lake that soothe Pitta's tendency toward excessive heating qualities. This gesture directs breath, awareness and energy into the pelvis and base of the body, soothing and nourishing the reproductive, urinary and eliminatory systems. Jalashaya mudra instills a refreshing quality on the inhalation, which supports relief from inflammation. On the lengthened exhaling breath, this gesture induces a calming effect, supporting deep relaxation that helps to release stress. Jalashaya mudra cultivates a sense of softness and ease, which can help soothe Pitta's tendency toward excessive judgment, criticism and hyperperfectionism.

Systems Balanced:

 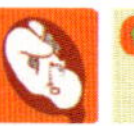 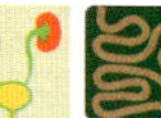 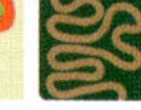

Elements Activated:

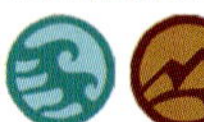 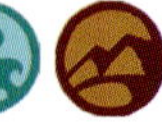

Doshas Balanced:

Prana Vayus Nourished:

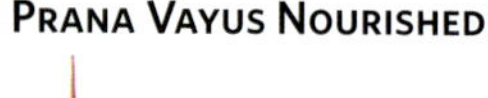

Chakras Balanced:

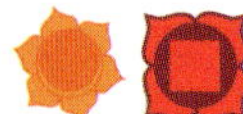

Scale from Calming to Energizing:

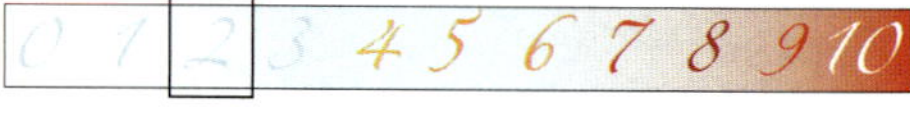

Guided Meditation: Lake of Serenity

- As you hold Jalashaya mudra, take several natural breaths to attune to all the feelings and sensations evoked by this gesture.
- Notice how your breath is gently directed into your pelvis and the base of your body, allowing you to experience greater ease and serenity.
- To deepen your sense of serenity, visualize yourself near a calm lake, surrounded by shady green trees and wildflowers swaying in a soft breeze.
- Take several breaths to sense yourself within this scene; your lake is just slightly cool and refreshing; the sandy bottom is shallow, clear and clean, inviting you to enter in complete comfort and safety.
- As you bathe effortlessly in your lake of serenity, you receive all of its essential nourishing qualities.
- Begin by absorbing the quality of release, taking several breaths to sense yourself letting go, allowing things to simply be, without needing to change or control anything.
- As you allow things to simply be, stress and tension begin to dissolve naturally, and you take some time to sense your breathing becoming even more calm and serene.
- With a greater sense of calm and serenity, contentment unfolds naturally, taking several breaths to sense that you already possess everything you need for your life journey.
- Resting contentedly, you naturally develop appreciation for all of life's simple things, allowing you to savor the present moment more completely.
- More attuned to the present moment, you sense your oneness with the natural world, taking all the time you need to experience all of creation as a seamless unity.
- Within this experience of oneness, you naturally sense your communion with all beings, taking several breaths to allow empathy and compassion to unfold naturally.
- With a greater sense of compassion and unity, you envision cooperation and harmony within all of your activities, unfolding your talents and abilities while serving the world open-heartedly.
- Now, take several breaths to bathe in all of your lake's nourishing qualities, allowing you to rest in complete inner peace and absolute serenity.
- As you rest deeply, repeat the following three times, aloud or silently: **"Bathing in the calm waters of my inner being, I experience absolute serenity."**
- Now, slowly release the gesture, taking several breaths to simply rest.
- When you are ready, open your eyes, returning slowly and gently, bathed in a sense of deep serenity.

Annamaya kosha (physical body)

- **Directs breath and awareness into the pelvis and base of the body, creating a massaging effect that increases circulation to the reproductive, urinary and eliminatory systems.**
- **Facilitates deep abdominal breathing, whose calming effects reduce stress and blood pressure.**
- **Lengthens the exhalation, helping to renew the residual air in the lungs.**
- **Instills a sensation of refreshment on the inhaling breath, which may help to reduce the discomfort of inflammation.**
- **The enhanced breathing in the lower back helps to release tension from this area.**
- **The cooling and calming effects of this gesture are generally helpful for Pitta imbalance.**

Pranamaya kosha (energy body)

- **Activates Apana vayu, the downward moving current of energy.**
- **Opens and balances the first and second chakras, centers of safety and self-nourishment.**

Manomaya kosha (psycho-emotional body)

- **Instills calm and serenity.**
- **Cultivates compassion and empathy.**

Vijnanamaya kosha (wisdom body)

- **As we release into our inner lake of serenity, we experience the peace of our true being.**

Anandamaya kosha (bliss body)

- **As we deepen our sense of relaxation and serenity, feelings of inner nourishment and deep contentment arise naturally.**

49 Ratna Prabha Mudra

Gesture of the Radiant Jewel

For Balancing Kapha Dosha

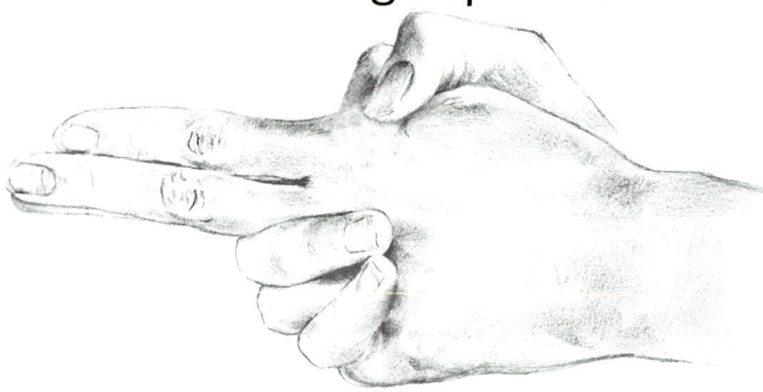

Awakening the light of radiant vitality,
I naturally unfold all of my possibilities.

Core Quality

Vitality

Especially Helpful For

- Balancing Kapha dosha by enhancing energy, enthusiasm and vitality.
- Activating digestion.
- Helping to clear congestion from the lungs and sinus passages.
- Increasing mental clarity.

Mudras with Similar Effects

Vajra, Kubera, Surya, Vajrapradama

Cautions

Those with hypertension should carefully monitor the effects. Surya mudra, which is less energizing, can be used as a substitute.

Instructions

1. Interlace all the fingers to the outside, with the right thumb on top.
2. Extend the index and middle fingers straight forward, joined along their length.
3. Rest the wrists onto the upper abdomen, with the fingers pointing forward.
4. Relax the shoulders back and down, with the elbows held slightly away from the body and the spine naturally aligned.

The *Kapha* constitution, composed of the earth and water elements, is characterized by stable joints, good overall health and a generally balanced level of energy. At the psycho-emotional level, Kapha possesses the qualities of reliability and amiability, allowing them to face adversity with ease. When out of balance, Kaphas tend toward congestion at both the physical and psycho-emotional levels. At the physical level, this congestion is often located in the lungs, the seat of Kapha, and can manifest as excessive mucus throughout the respiratory system. Kaphas also have a tendency toward water retention and sluggish digestion. At a psycho-emotional level, Kapha imbalance may manifest as dullness, lethargy and excessive attachment. Individuals with Kapha imbalance may become unmotivated, stuck in the past and unable to envision their own potential and possibilities. Kaphas can also become emotionally congested and have difficulty in expressing feelings, which can manifest as depression. The tendency toward congestion at the physical and psycho-emotional levels can make Kaphas more prone to obesity.

Ratna means "jewel," and *prabha* means "luster" or "radiance." *Ratna Prabha* is therefore a "radiant jewel." Ratna Prabha mudra awakens the jewel of our inner being, instilling energy and vitality that is helpful for reducing the lethargy associated with Kapha imbalance. This gesture strongly expands the breath at the front of the lungs, helping to clear congestion. This mudra also directs energy and awareness into the solar plexus, the seat of the fire element, enhancing physical digestion and also increasing enthusiasm and vitality. Ratna Prabha mudra builds self-esteem, instilling a clearer sense of life purpose, along with the energy to manifest our life vision more completely.

Systems Balanced:

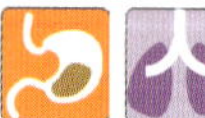
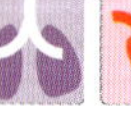

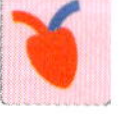

Elements Activated:

Doshas Balanced:

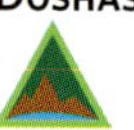

Prana Vayus Nourished:

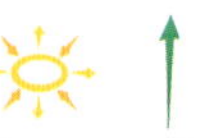

Chakras Balanced:

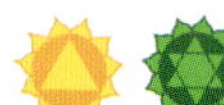

Scale from Calming to Energizing:

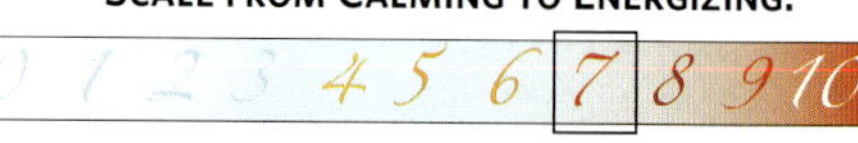

Guided Meditation: **Radiant Jewel of Vitality**

- ॐ As you hold Ratna Prabha mudra, take several natural breaths to attune to all the feelings and sensations awakened by this gesture.
- ॐ Notice how your breath is naturally directed into your solar plexus and chest, enhancing energy and instilling a sense of vitality.
- ॐ Visualize the source of this vitality as a brilliant jewel at the center of your solar plexus. Take some time to notice its color, shape, size and clarity, allowing its luminosity to radiate throughout your being.
- ॐ With each inhalation, the light of your inner jewel shines more brightly, and with each exhalation, you open to receive its luminous qualities.
- ॐ Begin by allowing this light to bathe your digestive system with vital energy, supporting it in breaking down food, thereby allowing you to absorb nutrients more efficiently.
- ॐ Now, the light of your inner jewel fills your respiratory system, clearing away any congestion, allowing your breath to flow freely and easily while naturally expanding your lung capacity.
- ॐ With your body and breath bathed in the light of vitality, your inner jewel naturally illuminates your mind with enthusiasm and self-esteem.
- ॐ Take several breaths to embody this enhanced enthusiasm and self-esteem, envisioning your senses opening to receive all of the colors, sights, sounds, flavors and textures of life more vibrantly.
- ॐ As the light of your inner jewel infuses your body, mind and senses, you explore new frontiers and opportunities, sensing your life as a field of infinite possibilities.
- ॐ Take several breaths to allow this radiant light to illuminate all of your possibilities while providing the energy to manifest them completely.
- ॐ Affirm your vital energy, as you repeat the following three times, aloud or silently: **"As my inner jewel shines forth radiantly, I live with enthusiasm and vitality."**
- ॐ Slowly release the gesture, taking several breaths to experience your inner brilliance.
- ॐ When you are ready, open your eyes, returning slowly and gently, integrating greater enthusiasm and vitality into all of your activities.

Annamaya kosha (physical body)

• Directs breath and awareness into the solar plexus and chest, expanding breath capacity and reducing lung congestion.
• The enhanced movement of the diaphragm increases circulation to the digestive system.
• Increases metabolism, which may be helpful for weight loss.
• Opens the back ribs, massaging the area of the kidneys and adrenal glands, thereby enhancing energy.
• The stimulating and energizing effects of this gesture are generally helpful for Kapha imbalance.

Pranamaya kosha (energy body)

• Activates Samana and Prana vayus, the horizontal and upward moving currents of energy.
• Opens and balances the third and fourth chakras, centers of personal power and unconditional love.

Manomaya kosha (psycho-emotional body)

• Cultivates enthusiasm, vitality and self-esteem.
• Opens the emotional body so that feelings can be experienced and digested more easily.

Vijnanamaya kosha (wisdom body)

• Cultivates mental clarity and energy, which are helpful in clarifying our life purpose and manifesting it more easily.

Anandamaya kosha (bliss body)

• With greater energy and vitality, feelings of enthusiasm and inner brilliance arise naturally.

Chapter Nine

Nourishing the Body with Vital Energy

MUDRAS FOR THE PRANA VAYUS

The *Pranamaya kosha* is the energy dimension of our being, composed of *prana*, the life force energy. This dimension is more subtle than the physical body and cannot be perceived directly through the five senses. The subtle body is composed of three systems, each of which plays a specific role in balancing the overall flow of energy throughout our entire subtle anatomy. These three systems are:

The Nadis - These are the minute channels that distribute subtle energy throughout our being (see Chapter 11 for details).

The Chakras - These are the seven major energy centers that receive, store, transform, purify and channel subtle energy to specific areas of the body (see Chapter 10 for details).

The Prana Vayus - These five main currents of subtle energy are the focus of this chapter. Their principal function is to nourish the systems of the physical body. Each system of the body depends on the regular flow of one or more of the prana vayus for its energetic nourishment. When the flow of vital energy is optimal, our physiology functions smoothly and efficiently. Chronic blockages in the flow of energy within these currents result in energy deficiencies that may lead to imbalance in the physical body.

Mudras are a primary vehicle for reestablishing the optimal flow of energy within the prana vayus. Specific gestures activate each prana vayu individually by directing breath to the systems and areas of the body related to each current of energy. Mudras also allow us to sense the flow of the prana vayus more palpably, so that we are able to perceive balance and imbalance more easily. Certain mudras, such as Hakini, balance and integrate all of the prana vayus simultaneously, naturally nourishing all of the systems of the body.

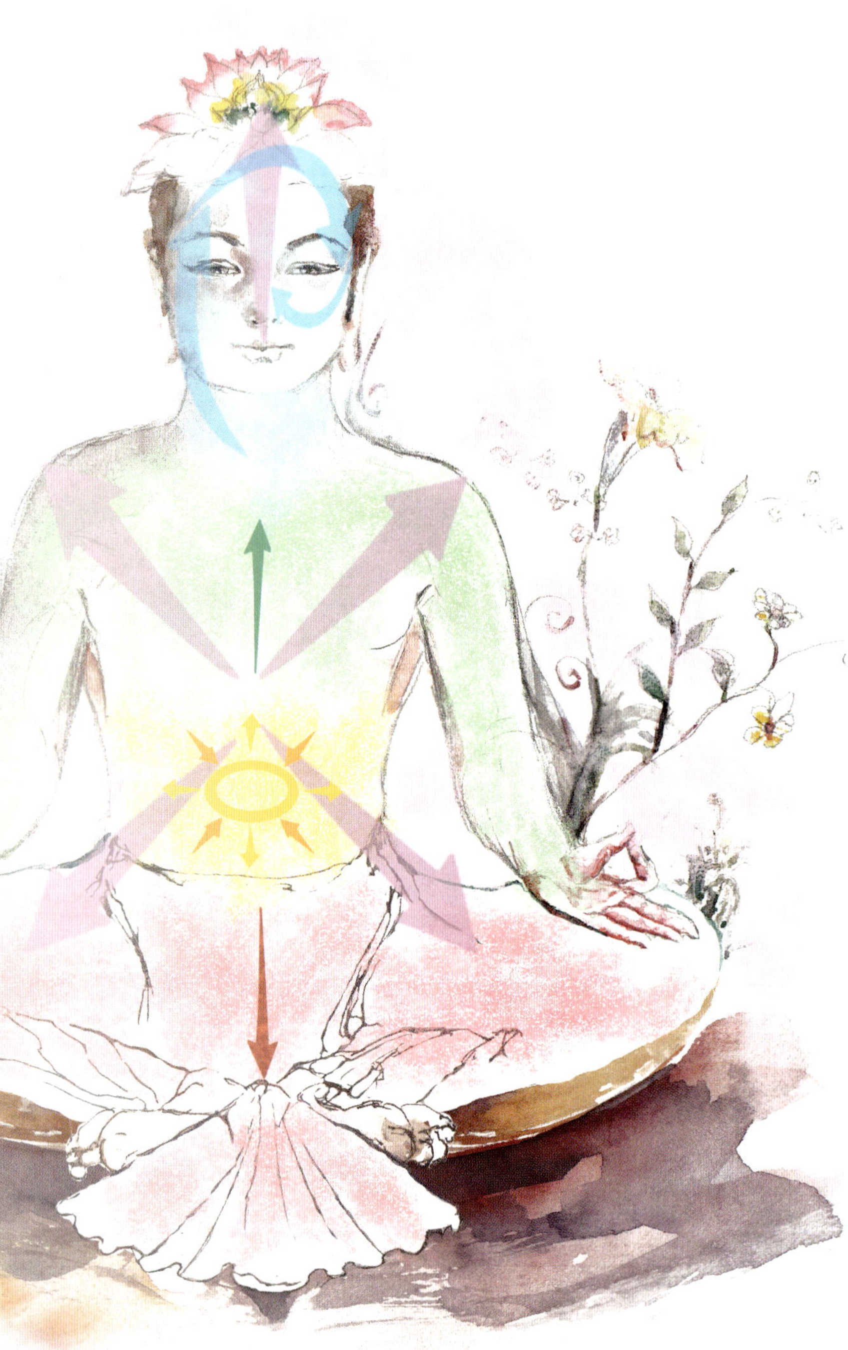

The Prana vayus play an important role in our health by nourishing the systems of the body with vital energy.

Principal Mudra for Activating Each Prana Vayu	Symbol for Each Prana Vayu	Direction of Energy Location in the Body Systems Nourished	Point of Origin & Trajectory of the Breath	Color Related Chakras Related Elements
Apana 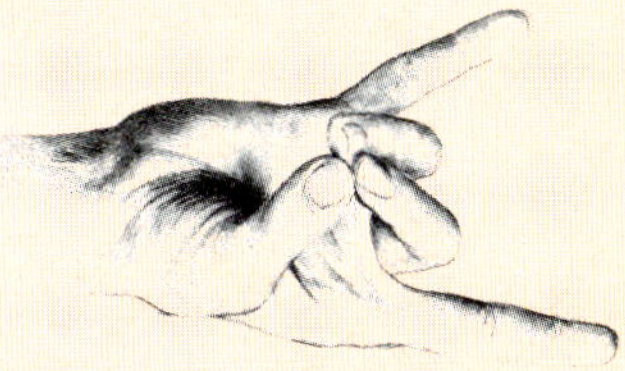	Apana 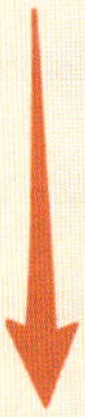	Downward Pelvis, base of the body, legs & feet Eliminatory, urinary & reproductive systems	Arises at the level of the navel & moves downward on the exhalation.	Red earth First & second chakras Earth & water elements
Prana 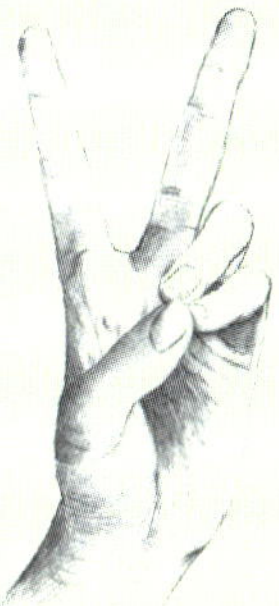	Prana 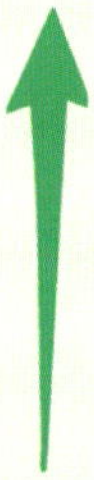	Upward Entire upper torso Cardio-respiratory & immune systems	Arises at the level of the navel & moves upward into the chest on the inhalation.	Light green Fourth chakra Air element
Matangi 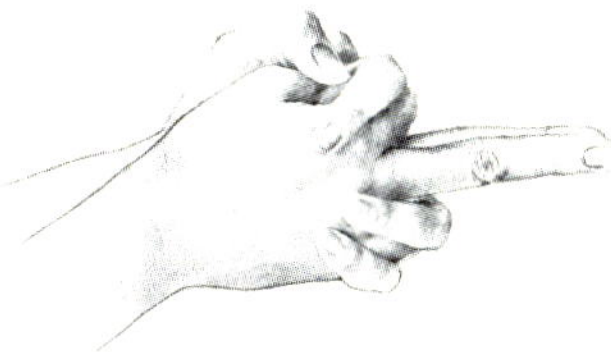	Samana 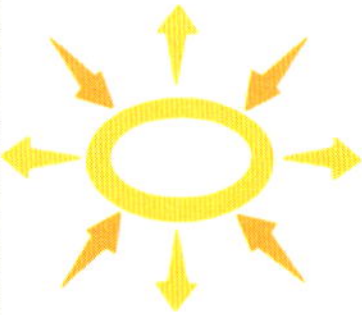	Inward & outward horizontally Solar plexus Digestive system	Arises at the center of the solar plexus, expanding outward on the inhalation, & drawing back toward the center on the exhalation.	Golden sunlight Third chakra Fire element
Linga 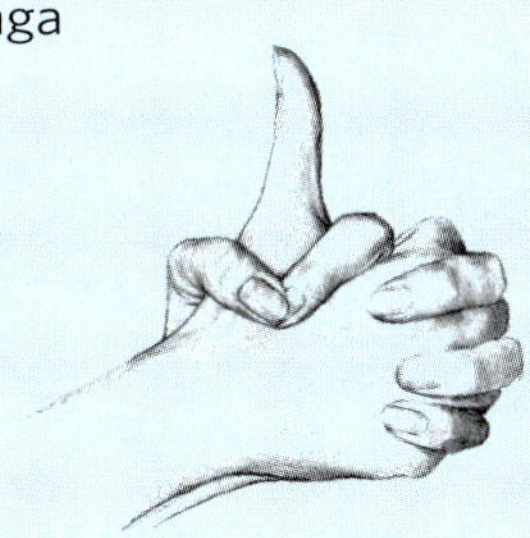	Udana 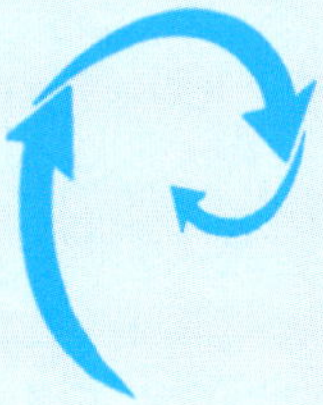	Upward & circulating Neck, throat & head Central nervous system, endocrine system & senses	Arises at the collarbones & flows upward into the neck & head on the inhalation, then circulates through the head and senses on the exhalation.	Sky-blue Fifth chakra Space element
Anushasana 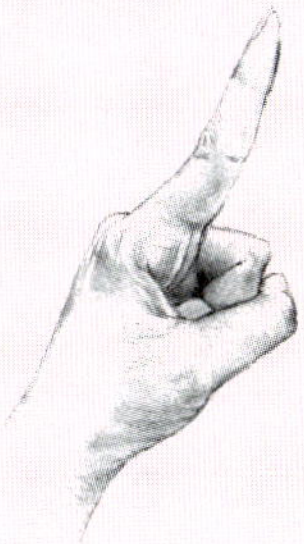	Vyana 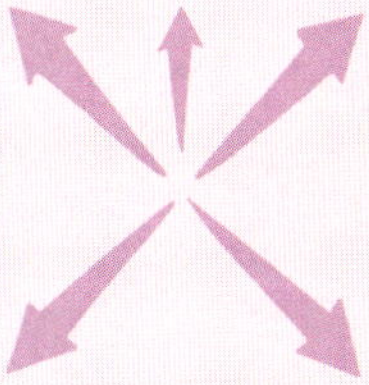	From center to periphery Entire body, especially extremities Circulatory, lymphatic & peripheral nervous systems	Energy is concentrated at the center of the body on the inhalation, & radiates outward toward the extremities on the exhalation.	Violet Second through sixth chakras Space, air, fire & water

50

Apana Mudra

Gesture of the Downward Current of Purifying Energy
For Activating Apana Vayu

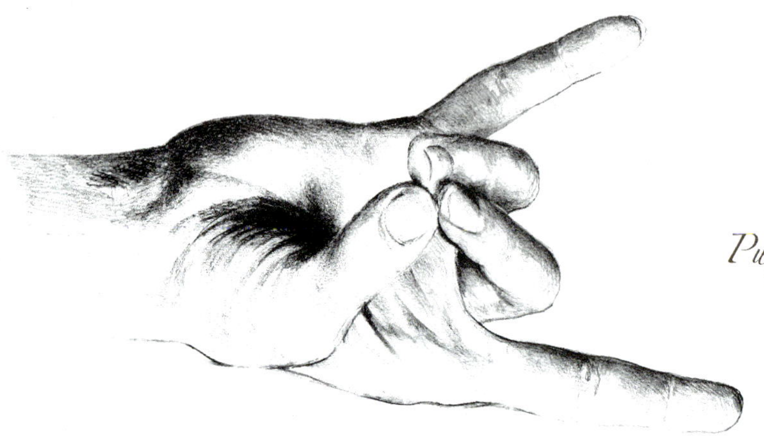

The downward current of energy
Purifies my body and mind completely.

Core Quality
Purifying Current of Energy

Especially helpful for
- Supporting all eliminatory processes.
- Constipation and menstrual cramping.
- Lowering blood pressure.
- Relieving stress and anxiety.
- Releasing attachment.

Mudras with similar effects
Prajna Prana Kriya, Pranidhana, Apanayana

Cautions
Those with low blood pressure should carefully monitor the effects.

All gestures that activate Apana vayu should be used cautiously during pregnancy, without extended holding.

Instructions
1. Touch the tips of the middle and ring fingers of each hand to the thumbs of the same hand.
2. Extend the index and little fingers.
3. Rest the backs of the hands onto the thighs or knees.
4. Relax the shoulders back and down, with the spine naturally aligned.

Apana means "air moving downward," and *Apana vayu* is the downward moving current of energy, which originates at the level of the navel and moves downward to nourish and purify the pelvis and pelvic floor. Its essential function is to support all processes of elimination. Apana vayu is especially important for the health of the eliminatory, urinary and reproductive systems. As these systems are nourished with vital energy, they are able to purify the body more efficiently. This purifying current also has a relaxing effect, closely associated with the lengthened exhaling breath, which helps to release stress and tension, thereby reducing blood pressure. At a psycho-emotional level, the free flow of Apana vayu enhances our sense of grounding, allowing us to live with a greater sense of security. Apana vayu also cultivates a feeling of release, supporting us in letting go of all we no longer need in order to live with greater lightness and ease.

Apana mudra directs breath, awareness and energy into the lower body, activating the downward moving current of Apana vayu. By making this downward current more palpable, this gesture helps us to perceive energetic blockages in the pelvis and base of the body, thereby supporting their release. Apana mudra lengthens the exhaling breath, enhancing Apana vayu's purifying effects as well as its calming and grounding qualities. This gesture also facilitates a sense of relaxation and release at the level of our thoughts and feelings, making it helpful for the treatment of anxiety. At the spiritual level, Apana mudra supports the cultivation of the quality of *vairagya*, non-attachment.

Systems Balanced:

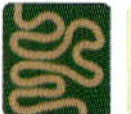 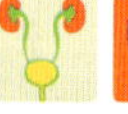 

Elements Activated:

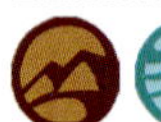 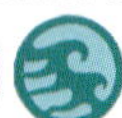

Doshas Balanced:

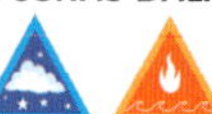

Prana Vayus Nourished:

Chakras Balanced:

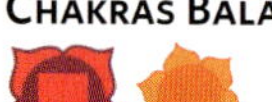

Scale from Calming to Energizing:

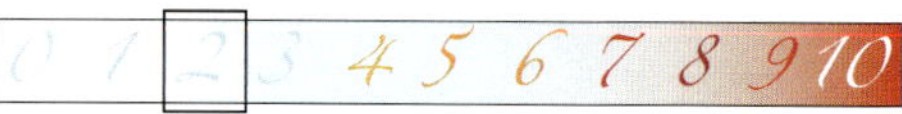

Guided Meditation: Purifying Downward Current of Energy

- As you hold Apana mudra, take several natural breaths to attune to all the feelings and sensations evoked by this gesture.
- Notice how your breath is directed downward from your navel to the base of your body, cultivating a sense of grounding.
- Sense your exhalation lengthening naturally, allowing all tension from your body to be released down and out into the earth beneath.
- Take several breaths to attune to the downward current of Apana vayu, a red earth-colored energy, which carries away all that is no longer needed from your body.
- Begin by taking some time to sense this downward current of energy massaging your large intestine internally, nourishing your eliminatory system to support its optimal functioning.
- For your next few cycles of breath, experience the downward current flowing through your urinary tract, from your kidneys to your bladder, supporting this system in removing excess liquids smoothly and easily.
- Sense the current of Apana vayu nourishing your reproductive organs, supporting the movement of fluids that bring new life into being, optimizing this system's health and vitality.
- Now, take several breaths to experience the current of red earth energy purifying your entire physical being, releasing all that you no longer need, down and out into the earth beneath.
- With your physical body nourished and purified, Apana vayu now infuses your thoughts and feelings with a sense of relaxation and release.
- Take some time to sense how each exhalation supports the release of all limiting thoughts, feelings and beliefs that no longer support your journey, naturally purifying your psycho-emotional being.
- Affirm your sense of release as you repeat the following three times, aloud or silently: **"Purified by the downward current of energy, I release all that no longer supports my journey."**
- Now, slowly release the gesture, taking several breaths to sense complete purification.
- When you are ready, open your eyes, returning slowly and gently, with a greater sense of release in your mind and body.

Annamaya kosha (physical body)

• Directs breath and awareness to the pelvis and base of the body, creating a massaging effect that increases circulation to the eliminatory, urinary and reproductive systems.
• Cultivates a lengthened exhalation, which activates the relaxation response, releasing muscular tension, and reducing stress and blood pressure.
• Increases comfort in the entire pelvic area, which may help alleviate constipation and the discomfort of menstrual cramping.
• The grounding effects of this gesture are generally helpful for Vata imbalance.
• The calming effects are generally helpful for Pitta imbalance.

Pranamaya kosha (energy body)

• Activates Apana vayu, the downward moving current of energy.
• Opens and balances the first and second chakras, centers of safety and self-nourishment.

Manomaya kosha (psycho-emotional body)

• Facilitates the release of stress and tension from the mind and emotions.
• Cultivates a sense of grounding and support.

Vijnanamaya kosha (wisdom body)

• The extended pause at the end of the exhalation allows us to experience the inner silence and absolute serenity that are reflections of our true being.

Anandamaya kosha (bliss body)

• As we experience Apana vayu more completely, a sense of complete release arises naturally.

51 Prana Mudra

Gesture of the Upward Current of Vital Energy

For Activating Prana Vayu

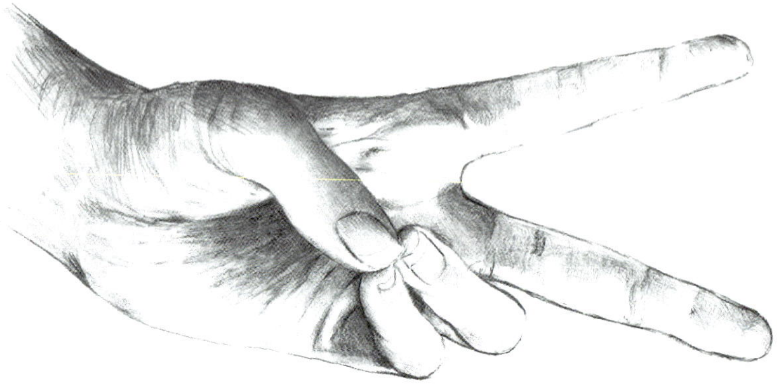

Nourished with uplifting energy,
I embrace life wholeheartedly.

Core Quality

Uplifting Current of Energy

Especially helpful for

- Supporting the health of the cardio-respiratory and immune systems.
- Increasing breath capacity.
- Enhancing vitality, optimism and enthusiasm.

Mudras with similar effects

Dirgha Svara, Vajrapradama, Medha Prana Kriya, Padma

Cautions

Those with hypertension should carefully monitor the effects.

Instructions

1. Touch the tips of the thumbs to the tips of the ring and little fingers.
2. Extend the middle and index fingers straight out in a "V" shape.
3. Rest the backs of the hands onto the thighs or knees, or hold the hands out to the sides of the body, palms facing forward at shoulder height, for increased energy.
4. Relax the shoulders back and down, with the spine naturally aligned.

Prana means "vital energy," and *Prana vayu* is the upward moving current of energy that originates at the level of the navel and rises upward to nourish the chest, heart, lungs, side ribs and upper back. This uplifting energy is closely associated with the inhaling breath, which naturally instills a sense of vitality and enthusiasm. The main function of Prana vayu is to support and nourish the cardio-respiratory system. Prana vayu also increases circulation to the area of the thymus gland, supporting immune system health. At a psycho-emotional level, this upward moving current instills optimism, trust and confidence, along with a feeling that we can meet and overcome challenges more easily. Prana vayu facilitates the opening of the subtle heart, enhancing our sensitivity and supporting us in welcoming and experiencing all of our feelings. This opening creates space for seeing and releasing limiting beliefs that keep us from living with greater enthusiasm and vitality.

Prana mudra activates and enhances the flow of Prana vayu, expanding and opening the entire thoracic area, optimizing breath capacity. As breathing is enhanced, this gesture supports us in deepening our awareness of each of the areas of the lungs and each of the four phases of the breathing process: inhalation, natural retention, exhalation and natural suspension. This gesture also directs the breath to the area of the upper sternum, where the thymus gland is located, supporting the optimal functioning of the immune system. Prana mudra activates the air element, awakening its essential qualities, including sensitivity, lightness, openness and gracefulness. As this gesture cultivates freer breathing, feelings of joy, optimism and enthusiasm awaken naturally, supporting us in living more vibrantly.

Systems Balanced:

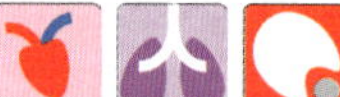

Prana Vayus Nourished:

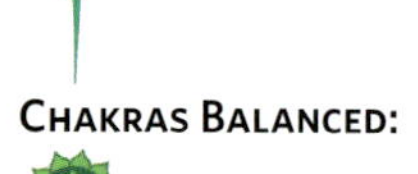

Elements Activated:

Chakras Balanced:

Doshas Balanced:

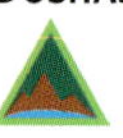

Scale from Calming to Energizing:

Guided Meditation: Vitalizing Upward Current

- As you hold Prana mudra, take several natural breaths to attune to all the feelings and sensations awakened by this gesture.
- Notice how your breath is directed upward into your chest, cultivating an experience of uplifting energy that allows you to breathe more freely.
- Take some time to sense how your inhalation is lengthened naturally, serving as a vehicle for Prana vayu, the upward moving current of vital energy.
- Sense this uplifting current as the color of a light green meadow, filling your upper torso with nature's own vitality, nourishing your heart and lungs completely.
- As you breathe in greater vitality, each area of your lungs is infused with life giving energy.
- Begin by taking several breaths to sense the upward moving current of energy nourishing the front of your lungs completely, providing the vitality to meet life confidently.
- Now, take some time to sense your current of vital energy infusing the back of your lungs, releasing all tension from this area of your being, allowing you to live and breathe with greater lightness and ease.
- Next, sense the upward moving current of energy expanding your lungs horizontally, allowing you to embrace life completely in a natural balance of giving and receiving.
- Now, take some time to sense all areas of your lungs integrated and breathing evenly, fully vitalized by the upward moving current of energy.
- With your breath flowing freely, experience this light green current nourishing your heart softly and gently, supporting it in functioning smoothly and rhythmically.
- Sense this current of vitality nourishing your thymus gland, behind your upper sternum, enhancing circulation to this area of your being, supporting your immune system in functioning optimally.
- With your entire upper torso bathed in light green energy, allow the upward moving current to permeate your thoughts and feelings, enhancing your level of enthusiasm, optimism and vitality.
- Nourished with uplifting energy, you naturally live more vibrantly, appreciating each moment of life as a precious gift to be embraced completely.
- Affirm your vital energy as you repeat the following three times, aloud or silently: **"Nourished by the upward current of energy, I live with enthusiasm and vitality."**
- Slowly release the gesture, taking several breaths to sense your enhanced vitality.
- When you are ready, open your eyes, returning slowly and gently, bringing greater enthusiasm and vitality to all of your activities.

Annamaya kosha (physical body)

• Directs breath and awareness into the chest, creating a massaging effect that enhances circulation to the cardio-respiratory system.
• Enhances breath capacity.
• Directs breath and awareness to the upper sternum, increasing circulation to the area of the thymus gland.
• Gently increases heart rate and blood pressure, vitalizing the entire body.
• The energizing effects of this gesture are generally helpful for Kapha imbalance.

Pranamaya kosha (energy body)

• Activates Prana vayu, the upward moving current of energy.
• Opens and balances the fourth chakra, center of unconditional love.

Manomaya kosha (psycho-emotional body)

• Helps to open the emotional heart, cultivating positive feelings while dissolving negativity.
• The uplifting effect may be helpful for depression.
• Focuses the mind, enhancing concentration and alertness.

Vijnanamaya kosha (wisdom body)

• The enhanced enthusiasm and vitality are an essential support for transforming challenges into opportunities along our spiritual journey.

Anandamaya kosha (bliss body)

• As the heart center opens, feelings of joy and radiant vitality awaken naturally.

52

Matangi Mudra

Gesture of the Goddess of Transformation

For Activating Samana Vayu

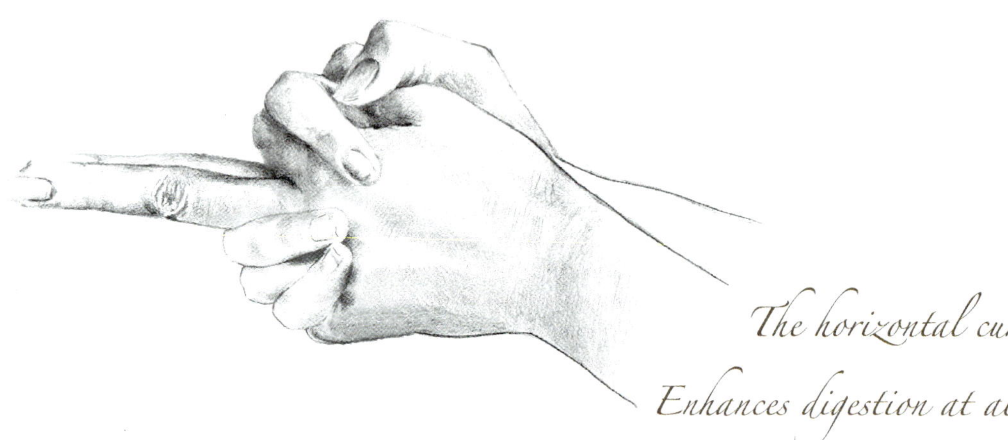

The horizontal current of energy
Enhances digestion at all levels of my being.

Core Quality

Radiating Current of Energy

Especially helpful for

- Enhancing digestion and assimilation.
- Supporting circulation and lymphatic drainage from the lower extremities.
- Digesting life experiences more easily.
- Cultivating energy, self-esteem and determination.

Mudras with similar effects

Achala Agni, Brahma, Vajra, Pushan

Cautions

Contraindicated for hyperdigestive conditions, such as acidity. Pushan mudra, which is less energizing, can be used as a substitute.

Instructions

1. Interlace the fingers to the outside, with the right thumb over the left.
2. Extend the middle fingers, joining them along their length, and point them straight forward.
3. Rest the wrists against the solar plexus.
4. Relax the shoulders back and down, with the elbows held slightly away from the body and the spine naturally aligned.

Samana means "equal," and *Samana vayu* is the horizontal current of energy, which expands outward from the center of the solar plexus on the inhalation and moves inward toward the center of the body on the exhalation. The essential function of Samana vayu is supporting digestion within all dimensions of our being. This golden current of energy enhances the movement of the diaphragm, massaging the entire digestive system and increasing circulation to the digestive organs. The increased diaphragmatic movement also creates a pumping effect that facilitates circulation of blood and lymph from the lower body. This current of energy kindles the subtle digestive fire, called *agni*, that optimizes digestion and assimilation of nutrients while supporting the removal of toxins. At the psycho-emotional level, the free flow of Samana vayu supports the digestion and assimilation of life experiences, thereby liberating vital energy, allowing us to clarify and manifest our life purpose.

Matangi is the "goddess of transformation," and Matangi mudra activates and enhances the flow of Samana vayu by directing breath, awareness and energy into the solar plexus. This gesture enhances the horizontal expansion and relaxation of the diaphragm, optimizing respiration, especially at the base of the lungs, which has the greatest surface area for the exchange of oxygen and carbon dioxide. Matangi mudra cultivates inner heat, reducing lethargy and providing enhanced energy for all of our activities. This gesture also supports the digestion of sensory impressions, allowing us to better conserve and channel our life force energy. The extended middle fingers represent clear direction along our life journey as well as the determination to overcome all obstacles that we meet.

Systems Balanced:

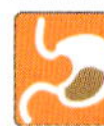

Prana Vayus Nourished:

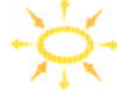

Elements Activated:

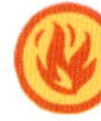

Chakras Balanced:

Doshas Balanced:

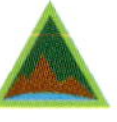

Scale from Calming to Energizing:

Guided Meditation: Current of Radiant Energy

- As you hold Matangi mudra, take several natural breaths to attune to all the feelings and sensations awakened by this gesture.
- Notice how your breath is directed into your solar plexus, cultivating a sense of warmth and energy that radiates throughout the middle portion of your body.
- Sense how your solar plexus expands horizontally with each inhalation, and how it naturally softens inward on each exhalation.
- As your solar plexus expands and releases energetically in synchrony with your breathing, visualize the horizontal current of Samana vayu as a radiant golden energy that cultivates vitality at all levels of your being.
- Begin by taking several breaths to sense this golden current massaging each of your digestive organs energetically, enhancing their ability to transform food and absorb nutrients more efficiently.
- With your physical digestion functioning more efficiently, your golden glow of radiant energy allows you to transform experiences into opportunities for learning, taking in the lessons you need while releasing all that no longer supports your journey.
- As you transform emotional experiences more easily, you naturally cultivate the energy and vitality that allows you to unfold and manifest your life purpose completely.
- The balanced flow of horizontal energy also provides determination and resiliency, allowing you to overcome all obstacles along your journey.
- With the balanced flow of Samana Vayu, you conserve your life force energy wisely, providing for all your needs while participating fully in life for the benefit of all beings.
- Affirm your radiant energy, repeating the following three times, aloud or silently: **"The golden current empowers me with abundant energy and vitality."**
- Now, slowly release the gesture, taking several breaths to experience radiant energy.
- When you are ready, open your eyes, returning slowly and gently, with a greater sense of vitality in all of your activities.

Annamaya Kosha (Physical Body)

- Directs breath and awareness to the area of the solar plexus, cultivating a massaging effect that enhances circulation to the digestive system.
- The enhanced movement of the diaphragm creates a pumping effect that supports the return of venous blood and lymphatic fluid from the lower extremities.
- Enhanced movement of the diaphragm expands breath capacity, especially in the lower lungs.
- The increased diaphragmatic movement massages the mid back, enhancing circulation to the area of the kidneys and adrenal glands.
- The energizing effects of this gesture are generally helpful for Kapha imbalance.

Pranamaya Kosha (Energy Body)

- Activates Samana vayu, the horizontal current of energy.
- Opens and balances the third chakra, center of personal power.

Manomaya Kosha (Psycho-Emotional Body)

- Instills a sense of self-confidence and personal power.
- Cultivates a clear sense of direction and determination.
- Enhances our ability to fully digest and assimilate life experiences.

Vijnanamaya Kosha (Wisdom Body)

- Cultivates the mental clarity that allows us to envision our life purpose more easily.

Anandamaya Kosha (Bliss Body)

- With abundant energy and clear direction, a sense of inner radiance arises from within the solar plexus.

53

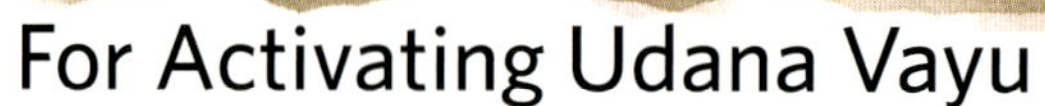

Linga Mudra

Gesture of the Symbol of the Creative Source

For Activating Udana Vayu

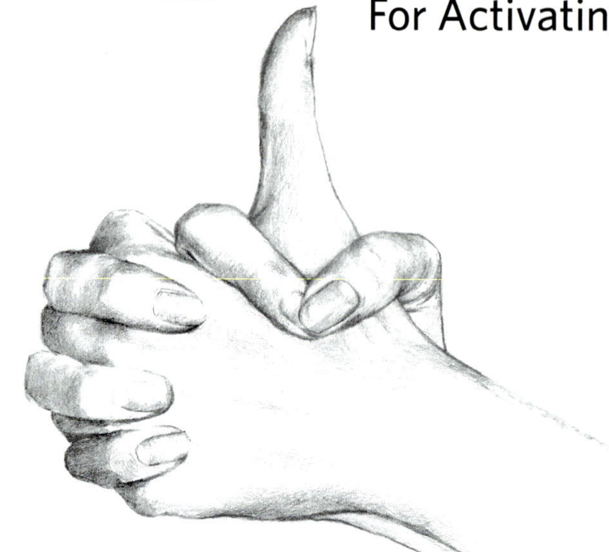

Attuned to the uppermost current of energy,
My senses open to all of life's beauty.

Core Quality

Clarifying Current of Energy

Especially helpful for

- Supporting the health of the endocrine and central nervous systems.
- Increasing energy and mental clarity.
- Revitalizing the senses.
- Aligning the cervical spine.
- Enhancing creativity and intuition.
- Supporting clear communication.

Mudras with similar effects

Kali, Shunya, Vishuddha, Garuda

Cautions

Contraindicated for thyroid conditions, hypertension, stroke, migraine or tension headaches. Shunya mudra, which is less energizing, may be used as a substitute.

Instructions

1. Interlace the fingers to the outside, with the right thumb on top.
2. Extend the left thumb straight up.
3. Rest the wrists against the solar plexus.
4. Relax the shoulders back and down, with the elbows slightly away from the body and the spine naturally aligned.

Udana means "upward," and *Udana vayu* is the uppermost current of energy, originating at the collarbones and rising upward to nourish the neck, throat and head. Its essential function is supporting the energetic health of the senses, endocrine and central nervous systems. The balanced flow of Udana vayu is essential for mental clarity and concentration. In addition, this uppermost current of energy nourishes the vocal cords, facilitating all forms of communication and creative expression. When this uppermost current is flowing smoothly and freely, it enhances the power of intuition, supporting us in attuning to our authentic inner voice and clarifying our life vision.

Linga is a sacred Indian symbol that represents the "creative source of the universe." Linga mudra activates and enhances the flow of Udana vayu by directing breath, awareness and energy into the neck and head. Linga mudra nourishes the throat area, supporting the health of the vocal cords, allowing us to communicate clearly and authentically. It also creates a massaging effect in the area of the thyroid gland at the front of the throat, activating metabolism. Linga mudra directs awareness and energy into the head, nourishing the brain and senses, supporting concentration and mental clarity. This gesture naturally facilitates *Ujjayi* breathing in which the throat is lightly contracted, creating a subtle sound that lengthens the breath, giving the mind a natural point of focus. The enhanced focus and mental clarity allow us to unfold all of our talents and possibilities more easily.

Systems Balanced:

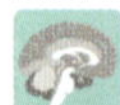 

Elements Activated:

Doshas Balanced:

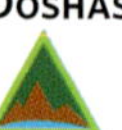

Prana Vayus Nourished:

Chakras Balanced:

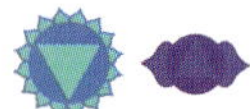 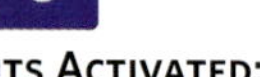

Scale from Calming to Energizing:

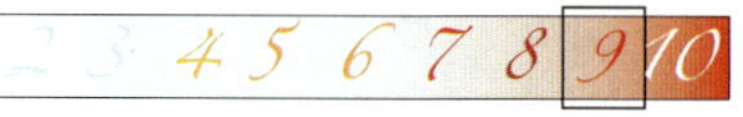

Guided Meditation: Awakening Clarity

- As you hold Linga mudra, take several natural breaths to attune to all the feelings and sensations awakened by this gesture.
- Notice how your breath is directed into your neck and head, activating the uppermost current of energy, Udana vayu, which cultivates a greater sense of clarity.
- With each inhalation, your breath rises upward from your collarbones into your neck and head, and with each exhalation, energy circulates gently throughout these areas.
- Take several breaths to sense this upward current of Udana vayu as a sky blue energy that nourishes your neck, head and senses completely.
- As the uppermost current of sky blue energy flows freely, a gentle smile spreads across your face, allowing your jaw, eyes and forehead to soften naturally.
- Take some time to sense how Udana vayu lengthens your cervical spine on the inhalation, and with each exhaling breath, tucks your chin back and in, naturally aligning your head.
- As Udana vayu nourishes your throat and neck, sense how it activates your thyroid gland, enhancing energy for all of your activities.
- Take several breaths to sense how this blue-sky energy radiates outward from your thyroid gland, vitalizing your entire being.
- As your thyroid gland is bathed in blue-sky energy, your throat and vocal cords are nourished naturally, allowing you to communicate clearly and easily.
- With your throat and neck nourished completely, the uppermost current of energy infuses each of your senses with vitality and clarity.
- Begin by sensing blue-sky energy permeating your nasal passages, allowing your olfactory sense to breathe in all of life's rich fragrances.
- The uppermost current now bathes the inside of your mouth, enhancing your ability to savor all of life's abundant flavors.
- Blue-sky energy now nourishes your eyes and sense of sight, allowing you to take in all the beauty of life.
- Now, Udana vayu infuses your sense of hearing, naturally enhancing your power of listening to all of life's melodies.
- As your senses are filled with clarity, you experience an enhanced ability to touch and be touched by life more sensitively.
- Take several breaths to experience all of your senses immersed in blue sky-energy, fully alive and functioning optimally.
- With your senses nourished completely, now allow blue-sky energy to gently bathe your brain, improving concentration and memory while instilling greater clarity.
- With greater clarity at all levels of being, you naturally envision the unfolding of all of your unique talents and possibilities.
- Affirm your growing clarity as you repeat the following three times, aloud or silently: **"As the infinite blue-sky fills my being, I experience life with greater clarity."**
- Slowly release the gesture, taking several breaths to rest in the sky blue current.
- When you are ready, open your eyes, returning slowly and gently, bringing greater clarity to all of your activities.

Annamaya kosha (physical body)

• Directs breath and awareness to the neck and throat, cultivating a massaging effect that enhances circulation to the area of the vocal cords and thyroid gland.
• Also directs breath and awareness to the head, gently stimulating the brain and senses.
• Supports correct alignment of the cervical spine.
• Enhances circulation to the area of the pituitary gland.
• The energizing effects of this gesture are generally helpful for Kapha imbalance.

Pranamaya kosha (energy body)

• Activates Udana vayu, the uppermost current of energy.
• Opens and balances the fifth and sixth chakras, centers of spiritual purification and wisdom.

Manomaya kosha (psycho-emotional body)

• Cultivates alertness, concentration and mental clarity.

Vijnanamaya kosha (wisdom body)

• As our center of communication is nourished, we attune to our inner voice, opening to intuition, providing guidance for our life journey.

Anandamaya kosha (bliss body)

• As energy flows more freely through the neck and head, we experience a sense of expansiveness.

54

Anushasana Mudra

Gesture of Direction

For Activating Vyana Vayu

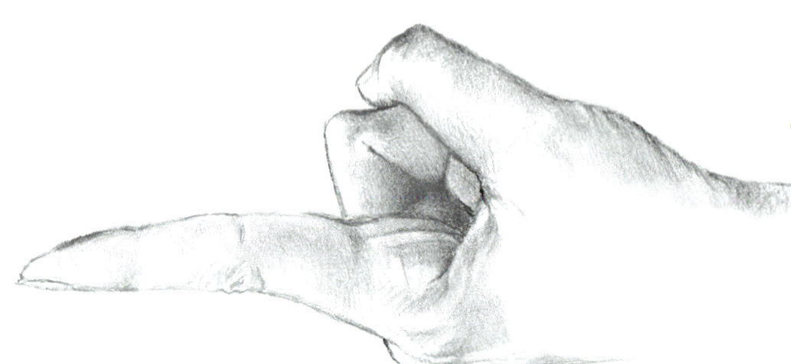

Attuned to the all-pervading current of energy,
All facets of my being are integrated
As a seamless unity.

Core Quality

All-Pervading Current of Energy

Especially helpful for

- Optimizing the health of the circulatory, lymphatic and peripheral nervous systems.
- Increasing circulation to the extremities.
- Supporting optimal posture.
- Increasing body awareness.
- Instilling a sense of integration and harmony.

Mudras with similar effects

Vyana Vayu, Hakini, Dharma Chakra

Cautions

None

Instructions

1. Make the hands into fists with the thumbs to the outside, resting on the second knuckle of the ring finger.
2. Extend the index fingers straight out.
3. Rest the backs of the hands onto the thighs or knees or, alternatively, hold the hands out to the sides of the body with the index fingers pointing upward.
4. Relax the shoulders back and down, with the spine naturally aligned.

Vyana means "pervading," and *Vyana vayu* is the current of vital energy that pervades the entire body. Its essential function is to support the optimal flow of energy from the center of our body outward toward the extremities. This violet current of energy moves inward toward the center of the body on the inhalation and radiates outward to the extremities on the exhalation. This energetic movement supports physical circulation of blood, lymph and nerve impulses. At a subtle level, this current supports the free flow of energy within the nadis, the subtle channels of spiritual energy. Vyana vayu also enhances coordination, facilitating balance and graceful movement. As it optimizes coordination and integration from center to extremities, Vyana vayu enhances body awareness and sensitivity. The overall effect of this all-pervading current is the integration of the whole body as a seamless unity, which naturally instills a greater sense of harmony.

Anushasana means "direction," "command" or "instruction," and Anushasana mudra awakens and enhances the all-pervading current of Vyana vayu. This gesture lengthens the inhalation, drawing energy into the center of the body. This mudra also lengthens the exhalation, supporting the movement of vital energy outward toward the extremities, thereby integrating the entire body. As Anushasana mudra cultivates greater awareness and sensitivity within the extremities, it brings warmth and tingling to the toes and fingers. The overall effect of this gesture is the integration between center and periphery, cultivating both a clearer sense of our center and an experience of unity and harmony.

Systems Balanced:

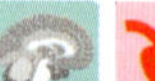
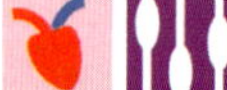

Elements Activated:

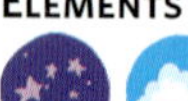
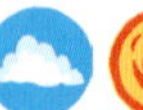

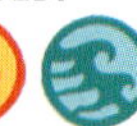

Doshas Balanced:

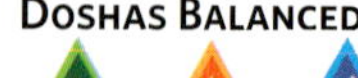

Prana Vayus Nourished:

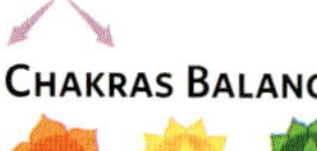

Chakras Balanced:

Scale from Calming to Energizing:

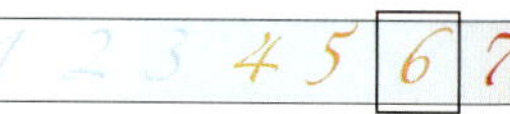

Guided Meditation: Awakening All-Pervading Energy

- As you hold Anushasana mudra, take several natural breaths to attune to all the feelings and sensations awakened by this gesture.
- With each inhalation, sense your breath naturally being concentrated into the center of your pelvis, connecting you more deeply with the energetic core of your being.
- With each exhaling breath, sense a current of violet energy radiating outward from your center toward your extremities.
- Take some time to attune to Vyana vayu, the all-pervading current of energy, flowing from center to periphery in synchrony with your rhythmic breathing, nourishing and integrating your entire being.
- As you inhale, sense this violet energy concentrated at the center of your being, and as you exhale, allow the all-pervading current to radiate down into your legs and feet.
- Take several breaths to allow your lower extremities to be fully nourished with vital energy and integrated with your entire being.
- With your next inhaling breath, connect to the center of your being, and as you exhale, sense Vyana vayu filling your abdomen, solar plexus, low and mid back.
- Take some time to allow the middle portion of your body to be infused with all-pervading energy.
- Now as you inhale, violet energy is concentrated at the center of your pelvis, and as you exhale, Vyana vayu radiates up into your chest, upper back, shoulders, arms and hands.
- Take several breaths to allow your chest and upper extremities to be fully nourished with life force energy, infusing these areas with warmth and vitality.
- With your next inhaling breath, sense violet energy being concentrated in your pelvis, and as you exhale, allow it to flow upward into your neck and head, naturally integrating these areas with your torso and extremities.
- Now, sense the all-pervading current infusing your entire being, from center to periphery, supporting circulation within your bloodstream, and optimal communication along all your nerve pathways.
- As your entire body is nourished from center to periphery, take several breaths to sense greater integration and harmony throughout your entire being.
- Affirm the all-pervading energy, repeating the following three times, aloud or silently: **"As the all-pervading current flows freely, I experience integration and harmony."**
- Now, slowly release the gesture, taking several breaths to sense complete integration from center to extremities.
- When you are ready, open your eyes, returning slowly and gently, experiencing greater harmony in all of your activities.

Annamaya kosha (physical body)

- Directs breath and awareness from the center of the body to the extremities, supporting the functioning of the peripheral nervous, circulatory and lymphatic systems.
- Enhances body awareness and a sense of integration and improved coordination.
- Supports optimal alignment of the entire skeletal system.
- The mildly energizing effects of this gesture are generally helpful for Kapha imbalance.
- The connection to the flow of subtle energy is generally helpful for Pitta imbalance.
- The enhanced concentration and gentle warmth in the extremities are generally helpful for Vata imbalance.

Pranamaya kosha (energy body)

- Activates the flow of Vyana vayu, the all-pervading current of energy.
- Releases blockages in the ayurvedic marmas, the energetic points located throughout the body.
- Opens and balances the second through sixth chakras.

Manomaya kosha (psycho-emotional body)

- Cultivates alertness and one-pointed concentration.
- Cultivates a sense of wholeness and integrity.

Vijnanamaya kosha (wisdom body)

- Instills a sense of overall integration and harmony, which are a reflection of our true being.

Anandamaya kosha (bliss body)

- As integration permeates our entire being, we naturally experience a sense of all-encompassing unity.

Chapter Ten

Balancing the Energy Centers

MUDRAS FOR THE CHAKRAS

The *chakras* are energetic centers that receive, store, transform and channel vital energy. There are seven principal chakras located along the subtle axis within the spinal column, beginning at the perineum and culminating at the crown of the head. Each of the energetic centers is represented by a lotus with a specific color and number of petals. The center of each lotus holds a symbol associated with one of the five elements, as well as a *bija mantra*, or "seed sound," that awakens each chakra's essential qualities. For example, the base chakra, *Muladhara*, has four red petals arranged around an ochre-colored square, representing the stability of the earth element. The root chakra's bija mantra, *LAM*, balances the flow of energy within the base chakra, naturally supporting the awakening of its essential qualities of stability, grounding and security.

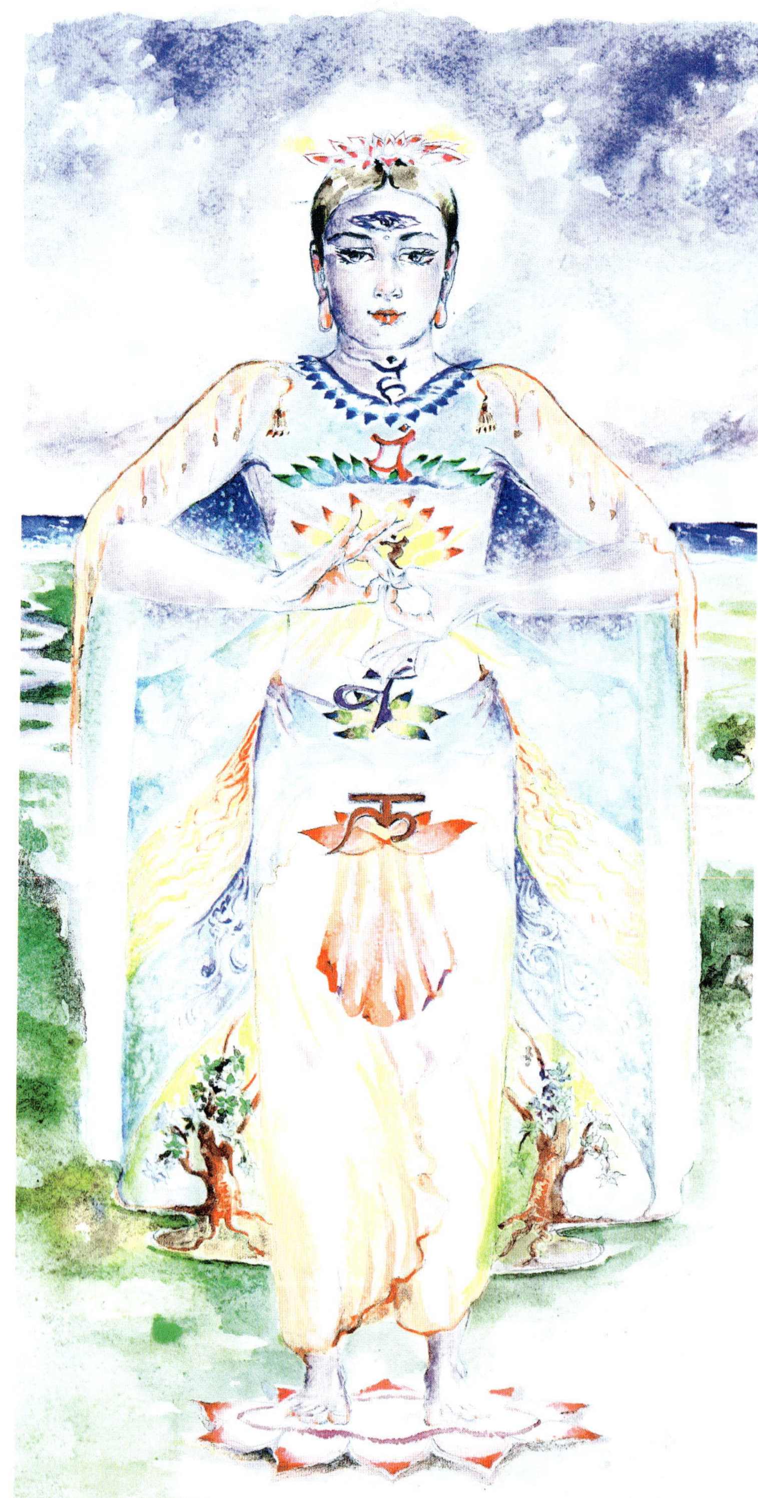

The Chakras are a road map for the journey of awakening.

Each of the chakras is also associated with a particular area of our body and a specific gland of the endocrine system. To the extent that the energy centers are balanced, these glands and body areas are nourished energetically. One of the ways to determine whether a particular chakra is balanced is to sense the free flow of energy within its respective body area. This can be done by visualizing the petals of a particular chakra opening with each inhalation and resting toward their center with each exhalation. To the extent that this movement is experienced as smooth and fluid, it is an indicator that the chakra is balanced.

This assessment of the chakras at the energetic level is complemented by assessing the extent to which each chakra's essential qualities are integrated into daily living. Each of the chakras encompasses several essential qualities. For example, the second chakra, *Svadhisthana*, focuses on self-nourishment, fluidity and the ability to experience pleasurable feelings, which form the foundation of healthy relationships. As we integrate these chakra qualities more completely into daily living, we naturally sense enhanced opening within the pelvis, the seat of Svadhisthana chakra.

Mudras play an important role, both in assessing the flow of energy within the chakras and in rebalancing them. Specific mudras direct breath, awareness and energy to each chakra individually, releasing energetic blockages and reestablishing the flow of vital energy. Mudras also support us in integrating the chakra's essential qualities, culminating in an overall experience of integration and harmony.

Mudra Core Quality	Chakra Name Name Translation Bija Mantra (seed syllable)	Number and Color of Petals Location Related Body Area	Related Body System Gland Main Health Conditions
Chinmaya Security	First Chakra, Muladhara Base of support LAM	Four red petals Perineum Base of body, legs & feet	Eliminatory Adrenals Chronic stress, anxiety
Svadhisthana Self-nourishment	Second Chakra, Svadhisthana Center of the self VAM	Six orange petals Four fingers below the navel Entire pelvic area	Reproductive Ovaries & testes Reproductive issues
Vajra Self-empowerment	Third Chakra, Manipura City of jewels RAM	Ten golden-yellow petals Center of solar plexus Entire solar plexus area	Digestive Pancreas Digestive issues
Padma Unconditional Love	Fourth Chakra, Anahata Unstruck YAM	Twelve green petals Center of the chest Entire upper torso	Cardio-respiratory, immune Thymus Cardio-respiratory & immune issues
Kali Purification	Fifth Chakra, Vishuddha Purification HAM	Sixteen sky-blue petals Throat center Entire neck & throat area	Endocrine Thyroid Thyroid problems, neck, throat & voice issues
Trishula Non-duality	Sixth Chakra, Ajna Center of command OM	Two violet petals Third eye Head & senses	Nervous Pituitary Neurological issues, problems with the senses
Ananta Unity Consciousness	Seventh Chakra, Sahasrara Thousand-petaled SO HAM	One thousand petals of crystal light Crown of the head Top of the head	All Pineal Separation as the source of all dis-ease
Dharma Chakra Integrating All the Chakras	Integration of All of the Chakras All Bija Mantras repeated in succession, followed by silence	Encompasses all petals All chakra locations Whole body	Integration of all body systems Integration of all glands For global healing

55

Chinmaya Mudra

Gesture of Embodied Knowledge
For Balancing the First Chakra

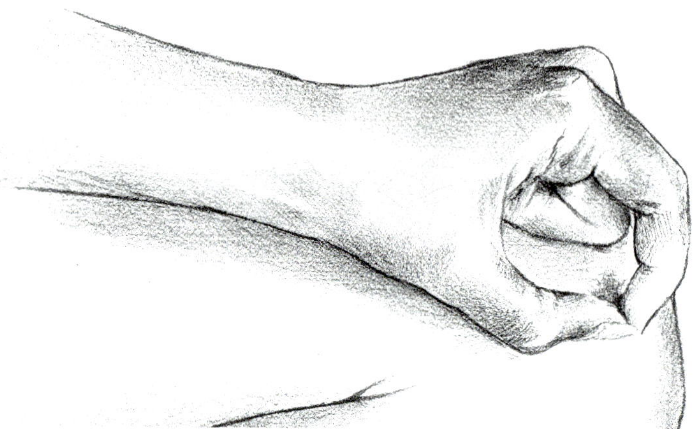

Fully supported by the earth,
I step forward in life safe and secure.

Core Quality
Security

Especially helpful for
- Balancing the first chakra by cultivating a sense of safety and security.
- Supporting the health of the skeletal system.
- Supporting optimal elimination.
- Reducing blood pressure.
- Reducing stress and anxiety.
- Enhancing a sense of grounding, embodiment and trust.

Mudras with similar effects
Adhi, Prithivi, Bhu, Murti, Rupa

Cautions
None

Instructions
1. Curl your fingers into a fist, with the thumbs outside.
2. Touch the tips of the index fingers to the tips of the thumbs, forming a circle.
3. Rest the hands with the palms down onto your thighs or knees.
4. Relax the shoulders back and down, with the spine naturally aligned.

The root chakra, *Muladhara*, which means "base of support," is located at the perineum. It is symbolized by a lotus with four red petals arranged around an ochre-colored square, representing stability and the four cardinal directions. The main theme of the first chakra is security. When the first chakra is balanced, we sense ourselves fully supported at all moments along our life journey. When this sense of support is not complete, we may experience fear and insecurity as well as a feeling that our basic survival needs are not provided for adequately. To balance the first chakra, we cultivate the qualities of grounding, embodiment, connection to the natural world and an enhanced sense of abundance. As we embody these qualities, we are able to perceive our needs for safety and security more objectively, allowing us to recognize that the nature of life is to support us abundantly. With a greater sense of support and trust, we begin to see that security is a natural reflection of our true being, thereby creating a firm foundation for our spiritual journey.

Chinmaya means "embodiment of knowledge." Chinmaya mudra directs breath, awareness and energy to the base of the body, the seat of the first chakra, deepening our connection to the earth and its qualities of grounding and stability. This gesture instills a sense of balance and alignment within the structure of the body. With enhanced grounding and a sense of support, we naturally inhabit our bodies more fully and comfortably. This gesture slows the breath, lengthening the exhalation, instilling a sense of serenity, which allows us to evaluate and meet our survival needs more objectively. As Chinmaya mudra cultivates embodiment, calm and stability, we naturally sense greater security as the foundation for our chakra journey.

Systems Balanced:

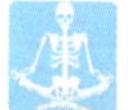 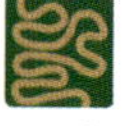

Elements Activated:

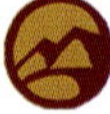

Doshas Balanced:

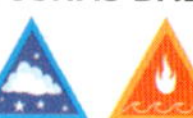

Prana Vayus Nourished:

Chakras Balanced:

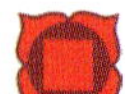

Scale from Calming to Energizing:

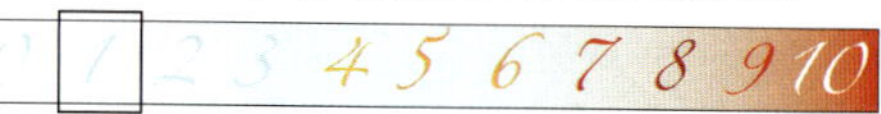

Guided Meditation: Embodying Complete Security

- As you hold Chinmaya mudra, take several natural breaths to attune to all the feelings and sensations evoked by this gesture.
- Notice how your breath is gently directed downward, toward the base of your body, the seat of Muladhara chakra, your center of absolute security.
- To connect with your root chakra more deeply, take several breaths to visualize an ochre-colored square surrounded by four red petals at the base of your body.
- By embodying the energy of each of these petals individually, you support the awakening of all of your first chakra's essential qualities.
- Begin by focusing your attention on the petal facing forward, associated with the quality of grounding.
- With each inhalation, sense this petal unfolding naturally, and with each exhaling breath, it softens inward.
- As you attune to this petal's rhythmic movement, take several breaths to sense your roots growing deep into the earth beneath, allowing you to experience complete grounding and stability.
- Now, focus on the petal facing right, associated with the quality of embodiment.
- With each inhalation, this petal unfolds completely, and with each exhaling breath, it rests inward naturally.
- As you attune to this petal's rhythmic movement, you inhabit your body more completely from the crown of your head to the soles of your feet, becoming fully present in all areas simultaneously.
- Next, focus on the petal facing left, associated with your connection to the natural world.
- With each inhalation, sense this petal unfolding smoothly and easily, and with each exhaling breath, notice how it relaxes inward naturally.
- As you attune to this petal's rhythmic movement, take several breaths to sense your deepening connection with all living things, experiencing a sense of oneness with your surroundings.
- Now, focus on the petal facing toward the back, associated with the quality of sustenance.
- With each inhalation, visualize this petal opening completely, and with each exhaling breath, sense it relaxing inward naturally.
- As you attune to this petal's rhythmic movement, open to receive all of the earth's rich bounty, recognizing that you are fully supported at each step of your journey.
- Now, sense all the petals of your lotus unfolding and softening in synchrony with your rhythmic breathing, taking some time to integrate all of your first chakra's essential qualities, allowing you to experience absolute security.
- Affirm your first chakra qualities, repeating the following three times, aloud or silently: **"Integrating the first chakra's essential qualities, I journey in absolute security."**
- Slowly release the gesture, taking several breaths to sense the lotus of your first chakra fully balanced.
- When you are ready, open your eyes, returning slowly and gently, with a greater sense of support and safety along your life journey.

Annamaya kosha (physical body)

- Directs breath and awareness to the base of the body, creating a massaging effect that releases tension and increases circulation to the eliminatory system.
- Cultivates a sense of stability within the musculo-skeletal system.
- Lengthens the exhalation, enhancing relaxation, thereby reducing stress, heart rate and blood pressure.
- The grounding effects of this gesture are generally helpful for Vata imbalance.
- The calming effects are generally helpful for Pitta imbalance.

Pranamaya kosha (energy body)

- Activates Apana vayu, the downward moving current of energy.
- Opens and balances the first chakra, center of safety.

Manomaya kosha (psycho-emotional body)

- Calms the body and mind, helping to reduce stress, fear and anxiety.
- Cultivates a sense of grounding, security and trust.

Vijnanamaya kosha (wisdom body)

- As the first chakra is balanced, we are able to face survival issues more objectively, eventually recognizing the inherent safety of our true being.

Anandamaya kosha (bliss body)

- As fear and anxiety are released, sensations of inner peace and harmony are awakened naturally.

56

Svadhisthana Mudra

Gesture of the Inner Dwelling Place

For Balancing the Second Chakra

Completely at home at the center of my being,
I experience deep nourishment and inner healing.

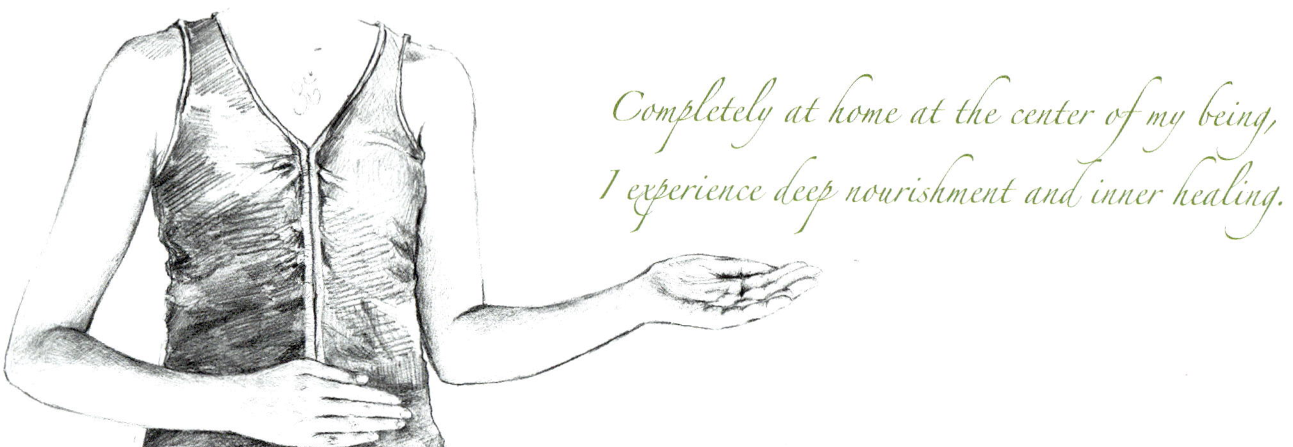

Core Quality

Self-nourishment

Especially helpful for

- Balancing the second chakra by cultivating self-nourishment.
- Supporting the health of the reproductive and urinary systems.
- Supporting balanced menstruation.
- Releasing tension from the sacrum and lower back.
- Enhancing our sense of being at home with ourselves.
- Supporting healthy relationships.
- Codependency and addiction.

Mudras with similar effects

Yoni, Shankha, Trimurti, Mira

Cautions

None

Instructions

1. Place the right hand, slightly cupped, over the lower abdomen, with the thumb resting just below the navel.
2. Cup the left hand and hold it facing upward at the level of the navel, and slightly angled to the left of the body, with the forearm parallel to the earth.
3. Relax the shoulders back and down, with the spine naturally aligned.

The second chakra, *Svadhisthana*, which means "one's own dwelling place," is located at the center of the pelvis. This energy center is represented by a lotus with six orange petals, arranged around a circle with a crescent moon at its base. The circle symbolizes our inherent wholeness, and the crescent moon represents the qualities of the water element, including femininity, receptivity and fluidity which are awakened as this chakra comes into balance. As the second chakra opens, we sense ourselves coming home to our own inner being, our inner source of nourishment and healing. When we are out of touch with our source of inner-nourishment, we may experience second chakra imbalances, including loneliness, feelings of abandonment and an inability to find pleasure and nourishment in our relationships. We support the blossoming of the second chakra by nourishing its essential qualities, including fluidity, the ability to savor life more completely, equanimity and serenity.

Svadhisthana mudra directs breath, awareness and energy into the pelvis, supporting our connection to our center of self-nourishment. The left hand opens to receive universal healing energy while the right hand channels this nourishment into the second chakra. This gesture cultivates a massaging effect in the lower abdomen and pelvis, supporting the health of the reproductive and urinary systems. This mudra lengthens the exhaling breath, instilling a sense of calm and serenity that helps to release stress and reduce anxiety. Svadhisthana mudra also awakens sensations of deep satisfaction and contentment that may be helpful for working with issues of codependency and addictions.

Systems Balanced:

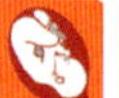

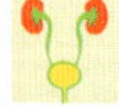

Elements Activated:

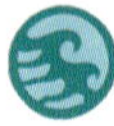

Doshas Balanced:

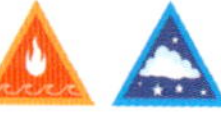

Prana Vayus Nourished:

Chakras Balanced:

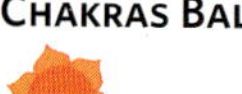

Scale from Calming to Energizing:

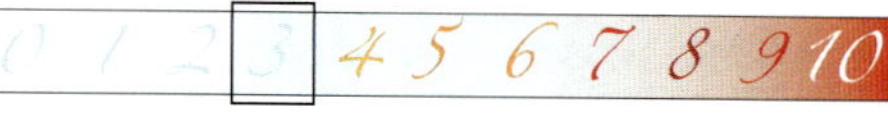

Guided Meditation: Coming Home to Yourself

ॐ As you hold Svadhisthana mudra, take several natural breaths to attune to all the feelings and sensations evoked by this gesture.

ॐ Notice how your right hand, held over the second chakra, at the center of your pelvis, instills a sense of comfort and inner nourishment.

ॐ Sense how your left hand is naturally open to receive universal healing energy, channeling it into Svadhisthana chakra, your inner dwelling place.

ॐ Take several breaths to attune to this nourishing energy, cultivating the sensitivity that will allow you to absorb all of your essential second chakra qualities.

ॐ With your next inhaling breath, attune to your inner dwelling place a, opening to receive the quality of fluidity. As you exhale, a sense of fluidity flows out from your Second chakra to nourish your entire being.

ॐ Nourished by the quality of fluidity, you naturally develop the ability to flow with all of life's cycles and seasons smoothly and easily.

ॐ Now, with your next inhaling breath, return to your inner home, and as you exhale, allow the quality of equanimity to naturally unfold.

ॐ For your next few breaths, sense your equanimity deepening naturally, allowing you to rest in the calm depths of your being, no matter what is happening in your surroundings.

ॐ With greater fluidity and equanimity, healthy relationships unfold naturally, allowing you to perceive that when you are at home within your own being, you are able to be with others in complete comfort and safety.

ॐ With your next inhalation, return to your inner dwelling place, and as you exhale, sense the integration of all of your Second chakra qualities, allowing a sense of deep self-nourishment to unfold naturally.

ॐ Take several breaths to allow self-nourishment to permeate your entire being, supporting you in caring for yourself and others lovingly at each step along your journey.

ॐ As you nourish yourself more completely and live in greater harmony, you naturally find pleasure in simple things, savoring the beauty of each moment of joyful living.

ॐ Affirm your self-nourishment, repeating the following three times, aloud or silently: **"At home within my being, I experience deep self-nourishment and healing."**

ॐ Slowly release the gesture, taking several breaths to integrate completely all of your Second chakra's nourishing qualities.

ॐ When you are ready, open your eyes, returning slowly and gently, more attuned to your inner source of nourishment and healing.

Annamaya kosha (physical body)

• Directs breath and awareness into the pelvis, creating a massaging effect that relaxes the entire pelvic area, optimizing circulation to the urinary and reproductive systems.
• May help to reduce the discomfort of menstrual cramping.
• The enhanced lower body breathing massages and releases tension from the sacrum and lower back.
• The soothing effects of this gesture are generally helpful for Pitta imbalance.
• The centering effects are generally helpful for Vata imbalance.

Pranamaya kosha (energy body)

• Activates Apana vayu, the downward moving current.
• Opens and balances the second chakra, center of self-nourishment.

Manomaya kosha (psycho-emotional body)

• Cultivates a sense of comfort and inner nourishment, a helpful antidote for second chakra issues such as codependency.
• Supports treatment of addictions and compulsions.

Vijnanamaya kosha (wisdom body)

• Awakens a deep sense of contentment, allowing us to be nourished by our true being, rather than seeking fulfillment and pleasure at the level of the personality.

Anandamaya kosha (bliss body)

• As inner nourishment increases, sensations of absolute comfort and bliss arise from within the pelvis.

57 Vajra Mudra

Gesture of the Diamond

For Balancing the Third Chakra

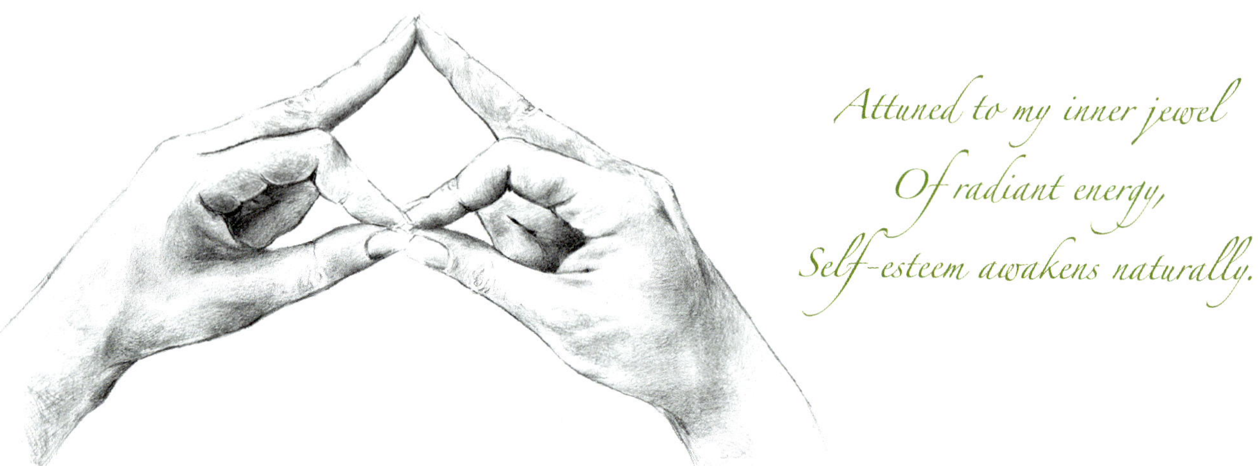

Attuned to my inner jewel
Of radiant energy,
Self-esteem awakens naturally.

Core Quality

Self-empowerment

Especially Helpful For

- Balancing the third chakra by cultivating self-empowerment.
- Enhancing digestion and assimilation.
- Building self-esteem.
- Enhancing energy and vitality, which may be helpful for depression.
- Clarifying life purpose.

Mudras with Similar Effects

Kubera, Matangi, Surya, Madhyama

Cautions

None

Instructions

1. Touch the tips of the thumbs to the tips of the index fingers of each hand.
2. Bring the thumbs and index fingers of each hand together.
3. Join the pads of the middle fingers together, forming a diamond shape.
4. Curl the little and ring fingers naturally inward toward the palms.
5. Hold the gesture at the solar plexus with the middle fingers facing forward.
6. Relax the shoulders back and down, with the elbows held slightly away from the body and the spine naturally aligned.

The third chakra, *Manipura*, which means "city of jewels," is located at the solar plexus. It is represented by a lotus with ten golden petals arranged around a circle with an upward facing triangle at its center. This triangle often contains a radiant golden sun as a symbol of the fire element and its qualities of warmth, luminosity and energy. The main theme of the third chakra is clarifying our life purpose and manifesting it completely. When the third chakra is balanced, we find a natural harmony between our own needs and our ability to serve the community. When this chakra is out of balance, we may experience a lack of personal power and self-esteem and a subsequent decrease in motivation and energy. Third chakra imbalance can also manifest as an inflated sense of self and a need for success at all costs which is a reflection of a deep sense of insufficiency. Third chakra balance is supported by integrating its essential qualities, including inherent self-esteem, clear life purpose, determination, vitality, conscious action and conservation of energy, resulting in inner and outer harmony.

Vajra means "diamond," referring to the diamond shape formed by the fingers in Vajra mudra. This gesture directs breath, awareness and energy into the third chakra, awakening our "inner diamond" of energy and vitality. This mudra enhances empowerment, determination and clarity, supporting the unfolding of all of our unique talents and possibilities. This gesture also enhances the movement of the diaphragm, creating a massaging effect that supports the health of the digestive system while increasing circulation to the area of the mid back, kidneys and adrenal glands.

Systems Balanced:

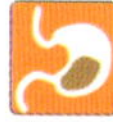

Elements Activated:

Doshas Balanced:

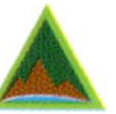

Prana Vayus Nourished:

Chakras Balanced:

Scale from Calming to Energizing:

Guided Meditation: Radiant Inner Jewel

- As you hold Vajra mudra, take several natural breaths to attune to all the feelings and sensations awakened by this gesture.
- Notice how your breath is naturally directed into your solar plexus, the seat of Manipura chakra, your center of personal power.
- Visualize your third chakra as a radiant jewel at the center of your being, each of whose facets represents one of Manipura chakra's essential qualities.
- Begin by awakening the facet of self-esteem, experiencing it as a light that shines radiantly from the center of your own being, releasing the need to seek approval externally.
- As inherent self-esteem shines brightly, your life mission is clarified, taking several breaths to envision all of your unique talents and possibilities unfolding naturally.
- With greater self-esteem and a clear vision for your journey, you receive the abundant energy that allows you to manifest your life purpose completely.
- As the facet of abundant energy shines brightly, the quality of determination awakens naturally, allowing you to meet challenges more confidently.
- With self-esteem, energy and confidence in your journey, you naturally cultivate the ability to act consciously, perceiving the effects of your actions on your surroundings in order to avoid harming while conserving your precious life force energy.
- Living consciously and with abundant energy, you experience inner and outer harmony, manifesting your own possibilities while cooperating with others for the benefit of all beings.
- Sense all the facets of your inner jewel shining forth brilliantly, integrating all of your third chakra's essential qualities, allowing you to journey forward with radiant vitality.
- Confident and filled with energy, repeat the following three times, aloud or silently: **"My inner jewel shines brilliantly, empowering me to manifest my life vision completely."**
- Now, slowly release the gesture, taking several breaths to sense all of your third chakra's radiant qualities.
- When you are ready, open your eyes, returning slowly and gently, empowered by the jewel of your inner being.

Annamaya kosha (physical body)

• Directs breath and awareness to the solar plexus, creating a massaging effect that enhances circulation to the digestive system.
• The enhanced diaphragmatic breathing in the mid back creates a massaging effect that increases circulation to the area of the kidneys and adrenal glands.
• The energizing and stimulating effects of this gesture are generally helpful for Kapha imbalance.

Pranamaya kosha (energy body)

• Activates Samana vayu, the horizontal current of energy.
• Opens and balances the third chakra, center of personal power.

Manomaya kosha (psycho-emotional body)

• The self-empowerment and self-esteem cultivated by this gesture may be helpful for depression.
• Instills the motivation and determination to overcome challenges.

Vijnanamaya kosha (wisdom body)

• Develops the ability to discern between the innate brilliance of our true being and external success achieved at the level of the personality.

Anandamaya kosha (bliss body)

• As we awaken the facets of the jewel of our inner being, clarity and radiance unfold naturally.

58 Padma Mudra

Gesture of the Lotus

For Balancing the Fourth Chakra

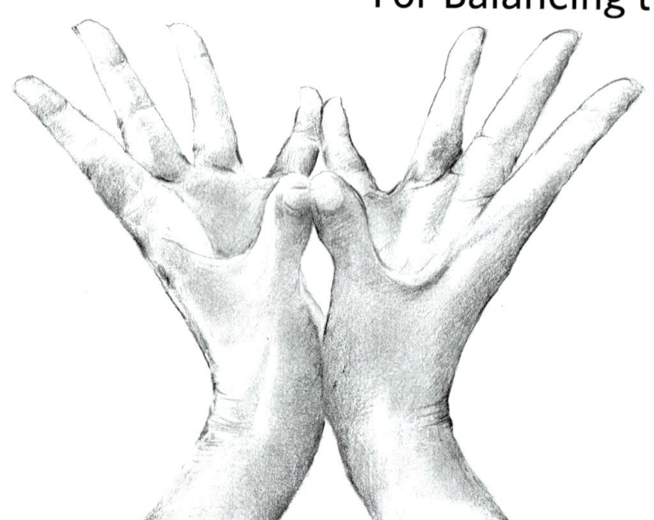

Nurturing the garden of my heart
Allows for the blossoming of
Unconditional love.

Core Quality

Unconditional Love

Especially helpful for

- Balancing the fourth chakra by unfolding the heart's essential qualities.
- Supporting the health of the cardio-respiratory and immune systems.
- Cultivating compassion and empathy.
- Supporting the treatment of depression.

Mudras with similar effects

Purna Hridaya, Karuna, Dirgha Svara, Vajrapradama, Hridaya

Cautions

For discomfort in the hands, Hridaya mudra is a possible substitute.

Instructions

1. Place the hands in prayer position in front of the heart.
2. While keeping the base of the palms, as well as the little fingers and thumbs together, open the middle, ring, and index fingers wide apart in the shape of an unfolding lotus.
3. Relax the shoulders back and down, with the elbows held slightly away from the body and the spine naturally aligned.

The fourth chakra, *Anahata*, which means "unstruck," is located at the center of the chest. Unstruck refers to the subtle sounds experienced in deep meditation as well as to the invincibility of our subtle heart which, unlike our emotional heart, cannot be "broken." Anahata chakra is represented by a lotus with twelve emerald-green petals arranged around a circle with a six-pointed star at its center. This star is composed of two triangles, one facing upward and the other facing downward, representing the integration of the upper and lower chakras. The heart chakra is related to the air element and its qualities of lightness, gracefulness and sensitivity. When the heart chakra is out of balance, we feel weighed down by life with a tendency to focus on the negative, both in terms of past memories and future possibilities. As the heart chakra opens, we are able to embrace and appreciate life with enthusiasm and optimism, allowing us to live in the present moment more fully. The opening of the heart chakra is supported by awakening its essential qualities of gratitude, compassion and communion, leading to unconditional love's full blossoming.

Padma means "lotus," and Padma mudra directs breath, awareness and energy into the front of the chest, instilling a sense of lightness and openness. This gesture supports the opening of the heart chakra by increasing our sensitivity to the heart's subtle sensations and feelings, bringing these to the surface to be experienced and embraced fully. As Padma mudra enhances our sensitivity, it supports us in opening our hearts to other beings with greater compassion and empathy. This mudra also directs breath and awareness to the thymus gland, supporting the health of the immune system.

Systems Balanced:

 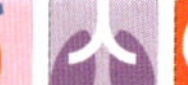 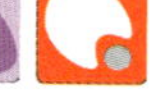

Elements Activated:

Doshas Balanced:

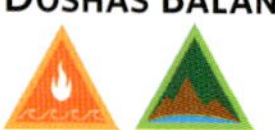

Prana Vayus Nourished:

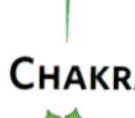

Chakras Balanced:

Scale from Calming to Energizing:

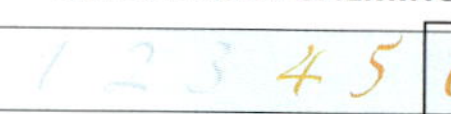

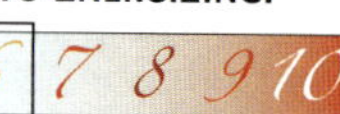

Guided Meditation: **Garden of the Heart**

- As you hold Padma mudra, take several natural breaths to attune to all the feelings and sensations awakened by this gesture.
- Notice how your breath is gently directed into your chest, the seat of Anahata chakra, your center of unconditional love.
- With each inhaling breath, the frontiers of your heart open gradually, and with each exhalation, you create a space in which to embrace all of your fourth chakra's essential qualities.
- Visualize your heart center as a fertile field for the blossoming of these qualities, a green meadow filled with wildflowers of all colors, shapes and varieties.
- Take some time to see yourself strolling through this meadow, allowing each flower that you meet to unfold one of your heart's essential qualities.
- The first flower you meet awakens the quality of lightness of being, your ability to move through life gracefully, savoring its sweetness without taking anything too personally.
- Take several breaths to envision yourself integrating lightness into all of your activities, allowing you to live with greater ease at each moment along your journey.
- As you continue through your garden with greater ease, you are drawn to the flower of gratitude, allowing you to see that everyone and everything you meet plays an essential role in revealing your life's deeper meaning.
- Take several breaths to sense the color, texture and fragrance of gratitude filling your being with deep appreciation for every moment of living.
- As gratitude fills your being, the flower of communion draws you to it naturally, allowing your heart to beat in synchrony with the heart of all beings.
- Take several breaths to absorb the color and fragrance of communion, envisioning all those with whom you share your journey living in greater harmony.
- As you continue through your garden with a greater sense of communion and harmony, you naturally perceive the flower of compassion unfolding naturally.
- As compassion unfolds, take some time to offer a heartfelt prayer for the happiness of all beings, recognizing that just like yourself, each one seeks love within the limits of their understanding.
- Now, embrace all the flowers of your heart as a single bouquet, allowing unconditional love to blossom naturally as the essential fragrance of your true being.
- Affirm your heart's qualities, repeating the following three times, aloud or silently: **"Awakening my heart's essential qualities, unconditional love blossoms naturally."**
- Slowly release the gesture, taking several breaths to sense the awakening of all of your heart chakra's essential qualities.
- When you are ready, open your eyes, returning slowly and gently, bringing the colors and fragrances of your inner garden into all of your activities.

Annamaya kosha (physical body)

• Directs breath and awareness to the chest, creating a massaging effect that enhances circulation to the area of the thymus gland.
• Expands the breath at the front and sides of the chest, creating a massaging effect for the lungs and heart.
• The mildly energizing effects and opening of the chest cultivated by this gesture are generally helpful for Kapha imbalance.
• The opening of the emotional heart is generally helpful for Pitta imbalance.

Pranamaya kosha (energy body)

• Activates Prana vayu, the upward moving current of energy.
• Opens and balances the heart chakra, center of unconditional love.

Manomaya kosha (psycho-emotional body)

• Expands the frontiers of the heart, supporting us in welcoming emotions so that they can be integrated more easily.
• Instills compassion and a sense of communion.

Vijnanamaya kosha (wisdom body)

• Teaches us to see through the eyes of the heart in order to respond with empathy and compassion rather than judgment or reaction.

Anandamaya kosha (bliss body)

• As the subtle heart opens, compassion, communion and universal love arise naturally.

59

Kali Mudra

Gesture of the Goddess of Spiritual Purification

For Balancing the Fifth Chakra

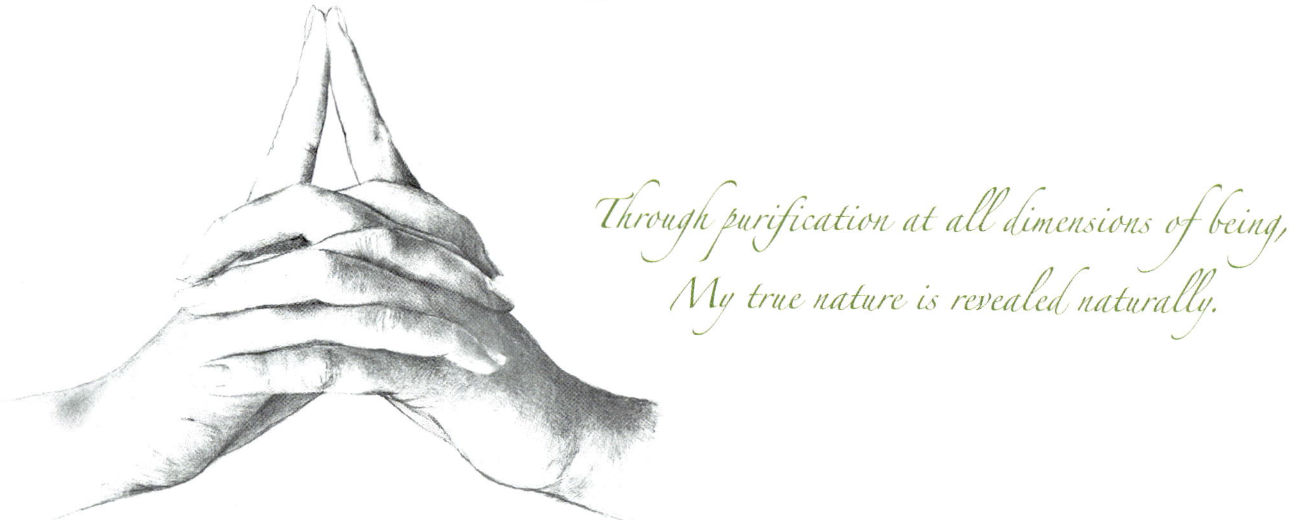

Core Quality

Spiritual Purification

Especially helpful for

- Balancing the fifth chakra through the process of spiritual purification.
- Releasing tension from the neck, shoulders, throat and vocal cords.
- Enhancing intuition, allowing us to receive spiritual guidance for our journey.

Mudras with similar effects

Garuda, Vishuddha, Shunya, Angushtha

Cautions

Contraindicated for hyperthyroid conditions. Shunya, which is less energizing, may be used as a substitute.

Instructions

1. Interlace the fingers to the outside, with the right thumb over the left.
2. Extend the index fingers straight upward and point them toward the throat center, with the hands held at the level of the sternum.
3. Relax the shoulders back and down, with the elbows held away from the body and the spine naturally aligned.

The fifth chakra, *Vishuddha*, which means "purification," is located at the level of the throat. This energy center is represented by a lotus with sixteen sky-blue petals arranged around a lustrous full moon. A drop of nectar, called *amrita*, the "nectar of immortality," hangs from the top of the moon. The main theme of this energy center is spiritual purification, the release of the limiting beliefs that keep us from experiencing the freedom of our true being. Vishuddha chakra is related to the space element and its qualities of vastness, expansiveness and subtlety. These qualities support the process of purification in which limiting beliefs can be seen and released. Through this process of release, we gradually align our thoughts, feelings and words and deeds with our authentic being, allowing us to communicate with clarity and integrity. This alignment is supported by the integration of all of the fifth chakra's essential qualities, including spiritual commitment, self-study, non-attachment, discernment, inner silence and limitlessness.

Kali is the "goddess of purification," who supports us in removing the limiting beliefs that keep us from aligning with our true being. She wields a sword and holds a human head as a symbol of attachment to the ego, which must be severed in order to attain spiritual freedom. Kali mudra directs breath, awareness and energy to the throat area, the seat of Vishuddha chakra, supporting the process of spiritual purification. This gesture facilitates the release of muscular tension from the neck, creating a space of openness in which limiting beliefs can be seen, explored and released more easily. This mudra increases circulation to the area of the thyroid gland, activating metabolism, which provides the energy for overcoming obstacles along our journey.

Systems Balanced:

Elements Activated:

Doshas Balanced:

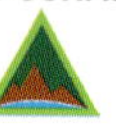

Prana Vayus Nourished:

Chakras Balanced:

Scale from Calming to Energizing:

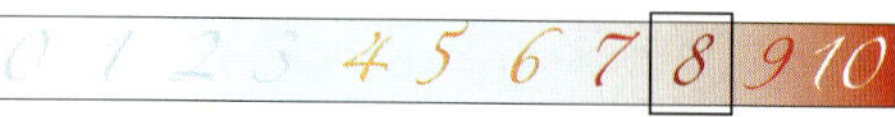

Guided Meditation: Pilgrimage of Purification

- As you hold Kali mudra, take several natural breaths to attune to all the feelings and sensations awakened by this gesture.
- Notice how your breath is gently directed into your throat and neck, the seat of Vishuddha chakra, your center of spiritual purification.
- With each inhaling breath, your throat center is bathed with soft blue energy, and with each exhalation, tension from your neck and throat is released naturally.
- As tension is dissolved, a process of purification occurs gradually, releasing all that limits your ability to align with your true being.
- To support your process of purification, you will embark on a pilgrimage, and at each stop along your journey, make an offering at a temple dedicated to one of the fifth chakra's essential qualities.
- Begin by visualizing yourself at the base of a great mountain range, in an area of rolling green hills and crystal clear streams, naturally inviting you to journey upward into the more subtle realms of your being.
- Your path begins comfortably and easily, and you soon arrive at a small temple dedicated to the quality of commitment to your spiritual journey.
- See yourself making an offering at the temple of commitment, taking several breaths to create an intention to make your spiritual journey your absolute priority.
- As your pilgrimage proceeds through green fields and flowering trees, you stop at the next temple, dedicated to the quality of self-study.
- As you make your offering at the temple of self-study, take several breaths to clearly perceive that spiritual awakening only proceeds with the release of the beliefs that keep you from aligning with your true being.
- Now, you journey higher still, until you reach the next temple dedicated to the quality of non-attachment, your ability to release more easily all that no longer supports your spiritual journey.
- See yourself making an offering at this temple, taking several breaths to envision yourself moving forward along your journey with greater simplicity, recognizing that all that is truly valuable already resides within your own being.
- Soon you come to a hilltop with the world spreading out before you, and there you see the temple dedicated to awakening the limitlessness of your true being.
- As you make an offering at the temple of limitless being, take several breaths to integrate the absolute knowing that you are inherently free, allowing you to continue your journey with greater lightness and clarity.
- Now, with your pilgrimage complete, you sit in meditation, sensing your mind silent and serene, knowing that the purification process will continue all the way to final awakening.
- Affirm your purification as you repeat the following three times, aloud or silently: **"Through spiritual purification, I clearly perceive the freedom of my essential being."**
- Slowly release the gesture, taking several breaths to integrate all of the fifth chakra qualities you have received along your pilgrimage.
- When you are ready, open your eyes, returning slowly and gently, ready to continue your spiritual journey with renewed clarity.

Annamaya Kosha (Physical Body)

• Directs breath and awareness to the throat and neck, enhancing circulation to the area of the thyroid gland, activating metabolism and energy.
• Facilitates fuller breathing in the uppermost portions of the lungs.
• Releases muscular tension from the neck and shoulders, supporting the alignment of the cervical spine.
• Releases tension from the throat and vocal cords, supporting speaking and singing.
• The energizing effects of this gesture are generally helpful for Kapha imbalance.

Pranamaya Kosha (Energy Body)

• Activates Udana vayu, the uppermost current of energy.
• Opens and balances the fifth chakra, center of spiritual purification.

Manomaya Kosha (Psycho-Emotional Body)

• Cultivates alertness that supports the process of exploring emotions.
• Instills a sense of openness that supports us in aligning with our voice of truth.

Vijnanamaya Kosha (Wisdom Body)

• Brings limiting beliefs to the surface and supports their release, gradually revealing our true being.

Anandamaya Kosha (Bliss Body)

• As tension is released from the throat, an experience of limitlessness and inner silence arises naturally.

60 Trishula Mudra

Gesture of the Trident

For Balancing the Sixth Chakra

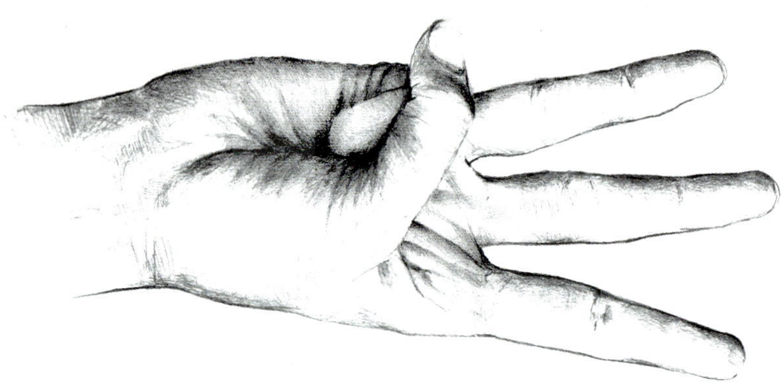

With eyes of clarity,
Life's doubts and challenges
Are resolved in a vision of unity.

Core Quality

Non-duality

Especially helpful for

- Balancing the sixth chakra by cultivating wisdom and clear seeing.
- Supporting the health of the nervous and endocrine systems.
- Improving mental clarity and concentration.
- Awakening a vision of unity beyond all dualities.

Mudras with similar effects

Dhyana, Jnana, Citta, Svadhyaya

Cautions

None

Instructions

1. Curl the little fingers inward to touch the base of the thumbs.
2. Place the pads of the thumbs onto the little fingers to secure them.
3. Extend the other three fingers straight out.
4. Rest the backs of the hands on the thighs or knees, or hold the hands out to the sides of the body at the level of the shoulders, with the fingers facing upward.
5. Relax the shoulders back and down, with the spine naturally aligned.

The sixth chakra, *Ajna*, which means "center of command," is located at the third eye, between the eyebrows. The main theme of this energy center is developing a vision of unity beyond all questions, doubts and dualities at the level of the personality. This vision of unity allows us to discern clearly between our limitless true Self and the limited personality. The process of moving beyond the play of opposites is represented by the lotus of the sixth chakra, with its two violet petals that are often placed on either side of an all-seeing eye of wisdom. Before the awakening of the third eye, we tend to see all of life as a play of opposites: success and failure, loss and gain that naturally create tension and conflict. As we move beyond duality through awakening wisdom and clarity, we come to see life's ups and downs as a process of exploration and learning that ultimately leads to a vision of unity.

Trishula means "trident," and is the symbol of *Shiva*, the deity that represents spiritual transformation through sustained discipline. The trident symbolizes Shiva's three eyes, the two physical eyes plus the eye of wisdom between the eyebrows. Trishula mudra gently directs breath, awareness and energy to the sixth chakra, facilitating the opening of the third eye, awakening the wisdom and one-pointed concentration that allow us to see beyond dualities. This gesture slows the train of thoughts, allowing us to witness them more easily rather than identifying with them and subsequently reacting unconsciously. In the silent space between thoughts cultivated by this gesture, we are able to perceive our true being as the unchanging background for all our thoughts, feelings and beliefs. Trishula mudra gradually leads us to this vision of clarity, revealing our essential nature as unity beyond all dualities.

Systems Balanced:

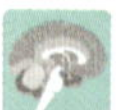 

Elements Activated:

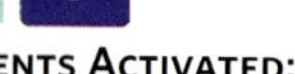

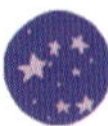

Doshas Balanced:

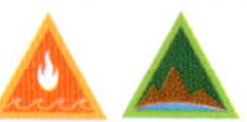

Prana Vayus Nourished:

Chakras Balanced:

Scale from Calming to Energizing:

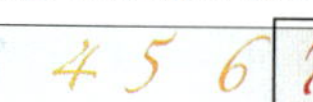 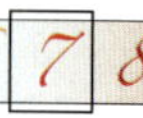 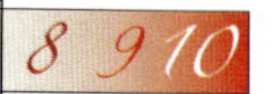

Guided Meditation: Seeing Beyond Duality

- As you hold Trishula mudra, take several natural breaths to attune to all the feelings and sensations awakened by this gesture.
- Notice how your awareness and breath naturally rest at your third eye, your center of clear seeing beyond all dualities.
- With each inhaling breath, subtle energy gently infuses Ajna chakra, and with each exhaling breath, your forehead, face and jaw naturally soften and relax.
- Take some time to visualize your sixth chakra's two violet petals unfolding and softening in synchrony with your rhythmic breathing.
- As the lotus of your sixth chakra unfolds naturally, you deepen your ability to see unity beyond life's dualities, allowing all doubts, questions and searching at the level of the personality to be resolved completely.
- To enhance your ability to see beyond dualities, bring to mind a question, doubt or issue in your life at the present time.
- Take several breaths to reflect on this question, acknowledging that there may be many ways of seeing beyond your habitual solutions at the level of your personality.
- To expand your horizons in relation to the issue you are exploring, begin by focusing your breath into your right nostril and right side of your body.
- Take some time to attune deeply to this right nostril breathing, noticing how the rational, logical aspect of your being is awakened naturally.
- From this logical perspective, envision one possible direction for the issue you are exploring, inquiring deeply as to how this direction would support your life journey.
- Now, direct your breath into your left nostril and left side of your body, taking some time to attune to the receptive, intuitive aspect of your being.
- From this more intuitive perspective, reflect on a different point of view, looking at this issue more holistically, taking into account everyone's perspectives and feelings.
- As you breathe through your left nostril, inquire within your being as to how this direction would support your life journey.
- Now, focus your breath into both nostrils and both sides of your body evenly while holding both possibilities within your third eye simultaneously.
- By simply remaining present, witnessing both possibilities, without judging or analyzing, you cultivate a space of non-duality in which insight can arise naturally.
- Take some time to allow insight to awaken from within your being, envisioning a path that integrates both your logical and intuitive polarities to reveal a vision of unity.
- Take several breaths to integrate this vision of unity, allowing your breath and awareness to rest at your third eye, experiencing clarity beyond all dualities.
- Affirm your vision of unity as you repeat the following three times, aloud or silently: **"Through the power of clear seeing, I awaken to the unity beyond all dualities."**
- Slowly release the gesture, taking several breaths to rest in the unity of your essential being.
- When you are ready, open your eyes, returning slowly and gently, continuing your journey with a greater sense of clarity.

Annamaya kosha (physical body)

• Balances the breath in both nostrils evenly, supporting equilibrium in the autonomic nervous system.
• Instills an experience of balance in both hemispheres of the brain.
• Traditionally said to balance the pituitary gland.
• Heightens our awareness of each of the five senses.
• The increased energy and enhanced awareness cultivated by this gesture are generally helpful for Kapha imbalance.
• The development of intuitive wisdom beyond dualities is generally helpful for Pitta imbalance.

Pranamaya kosha (energy body)

• Activates Udana vayu, the uppermost current of energy.
• Opens and balances the sixth chakra, center of wisdom.
• Balances Ida and Pingala nadis.

Manomaya kosha (psycho-emotional body)

• Facilitates one-pointed concentration.
• Cultivates emotional balance by creating space between thoughts.

Vijnanamaya kosha (wisdom body)

• Cultivates discernment between life's dualities and the vision of unity that is a reflection of our true being.

Anandamaya kosha (bliss body)

• With a vision of unity, sensations of bliss and clarity arise naturally.

61 Ananta Mudra

Gesture of Infinity

For Balancing the Seventh Chakra

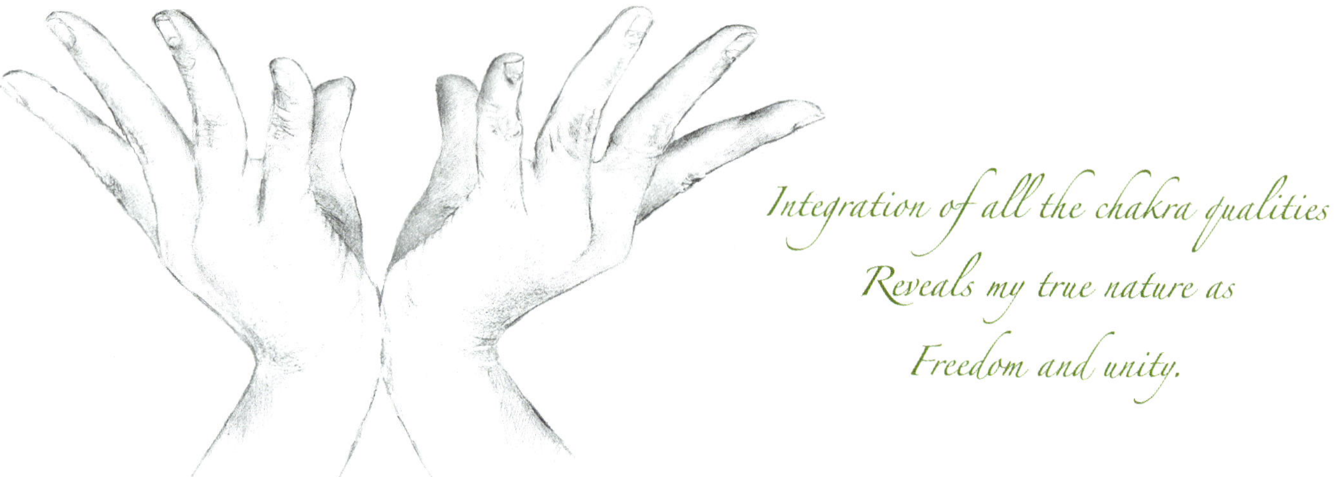

Integration of all the chakra qualities
Reveals my true nature as
Freedom and unity.

Core Quality

Unity Consciousness

Especially helpful for

- Unfolding the seventh chakra, revealing the nature of our true being as freedom and unity.
- Supporting optimal balance within all the systems of the body.
- Harmonizing the entire chakra system.
- Allowing us to experience glimpses of bliss.

Mudras with similar effects

Mandala, Bhairava, Shakata, Tejas

Cautions

Contraindicated for hypertension, headache and stroke. Mandala mudra can be used as a substitute.

Gain comfort with the other chakra mudras before practicing this gesture.

Instructions

1. Join the hands in prayer position in front of the heart.
2. Keep the base of the palms together and spread all the fingers and thumbs wide apart like an unfolding lotus.
3. Relax the shoulders back and down, with the spine naturally aligned.

The seventh chakra, *Sahasrara*, which means "thousand-petaled," is located at the crown of the head. This energy center is represented by a thousand-petaled lotus of crystal light, symbolizing the limitlessness of pure Consciousness. The journey of integration of all of the chakra qualities naturally leads to the unfolding of the seventh chakra. Through this opening, we experience our essential nature as limitless pure being beyond all conditioning. At this level, all sense of separation is released, allowing us to experience all of creation as a seamless unity. Pure Consciousness is experienced initially as glimpses during meditation. Eventually, we recognize pure Consciousness as the essence of our true being, always present as the silent background of all of our interactions and activities. As we align with our true being, life's challenges continue to arise, but instead of identifying with them personally, we simply resolve them objectively and compassionately.

Ananta means "infinite," and Ananta mudra resembles the thousand-petaled lotus of the crown chakra, evoking an experience of blissfulness that is a reflection of our limitless true Self. This gesture brings breath, awareness and energy to the crown of the head, expanding the silent space between thoughts, allowing us to merge more easily with our limitless true being. This gesture amplifies the light of Consciousness and supports us in channeling it into each of the energy centers, awakening and integrating each chakra's essential qualities. This experience of integration within our subtle anatomy is a powerful source of health and healing at all levels of being.

Systems Balanced:

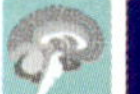 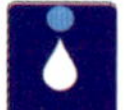

Elements Activated:

Doshas Balanced:

Prana Vayus Nourished:

Chakras Balanced:

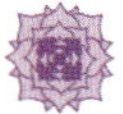

Scale from Calming to Energizing:

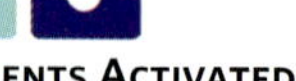

Guided Meditation: Awakening Pure Consciousness

- As you hold Ananta mudra, take several natural breaths to attune to all the feelings and sensations awakened by this gesture.
- Notice how your breath and awareness flow upward from the base of your body to the crown of your head, naturally resting at the seventh chakra, your center of pure Consciousness.
- As you attune to Sahasrara chakra, its crystal light harmonizes each of your energy centers individually, finally integrating them in an experience of unity.
- Begin by visualizing four red petals at the base of your body. With your inhaling breath, red energy ascends to the crown of your head, and as you exhale, crystal light descends, infusing your root chakra with the light of pure Consciousness.
- As the lotus of Muladhara chakra is illuminated with crystal light, it blossoms completely, supporting you in meeting your survival needs with a greater sense of security as the foundation for your spiritual journey.
- Now, attune to the six orange petals at the center of your pelvis. As you inhale, orange energy ascends to the crown of your head, and as you exhale, crystal light bathes your pelvic center.
- Sense the lotus of Svadhisthana chakra, bathed in the light of Consciousness, blossoming naturally, allowing your relationships to unfold with greater fluidity.
- Next, attune to the ten golden petals at your solar plexus. As you inhale, golden energy ascends to the crown of your head, and as you exhale, crystal light descends.
- As the lotus of Manipura chakra is illuminated with crystal energy, all of its petals unfold naturally, allowing you to clarify your life purpose and to manifest it completely.
- Now, attune to the twelve green petals within your heart chakra. As you inhale, emerald energy ascends, and as you exhale, crystal light permeates your heart center.
- Take some time to sense the lotus of Anahata chakra blossoming completely, allowing you to touch and be touched by all beings with compassion and empathy.
- Now, visualize sixteen sky-blue petals at your throat center. As you inhale, sky-blue energy ascends, and with your exhalation, crystal light purifies your throat and neck.
- As the lotus of Vishuddha chakra is filled with crystal light, its petals unfold naturally, allowing you to align with your authentic being and communicate your truth clearly.
- Your awareness now rests at your third eye, with its two violet petals. As you inhale, violet energy ascends, and as you exhale, crystal light infuses your center of wisdom.
- Take several breaths to sense the lotus of Ajna chakra infused with crystal light, blossoming completely, providing the wisdom and clarity to see beyond all dualities.
- Now, your awareness rests at the crown of your head, allowing crystal light to expand infinitely, harmonizing all of your chakras, allowing you to experience complete unity.
- Affirm your source energy as you repeat the following three times, aloud or silently: **"Resting in pure Conscious being, all of my chakras are harmonized naturally."**
- Now, slowly release the gesture, taking all the time you need to bring your awareness, chakra by chakra, back down to Muladhara, at the base of your body, sensing yourself completely integrated and grounded.
- When you are ready, open your eyes, returning slowly and gently, more deeply attuned to your essence as unity.

Annamaya kosha (physical body)

• Directs breath and awareness into the upper regions of the lungs, enhancing breath capacity in these areas.
• Enhances circulation to the area of the pineal gland.
• This gesture may be practiced by Kapha or Pitta, but only when they are in balance.

Pranamaya kosha (energy body)

• Activates Udana vayu, the uppermost current of energy.
• Opens and balances the seventh chakra, center of unity.
• Activates Sushumna nadi.

Manomaya kosha (psycho-emotional body)

• Cultivates lightness and joy.

Vijnanamaya kosha (wisdom body)

• As glimpses of unity expand gradually, they eventually permeate all of our interactions and activities.

Anandamaya kosha (bliss body)

• As the seventh chakra opens, there is an experience of luminosity, joy, openness and bliss that originates at the crown of the head and encompasses our entire being.

62 Dharma Chakra Mudra

Gesture of the Wheel of Truth

For Integrating the Chakras into Daily Living

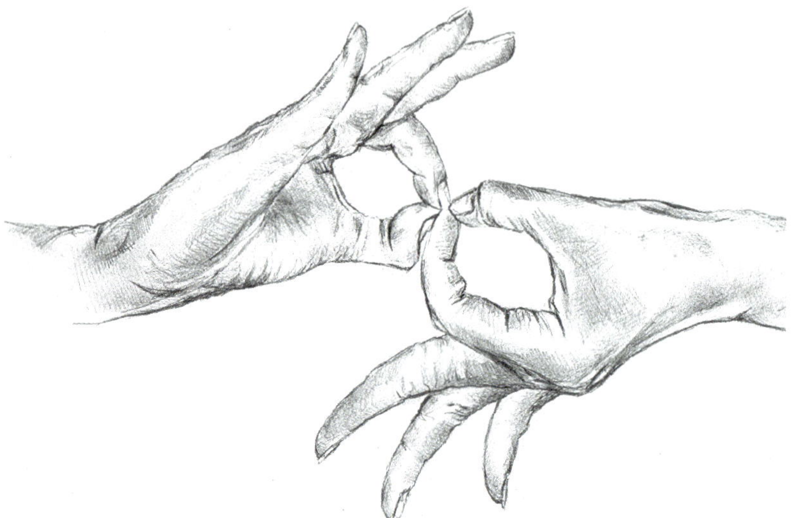

With all of my energy centers
Harmonized completely,
I integrate their qualities
Into daily living.

Core Quality

Integrating all the Chakras

Especially Helpful For

- Supporting us in manifesting all of the chakra qualities in daily living.
- Facilitating Full Yogic Breathing.
- Balancing all the systems of the body, especially the endocrine system.
- Cultivating an overall sense of wholeness and well-being.

Mudras with Similar Effects

Purna Jnanam, Hakini, Dharma Pravartana

Cautions

None

Instructions

1. Touch the tips of the thumbs to the tips of the index fingers of each hand.
2. Place the left palm in front of the solar plexus, and place the right palm above it, facing outward.
3. Touch the tips of the thumbs and index fingers together and gently extend all the other fingers.
4. Relax the shoulders back and down, with the elbows slightly away from the body, and the spine naturally aligned.

Dharma Chakra means "wheel of the law," and refers to the teachings of the Buddha, whose intention is to free all beings from rebirth and suffering. In relation to the chakras, Dharma Chakra refers to the truth of our being revealed gradually along the chakra journey. The journey of the chakras is usually conceived as an upward movement toward illumination. There is, however, a complementary and equally important aspect of this journey, which involves manifesting the qualities of each of the chakras into all of our interactions and activities. Through the integration of all of the chakra qualities, we naturally manifest our life's highest vision and deepest meaning. This manifestation of the chakra qualities into all of our interactions and activities, allows us to live with a sense of freedom and ease at each moment of our life journey.

Dharma Chakra mudra cultivates Full Yogic Breathing, supporting the integration of the entire chakra system. This gesture lengthens both the inhalation and exhalation while opening both nostrils evenly, cultivating balance in the mind and body. This mudra lengthens and aligns the spinal column, the seat of the chakras, allowing us to sense the location of each of the energy centers within the subtle body more palpably, thereby supporting the free flow of energy. Dharma Chakra mudra also cultivates the sensitivity that allows us to perceive any imbalances within our energy centers and rebalance them more easily. This gesture also instills a sense of harmony and equanimity that supports us in integrating all of the chakra qualities in daily living.

Systems Balanced:

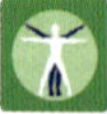

Elements Activated:

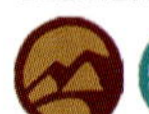
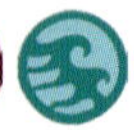

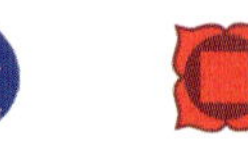

Doshas Balanced:

Prana Vayus Nourished:

Chakras Balanced:

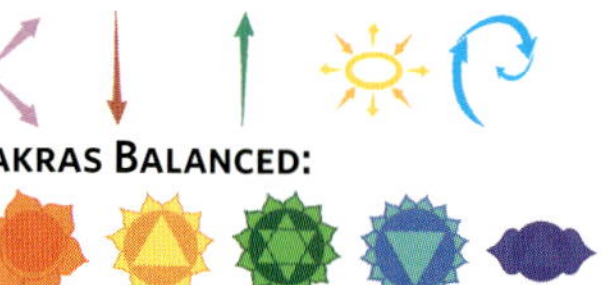

Scale from Calming to Energizing:

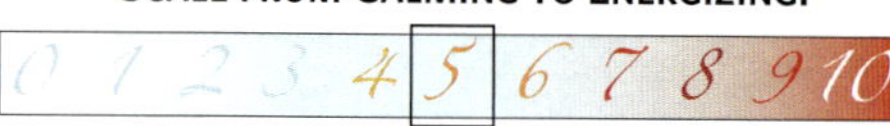

Guided Meditation: Manifesting Your Vision

- As you hold Dharma Chakra mudra, take several natural breaths to attune to all the feelings and sensations awakened by this gesture.
- Notice how your breath flows smoothly throughout your entire being, cultivating a sense of openness in which all of your chakras are integrated naturally.
- Through this integration, you clearly see that the ultimate intention of your journey is to manifest all of your chakra's essential qualities in daily living.
- Your journey of manifestation begins at the crown of your head, as you attune to the thousand petals of crystal light at Sahasrara chakra.
- As you bathe in crystal energy, take some time to allow a vision of your life's deepest meaning to arise naturally, providing inspiration for your journey.
- Inspired by a vision of your life's deepest meaning, crystal light descends to your third eye, illuminating the two violet petals of Ajna chakra, your center of clear seeing.
- At this level, you perceive all the details of your life mission clearly, envisioning the steps you will take to manifest your vision as a lived reality.
- The light of clarity now descends into your throat center, illuminating the sixteen sky blue petals of Vishuddha chakra.
- In order to express your vision clearly, take several breaths to release any limiting beliefs that keep you from communicating from your authentic being.
- Your light of clear communication now descends into your heart, infusing the twelve emerald-green petals of Anahata chakra.
- As emerald light permeates your being, you live in the world more compassionately, recognizing that everyone, just like yourself, seeks happiness within the limits of their understanding.
- Take several breaths to sense your heart of compassion beating in synchrony with the hearts of all beings.
- The light of your heart now descends into your solar plexus, illuminating the ten golden petals of Manipura chakra.
- As golden light radiates through your being, you affirm your inherent self-esteem, allowing you to unfold your life purpose while serving others consciously.
- Now, your golden light descends to fill the six orange petals of Svadhisthana chakra.
- As orange light bathes your being, you experience inner nourishment and healing, allowing you to live with greater fluidity while creating space for healthy relationships that support your journey.
- This light of fluidity now fills the base of your body, infusing the four red petals of Muladhara chakra, naturally cultivating greater stability and grounding.
- As red energy fills your being, your vision is transformed into a lived reality, manifesting your life's true meaning for your own awakening and for the benefit of all beings.
- Affirm your chakra journey, repeating the following three times, aloud or silently: **"Integrating all of the chakra qualities, my vision is manifest as a lived reality."**
- Slowly, release the gesture, taking several breaths to envision complete manifestation.
- When you are ready, open your eyes, returning slowly and gently, integrating all of your chakra qualities into daily living.

Annamaya kosha (physical body)

- Directs breath and awareness throughout the entire torso, facilitating Full Yogic Breathing, supporting the optimal functioning of all the systems of the body.
- Lengthens and aligns the spinal column.
- Balances the entire endocrine system.
- The balancing effects of this gesture are generally helpful for Vata, Pitta and Kapha imbalances.

Pranamaya kosha (energy body)

- Balances all five prana vayus with a special focus on Vyana vayu, the all-pervading current.
- Opens and balances all seven chakras.
- Balances all of the nadis.

Manomaya kosha (psycho-emotional body)

- Cultivates psycho-emotional balance.

Vijnanamaya kosha (wisdom body)

- As balance and integration increase, we experience perfect equanimity as a reflection of our true being.

Anandamaya kosha (bliss body)

- As we integrate all of the chakra qualities, we experience complete balance and harmony within all dimensions of our being.

Chapter Eleven

Balancing Energy Polarities

MUDRAS FOR THE NADIS

Nadi means "river" or "nerve." In relation to our subtle anatomy, nadis are the minute channels that distribute *prana*, "life force energy," throughout the body. The total number of nadis is often given as either 72,000 or 360,000. These numbers, rather than quantifying the total number of nadis, may be a symbolic way of saying that we are essentially composed of vital energy. Among the nadis, fourteen are described as especially important, and among these, three have particular significance. These are *Ida*, *Pingala* and *Sushumna* nadis, located on the left and right sides of the spine and within the spinal column itself, respectively.

A brief overview of the philosophy of *Tantra* is necessary for understanding the importance of these three main nadis. In Tantra, creation is seen as a manifestation of the union of male and female polarities, called *Shiva* and *Shakti*, representing Consciousness and Energy. The whole of life is an ongoing dynamic relationship between these polarities, establishing a field of learning in which we gradually come to recognize our essential nature as unity.

Within our subtle anatomy, Ida nạdi, running along the left side of the spine, represents Shakti, the lunar or feminine aspect of creation. Pingala nadi, running along the right side of the spine, represents Shiva, the solar or masculine aspect of creation. By balancing these two polarities, energy is naturally channeled into Shushumna nadi, the central channel of spiritual awakening, allowing us to experience unity beyond all dualities.

This journey toward unity through exploring and balancing our polarities is the essence of *Hatha Yoga*. The word *Hatha* reflects the importance of this solar-lunar balance: *ha* refers to the solar, active, energetic aspect of our being while *tha* refers to the lunar, receptive, cooling aspect. When these solar and lunar facets of our being are balanced and integrated, we experience the equilibrium that naturally leads to spiritual awakening.

The breath plays a key role in the harmonization of Ida and Pingala nadis, leading to the awakening of Sushumna nadi. Ida nadi is associated with the left nostril, left lung and left side of the body. Left nostril breathing activates the lunar channel that runs along the left side of the spine from the base chakra up to the left nostril. This energy is cooling and calming, related to moonlight and the receptive qualities of softness and intuition. Ida nadi is activated through the practice of Ida mudra.

Pingala nadi is related to the right nostril, right lung and right side of the body. It activates the solar channel that runs along the right side of the spine. This dynamic and vitalizing energy is related to sunlight, willpower and determination. Right nostril breathing and solar energy are activated by Pingala mudra.

When these two channels are balanced, the life force energy flows freely, harmonizing all of our polarities, allowing energy to be channeled into Sushumna nadi. As our awareness rests within Sushumna nadi, we experience the bliss of unity that comes from the union of Shiva and Shakti, Consciousness and Energy. This central channel is activated by Shakata mudra.

Ha - Shiva **Solar energy** **Pingala Mudra**	**Ha - Tha** **Integration of Solar & Lunar** **Shakata Mudra**	**Tha - Shakti** **Lunar energy** **Ida Mudra**
Focus: right nostril, right lung & right side of body	Focus: both nostrils, both lungs & sides of body	Focus: left nostril, left lung & left side of body
Warming & energizing, activating Pingala nadi	Balancing & harmonizing, activating Sushumna nadi	Cooling & calming, activating Ida nadi
Lengthens inhalation & pause after the inhalation	Lengthens both inhalation & exhalation as well as the pauses	Lengthens exhalation & pause after the exhalation
Related to the masculine, dynamic polarity	Balances dynamic & receptive polarities	Related to the feminine, receptive polarity
Focus on will & the role of individual effort	Spiritual awakening that integrates & transcends will & surrender	Focus on surrender & the role of Divine grace

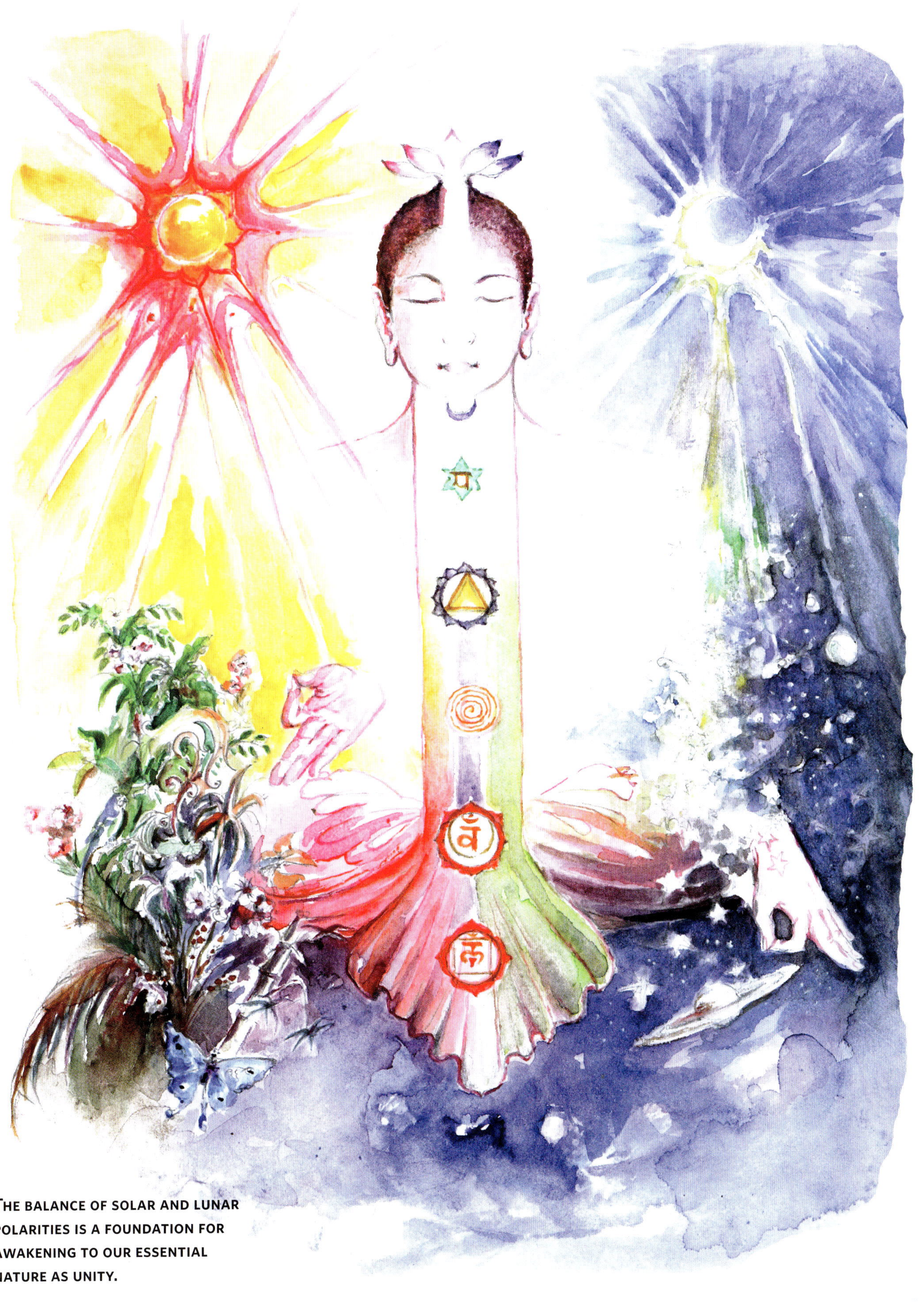

The balance of solar and lunar polarities is a foundation for awakening to our essential nature as unity.

63

Ida Mudra

Gesture of the Lunar Nadi

For Balancing the Lunar Channel of Energy

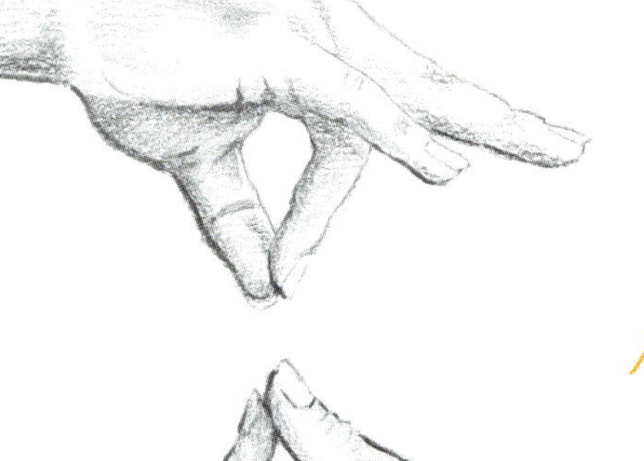

Bathing in soft moonlight energy,
I open to my receptive, feminine qualities.

Core Quality

Receptivity

Especially helpful for

- Awakening our lunar, feminine qualities, including softness, fluidity, pleasure and sensitivity.
- Reducing stress and blood pressure.
- Supporting the health of the reproductive and urinary systems.
- Helping to relieve inflammation.

Mudras with similar effects

Jala, Mira, Yoni, Svadhisthana

Cautions

None

Instructions

1. Touch the tips of the ring fingers to the tips of the thumbs of the same hand and extend the other fingers.
2. Place the left hand just below the navel, with the palm facing upward.
3. Place the right hand slightly above the left, palm down, so that the joined fingertips of the right hand are directly above the joined fingertips of the left hand, but not touching them.
4. Relax the shoulders back and down, with the elbows slightly away from the body and the spine naturally aligned.

Ida, which means "comfort," is the name for the lunar *nadi*, the subtle channel of cooling energy that runs along the left side of the spine, from *Muladhara chakra* at the base of the body up to the third eye, and then down to the left nostril. Ida nadi is associated with *chandra*, meaning "moon," and with calming colors such as light blue or silvery moonlight. Ida nadi encompasses our receptive, feminine qualities, including softness, self-nourishment, fluidity, sensitivity and the ability to find pleasure and joy in simply living. As we deepen our connection to Ida nadi, our awareness is naturally drawn inward, cultivating the intuition and inner listening that help to guide our life journey. With enhanced intuition and sensitivity, our powers of creativity awaken naturally, inspiring art, dance, painting or poetry that express the depths of our being. Moonlight energy also awakens us to the power of community in which decisions are made collectively. As we embody all of these lunar qualities, we live each moment of life with greater serenity and equanimity.

Ida mudra activates the free flow of energy within Ida nadi, naturally supporting us in connecting with our lunar, receptive qualities. This gesture brings breath, awareness and energy to the left nostril, left lung and left side of the body. Ida mudra calms and slows the breath while lengthening the exhalation, activating the parasympathetic nervous system, promoting deep relaxation and restoration, thereby reducing blood pressure. As relaxation deepens, our senses naturally turn inward, awakening intuition. This gesture cultivates a sense of self-nourishment, which promotes inner healing while releasing stress and anxiety. The rhythmic abdominal breathing supports the optimal functioning of the reproductive and urinary systems.

Systems Balanced:

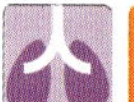 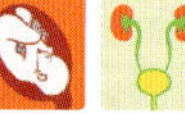

Elements Activated:

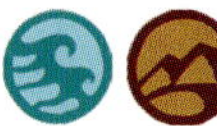 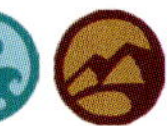

Doshas Balanced:

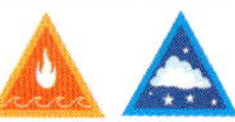

Prana Vayus Nourished:

Chakras Balanced:

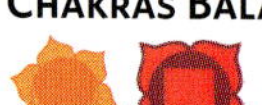

Scale from Calming to Energizing:

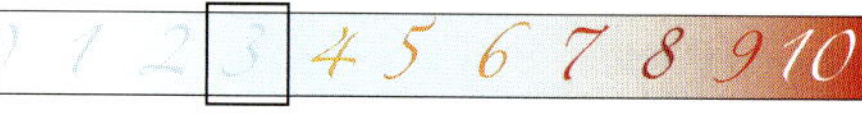

Guided Meditation: Nourished by Soothing Moonlight

- ॐ As you hold Ida mudra, take several natural breaths to attune to all the feelings and sensations awakened by this gesture.
- ॐ Notice how your breath is naturally directed into your left nostril while expanding your left lung and enhancing awareness of the entire left side of your body.
- ॐ For your next few breaths, sense the whole left side of your body expanding gently with each inhalation, and softening with each exhalation.
- ॐ As you deepen your awareness of the left side of your body, you naturally become more sensitive to your receptive, feminine qualities.
- ॐ You will awaken these qualities more completely by bringing awareness to Ida nadi, the lunar channel of soothing, refreshing energy.
- ॐ This channel of energy runs along the left side of your spine from your root chakra up to your third eye, then down to your left nostril.
- ॐ With each inhalation, cooling moonlight ascends, and with each exhaling breath, it flows back down to the base of your body, instilling a sense of soothing refreshment.
- ॐ Take some time to follow this upward and downward movement of silver moonlight energy, naturally cultivating a sense of calm and serenity.
- ॐ As you experience greater serenity, visualize yourself floating on a soft moonlit sea, naturally absorbing all of your receptive, feminine qualities.
- ॐ Begin by receiving the quality of fluidity, the ability to flow with life's cycles and seasons more easily.
- ॐ Take several breaths to sense the quality of fluidity moving up and down along the left side of your spine within Ida nadi.
- ॐ With greater fluidity, you absorb the quality of sensitivity, enhancing your ability to listen to your body's messages, naturally unfolding your powers of inner healing.
- ॐ As you integrate fluidity and sensitivity, the quality of intuition awakens naturally, providing inner guidance for your journey.
- ॐ As you breathe along Ida nadi, take some time to receive any messages from within your being that clarify your life's deeper purpose and meaning.
- ॐ With greater intuition and sensitivity, your essential creativity unfolds naturally, enhancing your ability to give birth to new possibilities that express your life's deeper meaning.
- ॐ Now, take some time to breathe up and down along Ida nadi, sensing the unfolding of all of your receptive qualities, allowing you to flow with life's stream more easily, experiencing pleasure even in simple things.
- ॐ Affirm your receptive qualities, repeating the following three times, aloud or silently: **"Bathing in soft moonlight energy, I flow with the rhythms of life more easily."**
- ॐ Slowly release the gesture, taking several breaths to bathe in soothing moonlight.
- ॐ When you are ready, open your eyes, returning slowly and gently, more attuned to the receptive qualities of Ida nadi.

Annamaya kosha (physical body)

- **Directs breath and awareness to the left nostril, left lung and left side of the body, activating the relaxation response.**
- **The lengthened exhalation further supports deep relaxation.**
- **Directs breath and awareness into the lower abdomen and pelvis, cultivating a massaging effect that enhances circulation to the reproductive and urinary systems.**
- **The refreshing effects of this gesture are generally helpful for Pitta imbalance.**
- **The calming effects are generally helpful for Vata imbalance.**

Pranamaya kosha (energy body)

- **Activates Apana vayu, the downward moving current of energy.**
- **Opens and balances the first and second chakras, centers of safety and self-nourishment.**

Manomaya kosha (psycho-emotional body)

- **Instills flexibility that allows us to flow with life more easily.**
- **Cultivates deep calm and serenity, which help to alleviate insecurity and anxiety.**
- **Instills a sense of self-nourishment.**

Vijnanamaya kosha (wisdom body)

- **The integration of our feminine, receptive qualities allows us to move inward to align with the subtle realms of our being.**

Anandamaya kosha (bliss body)

- **As we integrate our receptive qualities, we experience the bliss of feminine energy.**

64 PINGALA MUDRA

Gesture of the Solar Nadi

For Balancing the Solar Channel of Energy

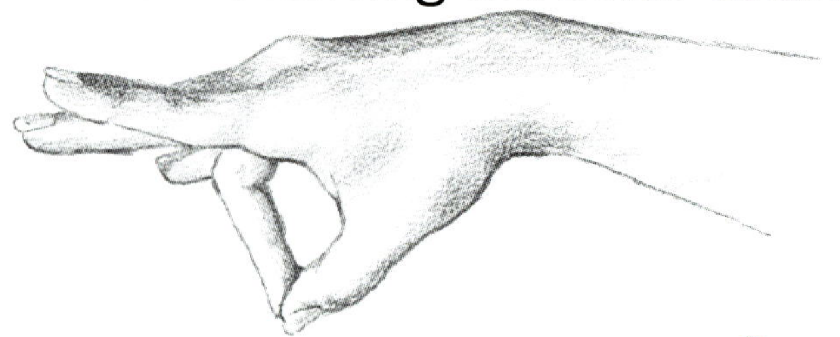

Awakening my radiant dynamic qualities, I experience abundant energy and vitality.

CORE QUALITY
Dynamism

ESPECIALLY HELPFUL FOR
- Awakening our solar, dynamic, masculine qualities, including assertiveness and determination.
- Stimulating digestion.
- Cultivating energy and vitality.
- Enhancing concentration.

MUDRAS WITH SIMILAR EFFECTS
Surya, Vajra, Kubera, Merudanda

CAUTIONS
Those with hypertension should carefully monitor the effects. Surya, which is less heating, may be used as a substitute.

INSTRUCTIONS
1. Touch the tips of the ring fingers to the tips of the thumbs of the same hand and extend the other fingers.
2. Place the right hand below the navel, with the palm facing upward.
3. Place the left hand above the right, palm down, so that the joined fingertips of the left hand are slightly above the joined fingertips of the right hand, but not touching them.
4. Relax the shoulders back and down, with the elbows slightly away from the body and the spine naturally aligned.

Pingala, which means "reddish" or "fiery," is the name for the solar *nadi*, the subtle channel of warming energy that runs along the right side of the spine, from *Muladhara chakra* at the base of the body up to the third eye, and then down to the right nostril. The energy within this channel is related to *surya*, meaning "sun." It is vitalizing and energizing and is associated with vibrant colors, such as orange, red or golden sunlight. Pingala nadi encompasses the dynamic, masculine qualities, such as rationality, logic, determination, assertiveness, detailed planning and a sense of control over one's own destiny. As we embody all of these qualities, we are able to clarify our life purpose and channel all of our talents to manifest it fully.

Pingala mudra activates the free flow of energy within Pingala nadi, naturally awakening all of the solar qualities. This gesture directs breath, awareness and energy into the right nostril, right lung and right side of the body. This mudra lengthens the inhalation as well as the pause at the end of the inhaling breath. This more energizing breath activates the sympathetic nervous system, naturally increasing metabolism, heart rate and blood pressure while instilling an overall feeling of vitality. Pingala mudra generates an overall feeling of warmth, especially in the right side of the body. This mudra enhances the breath in the area of the solar plexus, stimulating digestion. Pingala mudra increases alertness and concentration, supporting us in planning and defining our goals as well as envisioning the steps needed to achieve them. At the psycho-emotional level, this mudra instills a sense of empowerment and determination, giving us the strength and energy to manifest our life purpose completely.

SYSTEMS BALANCED:

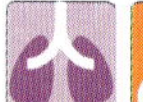
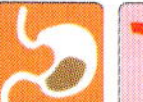

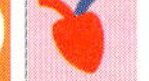

ELEMENTS ACTIVATED:

DOSHAS BALANCED:

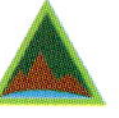

PRANA VAYUS NOURISHED:

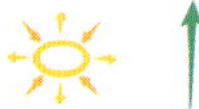

CHAKRAS BALANCED:

SCALE FROM CALMING TO ENERGIZING:

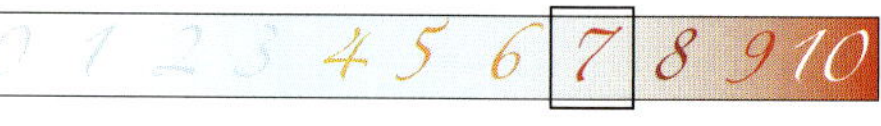

Guided Meditation: Radiant Sunlight Energy

ॐ As you hold Pingala mudra, take several natural breaths to attune to all the feelings and sensations awakened by this gesture.

ॐ Notice how your breath is naturally focused within your right nostril while expanding your right lung and enhancing awareness of the entire right side of your body.

ॐ For your next few cycles of breath, sense the whole right side of your body expanding with each inhalation, and releasing with each exhalation.

ॐ As you expand your awareness of the right side of your body, you naturally activate your dynamic, masculine qualities.

ॐ You will awaken these qualities more completely by focusing your awareness on Pingala nadi, the solar channel of energy and vitality.

ॐ This channel runs along the right side of your spine from your root chakra up to your third eye, then down to your right nostril.

ॐ With each inhalation, golden sunlight ascends along this channel, and with each exhaling breath, radiant energy flows back down to the base of your body.

ॐ Take some time to follow the upward and downward movement of radiant energy, naturally cultivating warmth and vitality.

ॐ To enhance this vitality, visualize yourself in a beautiful sunlit field, opening to receive the sun's rays in exactly the right quantity to activate all of your dynamic qualities.

ॐ Begin by awakening radiant self-esteem, enhancing your ability to unfold all of your talents and possibilities with a clear vision of your life's purpose and mission.

ॐ With greater clarity in relation to your life purpose and possibilities, your ability to plan logically is enhanced naturally, allowing you to define exactly what you want to achieve at each step of your journey.

ॐ With a clear vision and effective planning, you channel your energy one-pointedly toward that which you want to achieve, empowered with the determination to overcome obstacles confidently.

ॐ Along your journey of doing and achieving, you use your time and resources carefully, making the best of your opportunities while conserving your precious energy.

ॐ Even as you focus on your own goals, you also strive to achieve balance between your own needs and the overall good of the community, naturally unfolding your leadership abilities.

ॐ Take several breaths to envision your life journey, seeing clearly all the stages that allow you to transform your vision into a lived reality.

ॐ Now, bring your awareness back to Pingala nadi, sensing your breath moving along this channel of sunlight energy, supporting the integration of all of your dynamic qualities.

ॐ Affirm your solar qualities as you repeat the following three times, aloud or silently: **"Attuned to radiant sunlight energy, I manifest my life purpose completely."**

ॐ Slowly release the gesture, taking several breaths to fully integrate your radiant, solar qualities.

ॐ When you are ready, open your eyes, returning slowly and gently, infused with dynamic energy.

Annamaya kosha (physical body)

• Directs breath and awareness to the right nostril, right lung and right side of the body, increasing metabolism, heart rate and blood pressure.
• Directs the breath into the solar plexus, cultivating a massaging effect that enhances circulation to the digestive system.
• The warming, energizing effects of this gesture are generally helpful for Kapha imbalance.

Pranamaya kosha (energy body)

• Activates Samana and Prana vayus, the horizontal and upward moving currents of energy.
• Opens and balances the third chakra, center of personal power.

Manomaya kosha (psycho-emotional body)

• Cultivates enthusiasm and vitality.
• Facilitates logical thinking, clear planning and decision-making.

Vijnanamaya kosha (wisdom body)

• The integration of the masculine, dynamic qualities supports the commitment, energy and determination needed for spiritual transformation.

Anandamaya kosha (bliss body)

• As we awaken our dynamic qualities, we experience the radiance of our true being.

65

Shakata Mudra

Gesture of the Vehicle

For Balancing the Central Channel of Energy

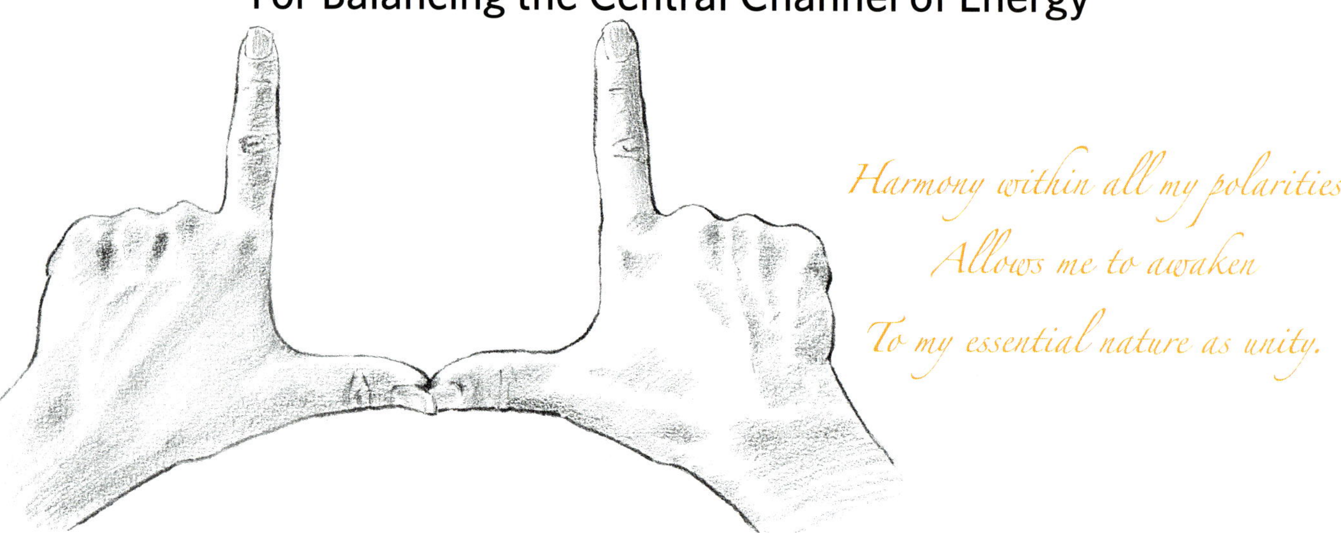

Harmony within all my polarities
Allows me to awaken
To my essential nature as unity.

Core Quality

Spiritual Unity

Especially helpful for

- Awakening Sushumna nadi, leading to an experience of freedom and unity.
- Supporting optimal alignment of the spine.
- Balancing the autonomic nervous system, supporting global healing.

Mudras with similar effects

Bhairava, Shivalingam, Merudanda

Cautions

Become comfortable with Ida and Pingala mudras before practicing Shakata mudra.

Instructions

1. Hold the hands, with the palms down.
2. Make the hands into loose fists, with the thumbs on the outside.
3. Extend the index fingers and thumbs straight out.
4. Touch the tips of the thumbs together, forming three sides of a square.
5. Hold the gesture below the navel or rest the hands on the lap.
6. Relax the shoulders back and down, with the elbows slightly away from the body and the spine naturally aligned.

Sushumna, which means "very gracious," is the central *nadi*, the main channel of subtle energy located within the spinal column. This channel is visualized as a column of crystal light, running from *Muladhara chakra* at the base of the body up to *Sahasrara chakra* at the crown of the head. The crystal light within this column is a reflection of our luminous essence as pure Consciousness. The awakening of Sushumna nadi occurs naturally as *Ida* and *Pingala* nadis, our lunar and solar channels, come into complete harmony. As our awareness and energy are awakened within the central channel, we experience the qualities of our essential being, including bliss, timelessness, limitlessness, wholeness and an all-pervading sense of unity. The experience of these qualities is initially temporary, but as the spiritual journey proceeds, they are integrated into all of our activities. As these qualities become our lived reality, all sense of limitation is released, allowing us to experience the freedom of our true being.

Shakata, which means "vehicle," refers to Sushumna nadi as the vehicle for *Shakti Kundalini*, the energy of spiritual awakening that remains dormant at the base chakra and gradually rises upward along the spiritual journey. Shakata mudra directs breath, awareness and energy into both nostrils, both lungs and both sides of the body evenly, balancing the autonomic nervous system, facilitating the harmony that supports spiritual awakening. The extended index fingers are symbolic of Ida and Pingala nadis, whose integration naturally awakens Shushumna nadi. This gesture creates space between thoughts and calms the emotional body, cultivating inner silence that allows us to rest in pure Consciousness for longer periods.

Systems Balanced:

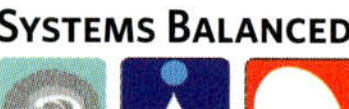

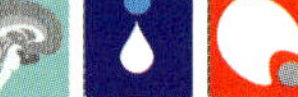

Elements Activated:

Doshas Balanced:

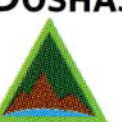

Prana Vayus Nourished:

Chakras Balanced:

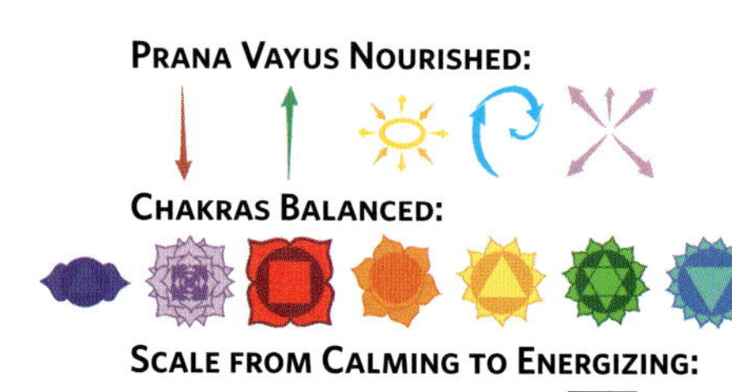

Scale from Calming to Energizing:

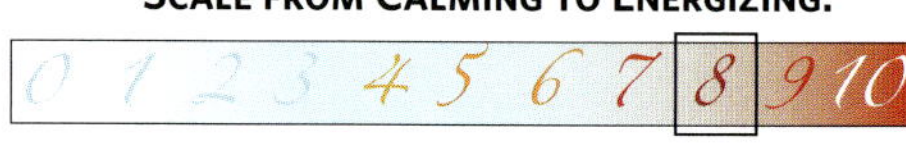

Guided Meditation: Awakening to Unity

- In preparation for exploring Sushumna nadi, your central channel of spiritual awakening, you will first balance the breath in your nostrils with the support of Ida and Pingala mudras.
- Begin by placing your hands in Ida mudra. Notice how your breath flows more smoothly through your left nostril, left lung and left side of your body.
- Take three cycles of breath to sense your receptive, lunar qualities awakening naturally.
- After completing your lunar breathing, place your hands in Pingala mudra. Notice how your breath flows more easily through your right nostril, right lung and right side of your body.
- Take three cycles of breath to sense your dynamic, solar qualities awakening naturally.
- When you are ready, release the gesture, resting your hands on your thighs or knees, taking some time to sense the balance of the receptive and dynamic facets of your being.
- Now, place your hands in Shakata mudra. Sense how your breath flows through both nostrils more evenly, deepening your sense of alignment and harmony.
- As you become more aligned within your being, your awareness turns inward naturally, allowing you to attune to Sushumna nadi, your central channel of subtle energy.
- Visualize this channel as a column of crystal light within your spine, running from Muladhara chakra at the base of your body all the way to Sahasrara chakra at the crown of your head.
- With each inhalation, sense crystal light ascending along Sushumna nadi, and with each exhaling breath, experience this energy descending to the base of your body.
- Take several breaths to sense crystal light energy flowing smoothly up and down along your central channel of spiritual awakening.
- As crystal light flows more freely, you naturally attune to your inner essence as limitless pure being, both integrating and transcending your lunar and solar polarities.
- Take several breaths to rest within this experience of unity, the essence of Sushumna nadi, allowing the present moment to expand infinitely.
- As you rest in timeless being, you merge completely with the crystal light of awakening.
- Affirm your awakening as you repeat the following three times, aloud or silently: **"As crystal light permeates my being, I experience my essence as unity."**
- Now, slowly release the gesture, taking several breaths to sense complete integration and harmony.
- When you are ready, open your eyes, returning slowly and gently, with a deeper connection to your essence as unity.

Annamaya kosha (physical body)

• Directs breath and awareness into both nostrils, both lungs, and both sides of the body evenly, supporting global healing.
• Fully expands all portions of the lungs, facilitating optimal breathing.
• Supports optimal postural alignment.
• The overall balance supports the health of the nervous, endocrine and immune systems.
• The energizing effects of this gesture are generally helpful for Kapha imbalance.

Pranamaya kosha (energy body)

• Balances Prana and Apana vayus while activating Samana, Udana and Vyana vayus.
• Opens and balances all seven chakras, with a focus on the sixth and seventh chakras, centers of wisdom and unity.

Manomaya kosha (psycho-emotional body)

• Instills a sense of openness in the mind and emotions.
• Cultivates one-pointed concentration.

Vijnanamaya kosha (wisdom body)

• The awakening of Sushumna nadi instills an experience of unity beyond the polarities of the personality.

Anandamaya kosha (bliss body)

• As light and energy move freely through the central channel, we experience the bliss and radiance of our true being.

Chapter Twelve

Invoking Universal Protection

MUDRAS FOR PROTECTION AND SAFETY

In order to experience complete protection, we need to cultivate safety and security at three main levels. First, we need to feel protected from external forces in the form of natural phenomena. Second, we need to sense protection from the negativity of other people and environments. The third level of protection is a sense of safety that develops as we release our own limiting thoughts, emotions and beliefs, allowing us to see ourselves and the world more objectively.

These three levels of protection are invoked by the Vedic mantra: "*Om Shantih, Shantih, Shantih; Hari Om.*" *Shantih* means "peace," referring to the peace we experience as we sense protection at each of these three levels of our being. The "*Hari Om*" that completes the mantra represents the ultimate protection that comes from complete trust in the Divine source. Each of the mudras in this chapter invokes one of these levels of protection.

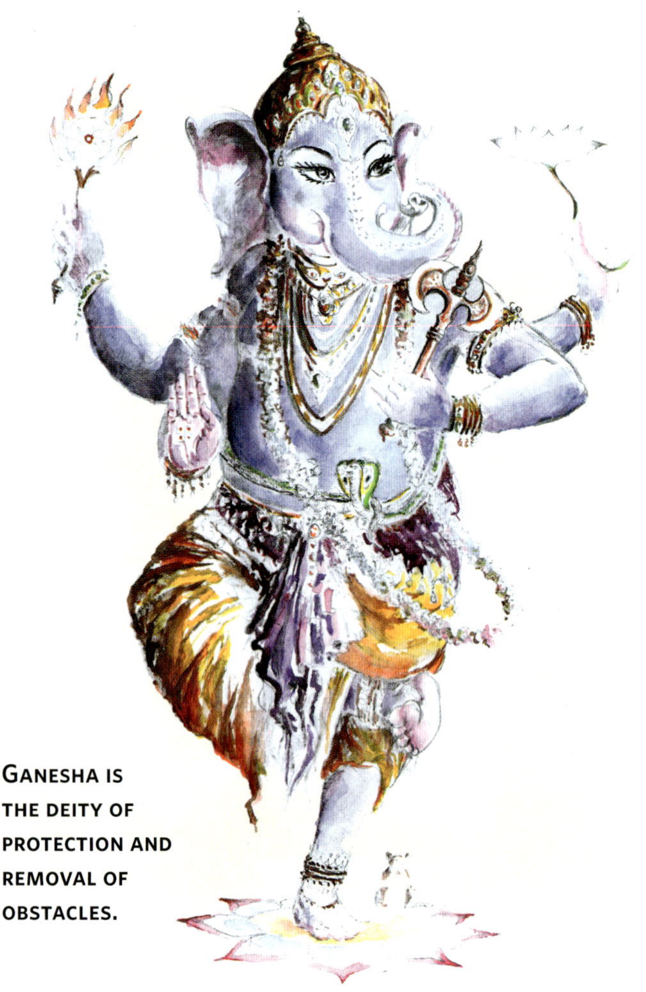

Ganesha is the deity of protection and removal of obstacles.

Adhidaivikam - Protection from Natural Phenomena

Adhi means "primordial," and *daiva* means "Divine." As we chant the first shanti, we invoke protection from all "acts of God," in the form of natural phenomena and events beyond our control. Vaikhara mudra serves as a powerful shield of protective energy against natural forces that could cause harm.

Adhibhautikam - Protection from External Energies

Bhauda refers to "other beings," and as we chant the second shanti, we invoke protection from people, animals or environments that could cause us harm. Svasti mudra invokes a powerful aura of protection from all forms of negativity, thereby supporting our health and well-being.

Adhyatmikam - Protection from Our Limiting Beliefs

Adhyatma refers to "our soul," and as we chant the third shanti, we invoke protection from our own limiting thoughts, emotions and beliefs, the colored lenses of our conditioning that create limitation and therefore suffering. Gupta mudra cultivates a sense of an inner sanctuary where we can experience the safety of our true being.

Pariraksanam - Highest Protection

Pariraksanam refers to the "absolute protection" invoked by "Hari Om," which follows the recitation of the three shantis. At this level, we recognize that our continual awareness of the Divine presence is our ultimate protection. Ganesha mudra invokes the energy of *Ganesha*, the elephant deity, for providing security, especially as we begin new projects.

Mudra	Quality
Vaikhara	*Adhidaivikam* *Protection from natural phenomena*
Svasti	*Adhibhautikam* *Protection from the negative energy of people & environments*
Gupta	*Adhyatmikam* *Protection from our own limiting thoughts, emotions and beliefs*
Ganesha	*Parirakshanam* *Highest Protection that comes from trust in the Divine*

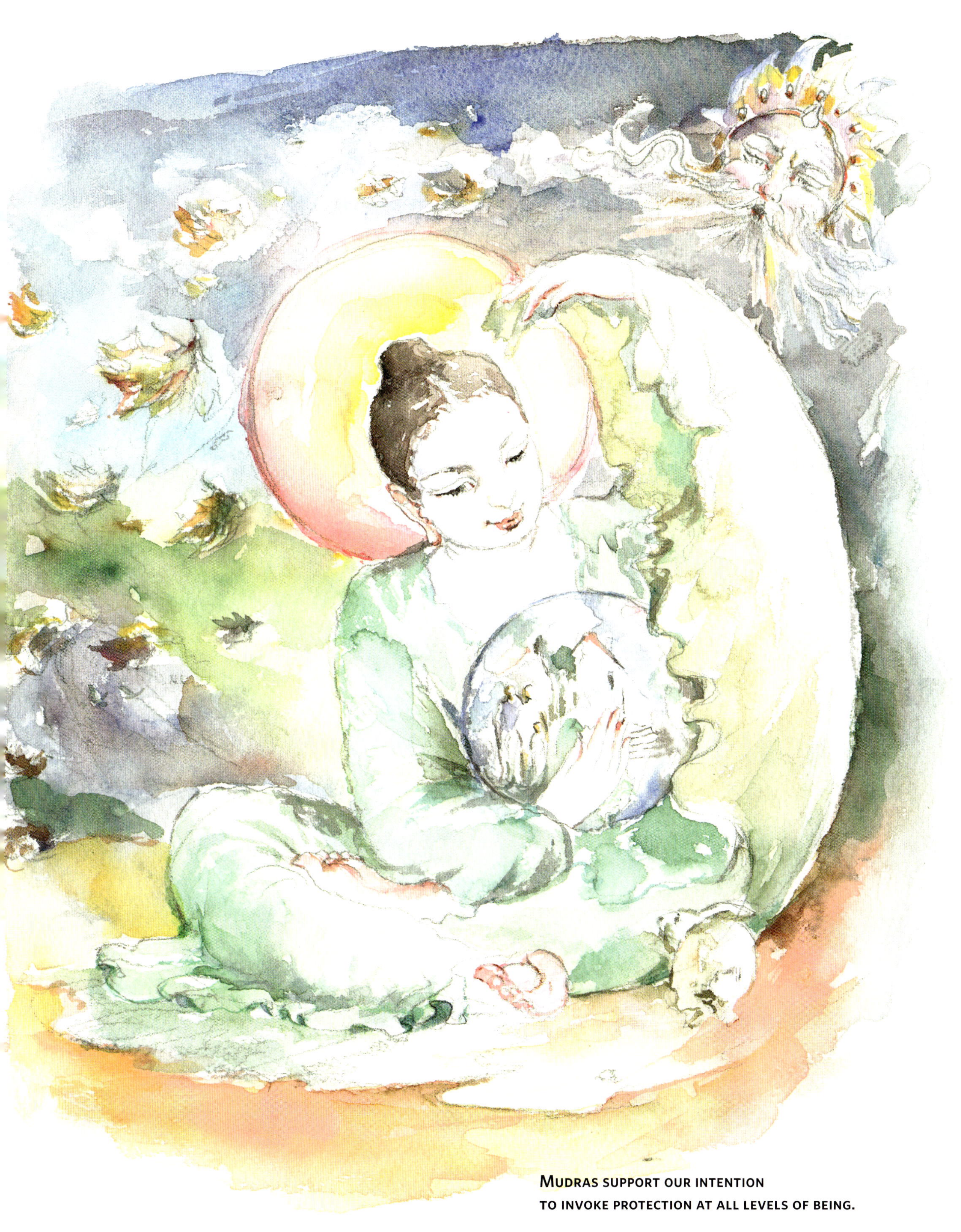

Mudras support our intention
to invoke protection at all levels of being.

66 Vaikhara Mudra

Gesture of the Protective Shield

For Protection from the Forces of Nature

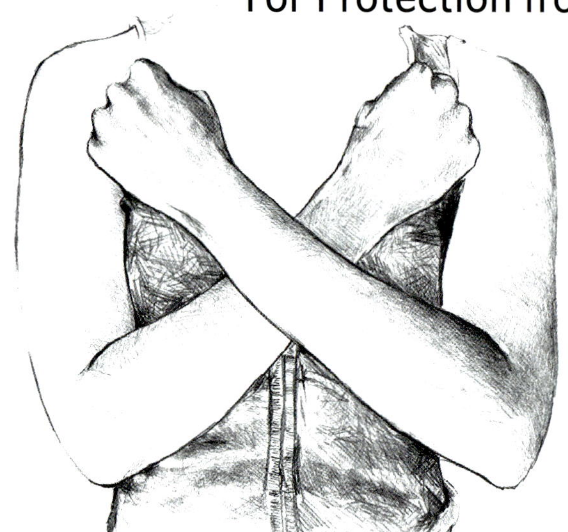

Attuned to creation's essential unity,
I experience absolute safety.

Core Quality

Protection from the Forces of Nature

Especially helpful for

- Instilling a sense of unity with the five elements that comprise our physical body.
- Discerning between safe and potentially harmful environments.
- Relaxing the muscles of the upper back.
- Supporting the health of the immune system.
- Cultivating a sense of empowerment.

Mudras with similar effects

Vajrapradama, Shivalingam, Vajra

Cautions

None

Instructions

1. Make your hands into fists, with the thumbs on the outside, resting on the second joint of the ring fingers.
2. Cross the arms in front of the chest, with the right arm closer to the body, placing the fists on either side of the chest, just below the shoulder joints.
3. Relax the shoulders back and down, with the spine naturally aligned.

Vaikhara means "solid and protective," like a coat of armor. Vaikhara mudra instills a sense of an energetic shield that protects us in the face of all challenges, especially those presented by natural phenomena. This gesture directs breath, awareness and energy into the chest, especially into the upper sternum where the thymus gland is located, supporting the health of the immune system. Vaikhara mudra lengthens the inhaling breath, enhancing alertness and providing the energy needed for dealing with emergencies quickly and efficiently.

As Vaikhara mudra enhances alertness, we become more aware of our surroundings, including the forces of nature in the form of the five elements. This gesture supports us in aligning with the protective qualities of each of the five elements. As we become more sensitive to the elements that are the matrix of all of creation, including our own bodies, we are able to discern more easily which environments are safe and which may be harmful. At the deepest level, Vaikhara mudra fosters a sense of our oneness with the natural world. As we recognize that we are composed of the same five elements that make up all of creation, we are able to embrace our unity with nature and honor its messages, sensing it as an extension of our own being rather than as a threat to our safety.

Systems Balanced:

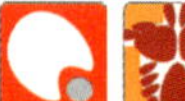
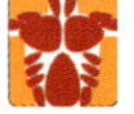

Elements Activated:

Doshas Balanced:

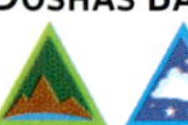

Prana Vayus Nourished:

Chakras Balanced:

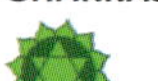

Scale from Calming to Energizing:

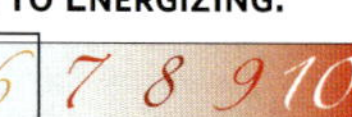

Guided Meditation: **Protective Qualities of the Elements**

ॐ As you hold Vaikhara mudra, take several natural breaths to attune to all the feelings and sensations evoked by this gesture.

ॐ Notice how your breath is naturally directed into your chest, instilling a sense of safety and protection.

ॐ Sense how your arms form a powerful shield of protective energy within all dimensions of being, especially from the forces of nature and the play of the five elements within your surroundings.

ॐ You will deepen your sense of safety by attuning to the protective qualities of the five elements that comprise all of creation, including your own body.

ॐ Begin by embodying the protective qualities of the earth, sensing yourself growing roots deep into its firm but yielding surface, cultivating stability, support and a sense of firmness.

ॐ As you deepen your connection to the earth's qualities, take several breaths to experience complete safety within your shield of protective energy.

ॐ Now, allow the protective qualities of water to bathe your being in the form of fluidity and flexibility, allowing you to flow with life's cycles and seasons more easily.

ॐ As you absorb water's qualities, you develop the adaptability to modify your plans and routines in accordance with nature's rhythms, naturally supporting your shield of protective energy.

ॐ Flowing through life with greater adaptability, you naturally open to receive the fire element's protective qualities of clarity and energy.

ॐ As you integrate the fire element's qualities, take several breaths to affirm the clarity that allows you to perceive situations of risk more easily, along with the energy to deal with them more efficiently.

ॐ As fire provides clarity and energy, the air element naturally infuses your being with its protective qualities of lightness and sensitivity.

ॐ With increased sensitivity, you respond to changes in your environment quickly while your enhanced lightness carries you to safety, naturally strengthening your shield of protective energy.

ॐ As the qualities of air lighten your being, you naturally attune to the space element's protective qualities of intuition and inner listening.

ॐ Listening intuitively, you deepen your ability to discern which environments and situations provide safety and which should be avoided completely.

ॐ Now, take several breaths to sense the integration of all of the elements' qualities within your being, naturally strengthening your shield of protective energy.

ॐ With all of the elements' qualities fully integrated, you experience your oneness with the natural world, providing the ultimate protection for your life journey.

ॐ Protected by the elements, repeat the following three times, aloud or silently:
"Attuned to all of the elements' protective qualities, I journey in complete safety."

ॐ Slowly release the gesture, taking several breaths to rest in the safety of your shield of protective energy.

ॐ When you are ready, open your eyes, returning slowly and gently, continuing your journey with a deeper sense of safety.

Annamaya kosha (physical body)

• Directs breath and awareness into the chest, enhancing circulation to the area of the thymus gland.
• Expands the breath in the upper back, relaxing the muscles between the shoulder blades.
• The mildly energizing effects of this gesture, together with the opening in the lungs, are generally helpful for Kapha imbalance.
• The enhanced sense of security is generally helpful for Vata imbalance.

Pranamaya kosha (energy body)

• Activates Prana vayu, the upward moving current of energy.
• Opens and balances the fourth chakra, center of unconditional love.

Manomaya kosha (psycho-emotional body)

• Cultivates a sense of security and protection.
• Enhances emotional stability.

Vijnanamaya kosha (wisdom body)

• As our sense of safety increases, we are able to glimpse the absolute security of our true being.

Anandamaya kosha (bliss body)

• With a greater sense of safety, unshakable trust in our journey arises naturally.

67

Svasti Mudra

Gesture of Well-being

For Protection from Negative Energy

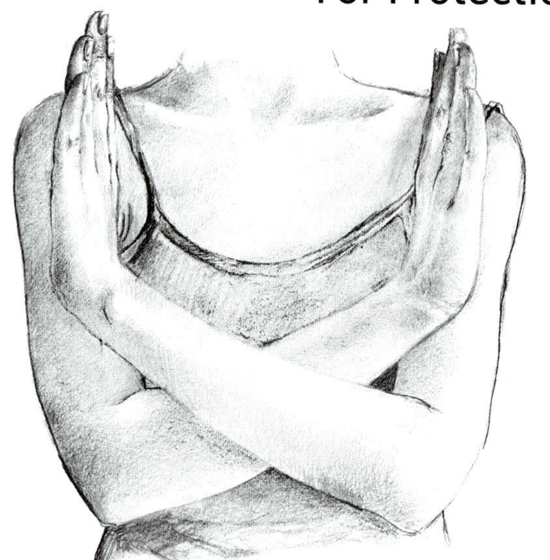

Deflecting all forms of negativity, I experience complete protection and safety.

Core Quality

Protection from Negative Energy

Especially helpful for

- Creating an aura of protection that deflects and neutralizes negativity.
- Relaxing the upper back and creating space between the shoulder blades.
- Optimal alignment of the spine.
- Supporting the health of the endocrine and immune systems.
- Cultivating healthy boundaries.
- Centering us in the present moment.

Mudras with similar effects

Vajrapradama, Purna Hridaya, Abhaya Varada

Cautions

None

Instructions

1. Place the hands in prayer position.
2. Cross the forearms with the right arm closer to the chest, so that the backs of the hands are facing each other, about six inches apart.
3. The fingers point upward.
4. Relax the shoulders, back and down, with the elbows held slightly away from the body and the spine naturally aligned.

Svasti means "well-being," "prosperity," "success" and "blessing." Svasti mudra cultivates an aura of protective energy within all dimensions of our being, especially from any negativity projected by others. This gesture is also helpful for neutralizing energy from negative environments. The crossed arms and upraised hands deflect negative projections, both from those who intend harm and from those who believe they are acting in our best interests, but lack the understanding to perceive our true needs. As we deflect these negative energies, we rest in our own center more easily, attuning to the wisdom of our inner being to guide our journey.

Svasti mudra directs breath, awareness and energy into the chest, side ribs and upper back, expanding breath capacity. As the breath fills the chest, it creates a massaging effect that enhances circulation to the thymus gland. Svasti mudra instills the courage and confidence needed to remain centered in the face of negative energy. This gesture also supports us in living with our heart open while maintaining healthy boundaries, further enhancing our ability to neutralize negativity. Additionally, this mudra brings breath to the back of the body, creating a massaging effect in the area of the kidneys and adrenal glands, giving us the energy to meet challenges more effectively. As it directs breath and awareness to the back of the body, this gesture also supports optimal postural alignment and the release of tension from the upper back, especially between the shoulder blades.

Systems Balanced:

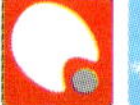
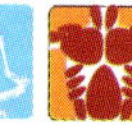
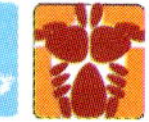

Elements Activated:

Doshas Balanced:

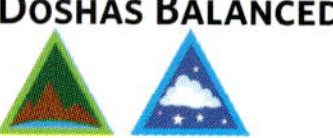

Prana Vayus Nourished:

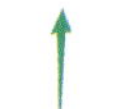

Chakras Balanced:

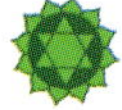

Scale from Calming to Energizing:

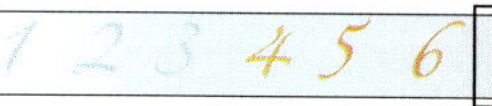

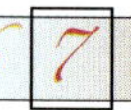
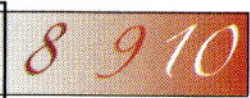

Guided Meditation: Aura of Protective Energy

- As you hold Svasti mudra, take several natural breaths to attune to all the feelings and sensations evoked by this gesture.
- Notice how your breath is directed into your chest, side ribs and upper back, creating an aura of protective energy that encompasses your entire being.
- Take several breaths to sense this aura expanding with your breathing, instilling a sense of complete protection from all forms of negativity.
- Begin by sensing protection from others' negativity, recognizing that, at the level of the personality, most people are focused on their own wants and needs, sometimes leading them to act unconsciously.
- As you inhale, sense the expansion of your aura of protective energy, and as you exhale, all negativity from others is deflected away from you naturally.
- Take several breaths to sense your aura of protection neutralizing other people's negativity.
- Negative energy can also come from those who believe they are acting for your benefit by trying to align your ways of seeing and being with their limiting beliefs.
- As you inhale, sense the expansion of your aura of protective energy, and as you exhale, all intentions that don't support your true well-being are deflected away from you naturally.
- Take several breaths to sense your aura of protection neutralizing completely other people's controlling energy.
- Negative energy can also infuse particular places and even cities because of their karmic history.
- As you enter these places, you may feel your energy depleted or weakened, and find yourself beginning to absorb their negative vibrations.
- As you inhale, sense the expansion of your aura of protective energy, and as you exhale, all negativity from these environments is deflected away from you naturally.
- Take several breaths to sense your aura of protective energy neutralizing any negativity that may be present in your surroundings.
- Now, take all the time you need to sense your aura of protective energy naturally neutralizing all forms of negativity, allowing you to journey forward in complete safety.
- Protected at all levels of being, repeat the following three times, aloud or silently: **"Within my aura of protective energy, all negativity is neutralized completely."**
- Slowly release the gesture, taking several breaths to sense complete protection.
- When you are ready, open your eyes, returning slowly and gently, safe and secure within your aura of protective energy.

Annamaya kosha (physical body)

• Directs breath and awareness to the entire rib cage, expanding breath capacity.
• Enhances circulation to the area of the thymus gland.
• Assists in developing optimal posture by strengthening the muscles of the upper back while creating space in the thoracic spine.
• The energizing effects and enhanced breathing cultivated by this gesture are generally helpful for Kapha imbalance.
• The centering and sense of safety cultivated are generally helpful for Vata imbalance.

Pranamaya kosha (energy body)

• Activates Prana vayu, the upward moving current of energy.
• Opens and balances the fourth chakra, center of unconditional love.

Manomaya kosha (psycho-emotional body)

• Cultivates emotional balance.
• Instills a sense of empowerment.
• Enhances our sense of safety.

Vijnanamaya kosha (wisdom body)

• Healthy boundaries support us in relaxing, allowing us to gain the clarity to recognize that our essential nature is absolute protection and safety.

Anandamaya kosha (bliss body)

• As we attune to our aura of protective energy, a sense of deep equanimity arises naturally.

68 Gupta Mudra

Gesture of the Inner Secret

For Protection from Our Limiting Beliefs

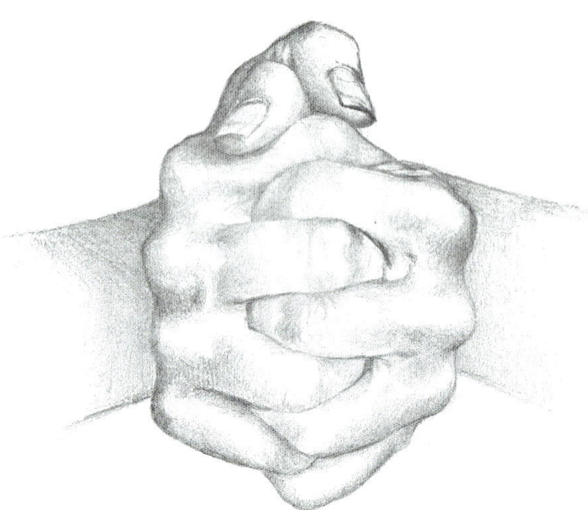

As limiting beliefs are released,
I rest in the sanctuary of my true inner being.

Core Quality

Protection from Our Limiting Beliefs

Especially helpful for

- Exploring and releasing limiting beliefs that keep us from experiencing the safety of our true inner being.
- Supporting the health of the digestive and eliminatory systems.
- Reducing stress, thereby supporting the functioning of the immune system.
- Relaxing the shoulders, neck, face and head, which may be helpful for neck pain and TMJ dysfunction.
- Enhancing a sense of centering and safety.

Mudras with similar effects

Shankha, Samputa, Kurma, Ishvara

Cautions

None

Instructions

1. Interlace the fingers loosely inward with the right thumb on top.
2. Gently join the base of the hands.
3. Rest the wrists against the abdomen.
4. Relax the shoulders back and down, with the elbows held slightly away from the body and the spine naturally aligned.

Gupta means "secret" or "hidden," and Gupta mudra cultivates a sense of entering an inner sanctuary of safety and security. Within the safety of this sanctuary, we are able to explore, integrate and eventually release our identification with the limiting beliefs that separate us from our true being. This gesture instills a sense of grounding that supports us in maintaining our equanimity as we explore our limiting beliefs, creating a space in which transformation can occur more easily. Gupta mudra further enhances this sense of an inner sanctuary by cultivating silence and inner peace that allows us to align with our authentic being.

Gupta mudra directs breath, awareness and energy to the base of the body, pelvis and solar plexus, expanding abdominal breathing and creating a massaging effect that supports digestion and elimination. This gesture relaxes the musculature of the entire body, especially the shoulders, neck, face and head. This relaxation of the face and head allows the jaw to soften completely, which may be helpful for TMJ. Gupta mudra integrates the left and right, male and female polarities of our being, instilling a sense of balance that allows us to rest more easily within our inner sanctuary. With enhanced digestion, greater relaxation and balanced polarities, Gupta mudra supports us in releasing all the limiting beliefs that keep us from resting within our sanctuary of serenity and safety.

Systems Balanced:

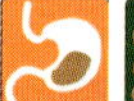
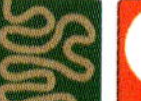
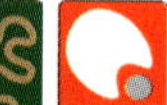

Elements Activated:

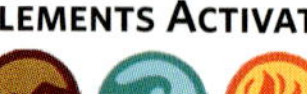

Doshas Balanced:

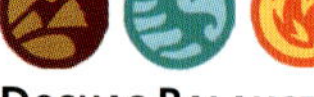

Prana Vayus Nourished:

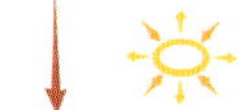

Chakras Balanced:

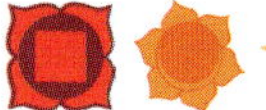

Scale from Calming to Energizing:

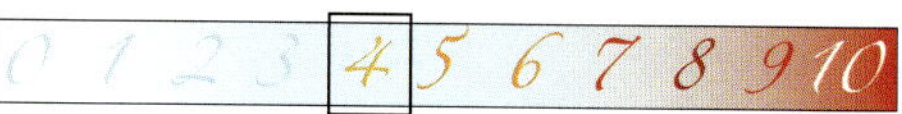

Guided Meditation: Sanctuary of Inner Safety

- As you hold Gupta mudra, take several natural breaths to attune to all the feelings and sensations evoked by this gesture.
- Notice how your breath is gently directed into your abdomen, cultivating a sense of warmth and ease, a feeling that you are entering your own inner sanctuary of safety.
- Take several breaths to rest within your sanctuary, deepening your connection with your inner being, inherently whole and complete, naturally enhancing your sense of protection and safety.
- To rest even more deeply within your inner sanctuary, it is important to release any limiting beliefs that cause disharmony in the world around you and within your own being.
- Begin by exploring your beliefs related to success and achievement. Striving for fulfillment is normal and healthy, but when it becomes an end in itself rather than a means, you sacrifice your inner peace, making it difficult to rest within your inner sanctuary.
- Take several breaths to sense the wholeness of your authentic being, recognizing that nothing in the world outside can add to or subtract from that which is inherently complete.
- Next, explore your limiting beliefs about how the world or other people should be. Having expectations is normal and healthy, but when they become rigid and demanding, you create conflict and disharmony that keeps you from experiencing the peace of your inner sanctuary.
- Take some time to recognize clearly that change always begins within your own being. As you focus on your own awakening, you naturally allow others to find their own time and space for transformation.
- Finally, explore your sense of individuality, which is an essential facet of your being. However, when your sense of "I" and "me" becomes all-encompassing, you create separation from others, fostering isolation and disharmony that make it difficult to rest within your inner sanctuary.
- Take several breaths to sense your essential oneness with all beings, allowing you to live and work in cooperation and harmony, naturally supporting your sense of protection and safety.
- With the gradual release of your limiting beliefs, take several breaths to sense yourself fully aligned with your authentic being, completely secure within your sanctuary of inner safety.
- Abiding in complete inner peace, repeat the following three times, aloud or silently: **"Resting within my inner sanctuary, I experience absolute protection and safety."**
- Slowly release the gesture, taking several breaths to rest in the safety of your authentic being.
- When you are ready, open your eyes, returning slowly and gently, sensing the absolute protection of your inner sanctuary.

Annamaya kosha (physical body)

- **Directs breath and awareness into the pelvis, abdomen and solar plexus, creating a massaging effect that enhances circulation to the digestive system.**
- **Relaxes the muscles of the shoulders, neck, face and jaw, which may be helpful for TMJ dysfunction and neck pain.**
- **The centering effects of this gesture are generally helpful for Vata imbalance.**
- **The calming effects are generally helpful for Pitta imbalance.**

Pranamaya kosha (energy body)

- **Activates Apana vayu, the downward moving current of energy.**
- **Gently activates Samana vayu, the horizontal current of energy.**
- **Opens and balances the first, second and third chakras, centers of safety, self-nourishment and personal power.**

Manomaya kosha (psycho-emotional body)

- **Instills a sense of protection and safety.**
- **Cultivates a sense of centering.**
- **Supports equanimity and conservation of energy.**

Vijnanamaya kosha (wisdom body)

- **As we release limiting beliefs, our true Self, whose very nature is safety, is revealed.**

Anandamaya kosha (bliss body)

- **Resting in our inner sanctuary, silence, peace and a sense of absolute protection arise naturally.**

69 Ganesha Mudra

Gesture of Elephant Deity

Protection for New Beginnings

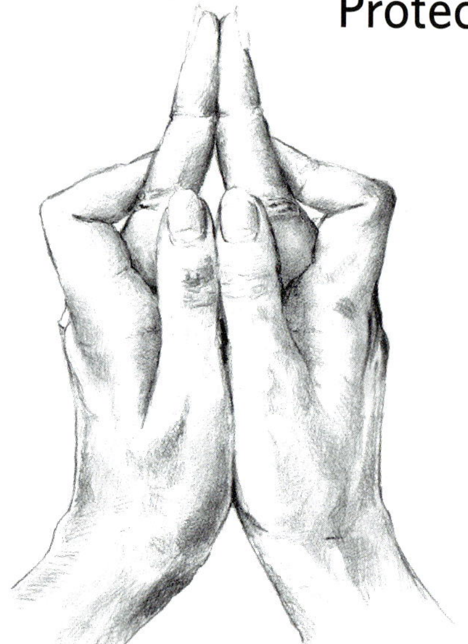

Attuned to Ganesha's protective energy, I sense support for all new beginnings.

Core Quality

Protection for New Beginnings

Especially Helpful For

- Invoking the universal energy of protection, especially for new projects.
- Facilitating healthy digestion and elimination.
- Balancing rest and activity, which supports us in planning, organizing and manifesting our plans and projects.

Mudras with Similar Effects

Vajra, Matangi, Kubera, Surya

Cautions

Those who experience discomfort in the hands may use Surya as a substitute.

Instructions

1. Interlace the fingers to the outside, with the right thumb on top.
2. Extend the middle fingers forward, and wrap the index fingers around them.
3. Place the thumbs side by side, joined along their length, onto the middle fingers.
4. Rest the wrists onto the solar plexus.
5. Relax the shoulders back and down, with the elbows held slightly away from the body and the spine naturally aligned.

Ganesha is a popular Indian deity who embodies universal protective energy. Each of Ganesha's attributes represents an essential protective quality. His great girth is associated with the ability to remove obstacles. His broad brow represents discernment. His large ears symbolize the ability to listen, so we can recognize challenges before they become insurmountable obstacles. His big belly represents the ability to digest life experiences fully, giving us the energy and vitality to overcome obstacles along our journey. His single tusk represents one-pointed concentration and the importance of focusing on one project at a time. His trunk is both strong and sensitive, giving us the ability to grasp both the obvious and the subtle details of any situation. Ganesha is often depicted with one foot solidly on the ground and the other raised in meditation, representing the ability to be fully present in the material world while remaining aligned with our spiritual being.

Ganesha mudra directs breath, awareness and energy into the base of the body, abdomen and solar plexus, creating a massaging effect that supports digestion and elimination. This gesture enhances our overall level of energy and vitality in order to manifest our plans and projects more easily. Ganesha mudra activates Samana vayu, further enhancing digestive health and vitality. The lengthened exhalation cultivated by this gesture also activates Apana vayu, supporting the health of the eliminatory system. At the psycho-emotional level, Ganesha mudra instills a sense of clear direction, which helps us to choose our projects carefully and to implement them with wisdom and clarity. The sense of balance instilled by this gesture helps us to maintain our grounding and objectivity while upholding our highest values and integrity.

Systems Balanced:

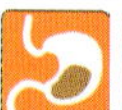
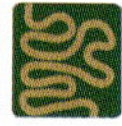

Elements Activated:

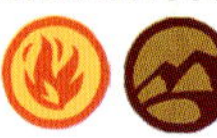
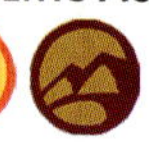

Doshas Balanced:

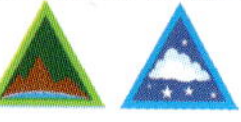

Prana Vayus Nourished:

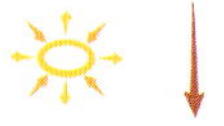

Chakras Balanced:

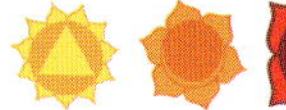
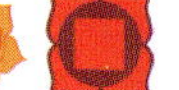

Scale from Calming to Energizing:

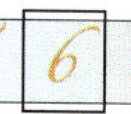

Guided Meditation: Protection for New Beginnings

- As you hold Ganesha mudra, take several natural breaths to attune to all the feelings and sensations awakened by this gesture.
- Notice how your breath is naturally directed into the base of your body, abdomen and solar plexus, cultivating a sense of grounding while instilling energy and vitality.
- This combination of grounding and vitality allows you to envision and manifest your life projects more easily.
- Whenever you begin a new project or phase in your life, it is helpful to invoke the protection of Ganesha, the elephant deity, who removes all obstacles along your journey.
- In order to awaken Ganesha's protective energy, bring to mind a project you are planning or working on at this time.
- Each aspect of Ganesha represents an important quality that will support you in organizing and manifesting your project.
- Begin by focusing on Ganesha's large ears, taking several breaths to integrate the quality of careful listening, your ability to receive advice from others while also attuning to the guidance of your own inner being.
- Now, bring your awareness to Ganesha's great girth, taking some time to absorb his power to overcome obstacles more easily, allowing you to move forward steadily along your journey.
- Next, focus on Ganesha's broad brow, taking several breaths to cultivate the discernment to perceive when you should continue on your path or when it is time to look at other possibilities.
- With enhanced discernment, you open to receive the power of Ganesha's trunk, both strong and flexible, allowing you to work with others easily while upholding your own values and integrity.
- Next, visualize Ganesha's single tusk, representing concentration and mindfulness, allowing you to focus on your project one-pointedly until it is complete.
- Now, bring your awareness to Ganesha's legs, one solidly rooted to the earth and the other raised in meditation, reminding you to remain fully grounded while aligned with your highest vision.
- As your project progresses, stress may increase. Ganesha's big belly reminds you to take time to digest all of your experiences completely, absorbing the lessons while releasing all you no longer need in order to conserve your precious energy.
- Finally, visualize an image of Ganesha as a whole, and embody his form completely, integrating all of his qualities, experiencing absolute protection along your journey.
- Protected by the elephant deity, repeat the following three times, aloud or silently: **"Embodying Ganesha's essential qualities, I am fully protected along my journey."**
- Slowly release the gesture, taking several breaths to rest in Ganesha's absolute protection.
- When you are ready, open your eyes, returning slowly and gently, sensing yourself fully supported in all your new plans and projects.

Annamaya kosha (physical body)

• Directs breath and awareness to the base of the body, abdomen and solar plexus, creating a massaging effect that improves circulation to the digestive and eliminatory systems.
• Lengthens the exhalation, supporting stress reduction.
• Balances the breath in both nostrils, creating a balance in the autonomic nervous system.
• The mildly energizing effects of this gesture are generally helpful for Kapha imbalance.
• The grounding and centering cultivated are generally helpful for Vata imbalance.

Pranamaya kosha (energy body)

• Activates Samana and Apana vayus, the horizontal and downward moving currents of energy.
• Opens and balances the first, second and third chakras, centers of safety, self-nourishment, and personal power.

Manomaya kosha (psycho-emotional body)

• Cultivates trust and determination.
• Instills clarity and a sense of direction.

Vijnanamaya kosha (wisdom body)

• Cultivates the discernment and objectivity that allows us to recognize which projects support the unfolding of our essential being.

Anandamaya kosha (bliss body)

• Instills a sense of unshakable confidence and absolute trust.

Chapter Thirteen

Strategies for Stress Reduction

MUDRAS FOR RESTORATION

Due to the fast pace of modern life and the constant sensory stimulation, stress and tension are ever present. The digital world is designed to make life easier, but in some ways, it has increased the level of stimulation, making life more stressful. Our digital environment is also a factor in unhealthy posture, sedentary lifestyle and a sense of isolation which all contribute to stress. Stress has always been a part of human life, and our body is well designed to cope with crises and emergencies, but in modern life, we seldom take the time for adequate rest and recovery. When stress becomes chronic, without sufficient time for restoration, stress-related symptoms can occur.

Early symptoms of chronic stress include irritability, hypertension, headache, fatigue, insomnia and digestive issues. These symptoms are warning signs that we need to make changes in our attitudes and lifestyle. Because of the pressure to succeed and the easy availability of over-the-counter remedies that give temporarily relief, many ignore these early warning signs. When ignored, stress can lead to more serious problems, including anxiety and depression, as well as digestive, circulatory and auto-immune issues. Relaxation and restoration are an essential part of the solution to our stressful modern lifestyles. There are four important steps for reducing stress and reestablishing balance.

1. The Art of Deep Relaxation - It is becoming increasingly clear that relaxation is an important foundation for health, but for many people, relaxing deeply and regularly is not easy. Mudras are an important support for restoration because they have the capacity to relax the entire musculature of the body almost instantly. Mudra practice also changes breathing patterns, allowing the breath to become calm and serene, thereby facilitating the relaxation response. Mudras also facilitate ease in the mind and emotions by creating space between thoughts while cultivating positive qualities, such as trust and self-esteem. Dvimukham mudra is one of the most effective gestures for facilitating deep relaxation.

2. Reducing Sensory Overload - It is very difficult to relax if we are constantly bombarded by sensory stimulus in the form of digital devices and social networking. Sensory overload can also be internal in the form of our accumulated memories, thoughts and feelings that tend to create a vicious cycle of worry and anxiety. Mudras have the ability to draw the senses inward naturally, reducing the amount of new sensory stimulus and creating a space in which accumulated sensory impressions can be processed and released. Kurma mudra is an excellent gesture for calming the senses and releasing accumulated sensory impressions.

3. Learning to Let Go - For everything we strive to achieve, a useful question is: "Is the juice worth the squeeze?" The larger our perceived needs and the stronger our drive to succeed, the more likely we are to pay the price of chronic stress. As we learn to relax, we gradually recognize that striving to meet our perceived needs may be bringing us more stress than happiness. As we open to a wider, more relaxed way of seeing, we are able to evaluate our needs more objectively which usually involves a process of simplifying. This letting go includes releasing attachment to material possessions as well as our need to control relationships and life in general. Pranidhana mudra facilitates a deep sense of release, supporting us in letting go of all that no longer supports our journey.

4. Developing Positive Attitudes - The first three steps help to reduce stress, but in order to manage our level of stress continuously, we need to change our attitudes and beliefs in order to see ourselves and life more positively. Mudras and affirmations are extremely helpful in cultivating more positive attitudes. Mudras also support the release of limiting beliefs and patterns of conditioning, allowing us to see life with fresh eyes, as a field of possibilities. Ushas mudra is one of the best gestures for cultivating a more positive attitude.

Mudra	Core Quality
Dvimukham	Deep Relaxation
Kurma	Reducing Sensory Overload
Pranidhana	Letting Go
Ushas	Cultivating a Positive Attitude

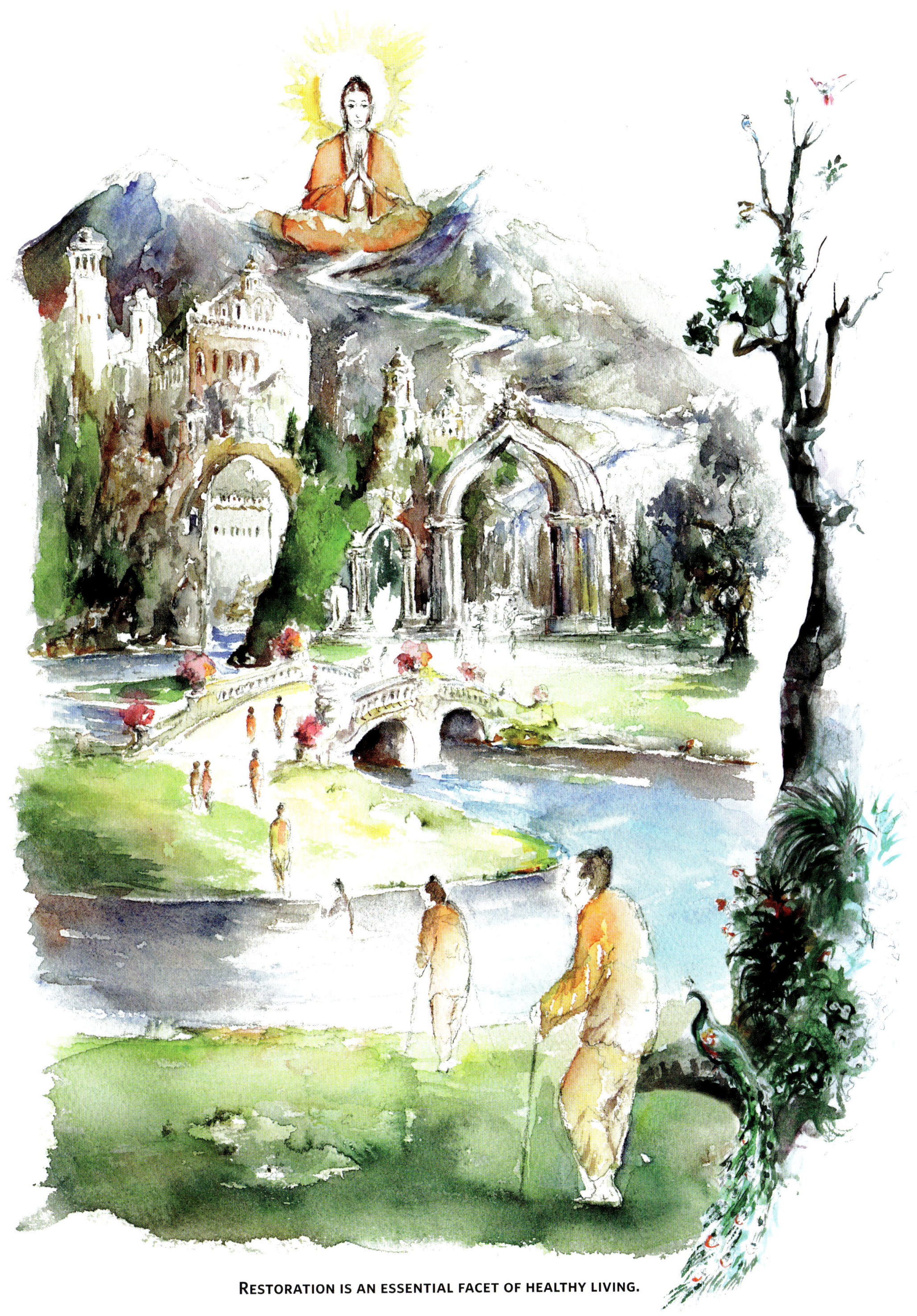

Restoration is an essential facet of healthy living.

70

Dvimukham Mudra

Gesture of Two Faces

For Facilitating Deep Relaxation

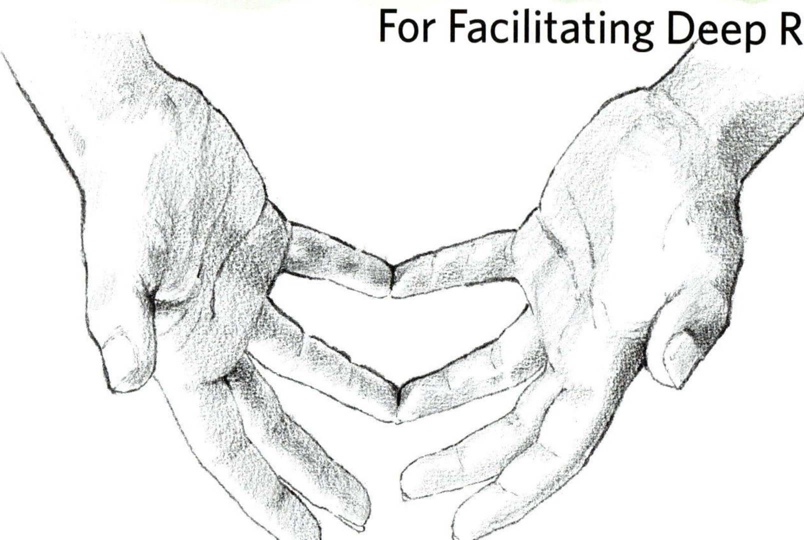

As waves of relaxation flow
Through my being,
I rest in complete serenity.

Core Quality

Deep Relaxation

Especially helpful for

- Facilitating deep relaxation.
- Supporting the health of the reproductive, urinary and eliminatory systems.
- Reducing stress and blood pressure.
- Supporting the treatment of anxiety.
- Supporting the treatment of insomnia.

Mudras with similar effects

Kanishtha, Chinmaya, Svadhisthana

Cautions

The deeply relaxing effects of this gesture may lower blood pressure; those with low blood pressure should proceed cautiously.

Instructions

1. Hold the hands facing upward below the navel.
2. Touch the tips of the little and ring fingers to the same fingers on the opposite hand.
3. Rest the hands below the navel, with the forearms resting against the abdomen or onto the lap.
4. Relax the shoulders back and down, with the spine naturally aligned.

Dvimukham means "two faces," and refers to the two sets of fingers that touch each other in this gesture. Symbolically, dvimukham refers to our own "two faces," our limited personality and our limitless true being. In order to relax deeply and completely, we need to release, at least temporarily, our concerns and worries at the level of the personality. This is challenging because the mind is constantly scanning our environment for threats and opportunities. Through cultivating relaxation consciously and taking time to relax regularly, we gradually release this constant vigilance, allowing restoration to become an essential facet of our daily activities. As we learn to relax more deeply, we gradually attune to our essential being that is inherently at ease, allowing us to experience deep relaxation as a homecoming.

Dvimukham mudra dramatically slows the breath, directing it down into the pelvis and lower abdomen, naturally activating the relaxation response. This gesture also lengthens the exhalation, further deepening our level of relaxation, thereby reducing stress and lowering blood pressure. The abdominal breathing cultivated by this gesture creates a massaging effect in the lower abdomen that enhances circulation to the reproductive, urinary and eliminatory systems, supporting their optimal functioning. The deeply relaxing effects of this mudra support the treatment of anxiety and all conditions in which stress is a factor. This gesture and the accompanying Guided Meditation are especially helpful for insomnia.

Systems Balanced:

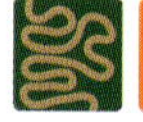 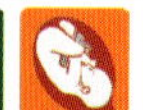 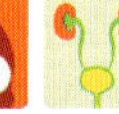 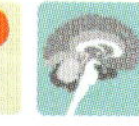

Elements Activated:

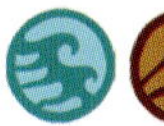 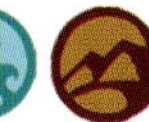

Doshas Balanced:

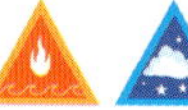

Prana Vayus Nourished:

Chakras Balanced:

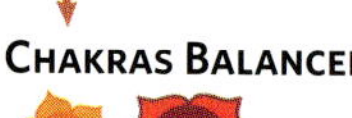

Scale from Calming to Energizing:

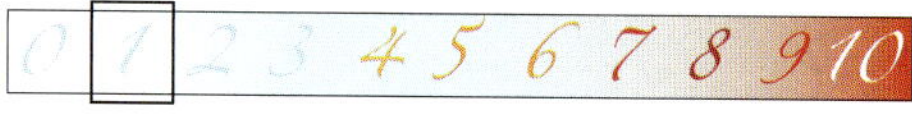

Guided Meditation: Waves of Tranquility

- As you hold Dvimukham mudra, take several natural breaths to attune to all the feelings and sensations evoked by this gesture.
- Notice how your breath is gently directed into your pelvis and lower abdomen, becoming slow and serene, allowing you to relax completely.
- To relax even more deeply, visualize yourself lying near a tranquil sea with gentle waves flowing softly, creating a soothing sound reflected in your rhythmic breathing.
- Now, these gentle waves of relaxation and ease flow up from this sea, caressing each area of your body individually, beginning with your lower extremities.
- With your next inhaling breath, sense soft waves of relaxation and ease bathing your feet and legs, and as you exhale, allow all tension from these areas to be naturally released.
- Take several breaths to experience the complete comfort of your soft, tranquil sea bathing your lower extremities.
- With your next inhalation, soft waves of relaxation bathe your pelvis, abdomen, low and mid back. As you exhale, all tension is released down and out through the soles of your feet.
- Take several breaths to rest in the growing relaxation and ease that encompass your entire lower body.
- Waves of relaxation and ease now flow gently upward with your inhaling breath to bathe your chest and upper back. As you exhale, a current of release carries all tension down and out of your body.
- Take several breaths to sense the comfort of your soft, tranquil sea bathing your body from your chest down to the soles of your feet.
- With your next inhalation, soft undulations flow up into your fingers and hands, all the way to your shoulders. As you exhale, sense all tension being released from your upper extremities,
- For your next few cycles of breath, sense the area from your shoulders, all the way to your feet, completely bathed in tranquility.
- Now, as you rest in the comfort of your soft, tranquil sea, sense your neck, head and senses relax naturally, allowing your forehead, eyes, jaw and mouth to become completely calm and serene.
- With your entire body relaxed and at ease, take all the time you need to allow your mind to rest completely within your soft, warm sea of tranquility.
- Affirm your absolute relaxation, repeating the following three times, aloud or silently: **"Bathed in gentle waves of comfort and ease, my entire being relaxes completely."**
- Slowly release the gesture, taking several breaths to rest in your tranquil sea of serenity.
- When you are ready, open your eyes, returning slowly and gently, bringing greater tranquility into all of your activities.

Annamaya kosha (physical body)

• Directs breath and awareness into the pelvis and lower abdomen, creating a massaging effect that enhances circulation to the reproductive, urinary and eliminatory systems.
• Cultivates slow abdominal breathing, with a focus on the lengthened exhalation, which facilitates relaxation and stress reduction, thereby lowering blood pressure.
• The calming effects of this gesture are helpful for anxiety.
• The relaxing effects are generally helpful for Pitta and Vata imbalances.

Pranamaya kosha (energy body)

• Activates Apana vayu, the downward moving current of energy.
• Opens and balances the first and second chakras, centers of safety and self-nourishment.

Manomaya kosha (psycho-emotional body)

• Calms the mind and instills a sense of inner peace.

Vijnanamaya kosha (wisdom body)

• As we relax more completely, we are able to glimpse the inherent serenity of our true being more easily.

Anandamaya kosha (bliss body)

• With deeper relaxation, inner silence, deep peace and well-being arise naturally.

71

Kurma Mudra

Gesture of the Tortoise

For Restoring the Senses

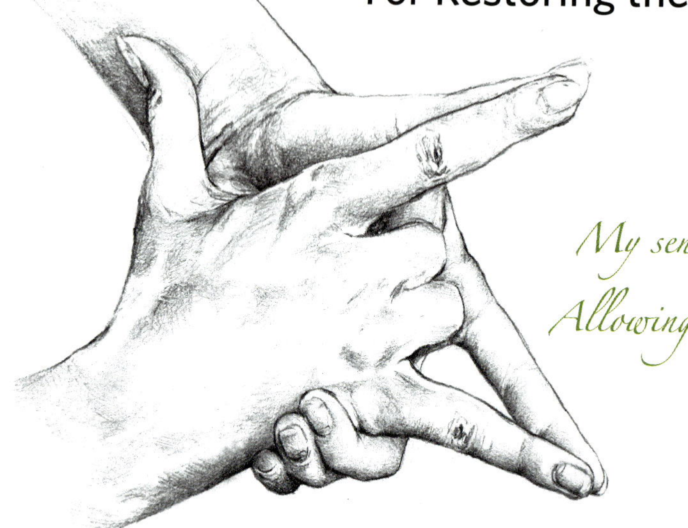

My senses rest inward, restored completely,
Allowing me to live with clarity and vitality.

Core Quality

Reducing Sensory Overload

Especially helpful for

- Supporting the senses in turning inward, reducing sensory overload.
- Reducing stress and blood pressure.

Mudras with similar effects

Shankha, Svadhisthana, Gupta, Ishvara

Cautions

For those with discomfort in the hands, Ishvara mudra is a good alternative.

Instructions

1. Curl the middle and ring fingers of the right hand into the right palm.
2. Place your right hand, palm down onto the palm of the left hand.
3. Place the extended right thumb onto the middle of the left wrist.
4. Join the pad of the right index finger to the pad of the left thumb.
5. Join the pad of the right little finger to the pad of the left index finger.
6. Wrap the middle, ring and little fingers of the left hand around the outer edge of the right hand.
7. Rest the wrists below the navel or on the lap, with the shoulders relaxed and the spine naturally aligned.

Kurma means "turtle," and Kurma mudra evokes several of the turtle's qualities that cultivate restoration and healing. The turtle is a master of conserving energy with one of the longest life spans in the animal kingdom. This longevity is partly due to its slow breathing. Kurma mudra cultivates this same slow breathing and conservation of energy. As our breath rate is decreased, our body and mind enter a state of deep restoration, almost as if going into hibernation. The turtle withdraws into its shell both for safety and restoration, and Kurma mudra produces a similar effect by naturally drawing our senses inward. This restoration is especially important for the brain and nervous system, which normally experience almost constant stimulus. As the senses rest, the mind and emotions become calm and serene, further supporting the process of restoration and healing.

Kurma mudra directs breath, awareness and energy into the pelvis and lower abdomen, eliciting the relaxation response, which naturally reduces heart rate and blood pressure. This gesture also lengthens the pauses between breaths, optimizing the absorption of oxygen and nutrients, further enhancing restoration. At a subtle level, the lengthened pauses between breaths allow *prana*, the life force energy, to be absorbed completely, thereby supporting restoration and healing. These lengthened pauses also instill a sense of inner silence, allowing us to attune to the inherent serenity of our true being. The deeply relaxing effects of Kurma mudra, together with the withdrawal of the senses, cultivate an experience of entering an inner sanctuary of restoration and healing, allowing us to return to our activities fully renewed.

Systems Balanced:

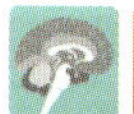
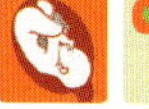
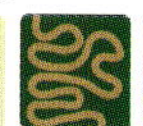
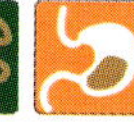
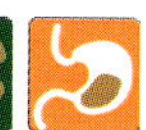
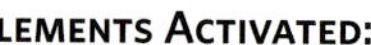

Elements Activated:

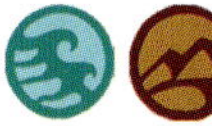
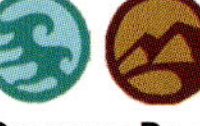

Doshas Balanced:

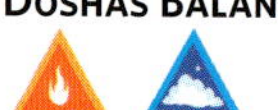

Prana Vayus Nourished:

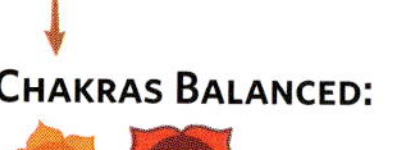

Chakras Balanced:

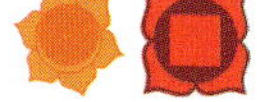

Scale from Calming to Energizing:

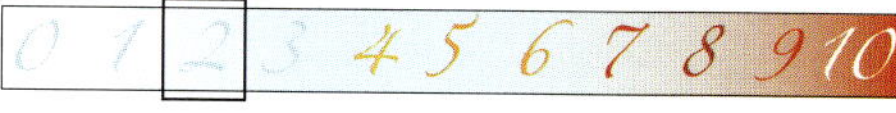

Guided Meditation: Restoring the Senses

- As you hold Kurma mudra, take several natural breaths to attune to all the feelings and sensations evoked by this gesture.
- Notice how your breath is gently directed into your pelvis and the base of your body, becoming smooth and deep, allowing you to relax completely.
- As you relax more deeply, you invite each of your senses to turn inward naturally, entering an inner sanctuary of restoration and healing.
- Begin by inviting your nose and sinus passages to relax deeply, taking several breaths to allow your sense of smell to be restored completely.
- Now, soften your throat, tongue, mouth and jaw, inviting your sense of taste to enter your sanctuary of restoration and healing, taking several breaths to savor the nourishment of your inner being.
- Your sense of sight now turns inward, taking several breaths to allow your eyes to be bathed in timeless healing, restoring them completely.
- Now, your sense of touch enters your sanctuary, taking several breaths to sense the nourishing embrace of your own inner being as it envelops you with healing energy.
- Finally, invite your sense of hearing to turn inward, taking several breaths to soften your outer and inner ears, resting completely in the silence of your inner sanctuary.
- As your senses rest deeply within your inner sanctuary, thoughts become slower, lighter and more serene, allowing all the dimensions of your being to be restored and healed completely.
- Affirm your inner healing as you repeat the following three times, aloud or silently: **"Resting in my inner sanctuary, I experience complete restoration and healing."**
- Slowly release the gesture, taking several breaths to allow your senses to completely rest.
- When you are ready, open your eyes, returning slowly and gently, restored completely within your sanctuary of inner healing.

Annamaya kosha (physical body)

• Directs breath and awareness to the pelvis and lower abdomen, creating a massaging effect that enhances circulation to the reproductive, urinary, eliminatory and digestive systems.
• Lengthens the exhalation, naturally reducing stress while cultivating deep rest for the nervous system and senses.
• The restorative effects of this gesture are generally helpful for Pitta and Vata imbalances.

Pranamaya kosha (energy body)

• Activates Apana vayu, the downward moving current of energy.
• Opens and balances the first and second chakras, centers of safety and self-nourishment.

Manomaya kosha (psycho-emotional body)

• Cultivates calm and inner silence.

Vijnanamaya kosha (wisdom body)

• Supports us in releasing the weight of the past and the expectations of the future, allowing us to live more fully in the present moment.

Anandamaya kosha (bliss body)

• As we rest in the calm depths of our being, we experience inner silence and timelessness.

72 PRANIDHANA MUDRA

Gesture of Surrender

For Learning to Let Go

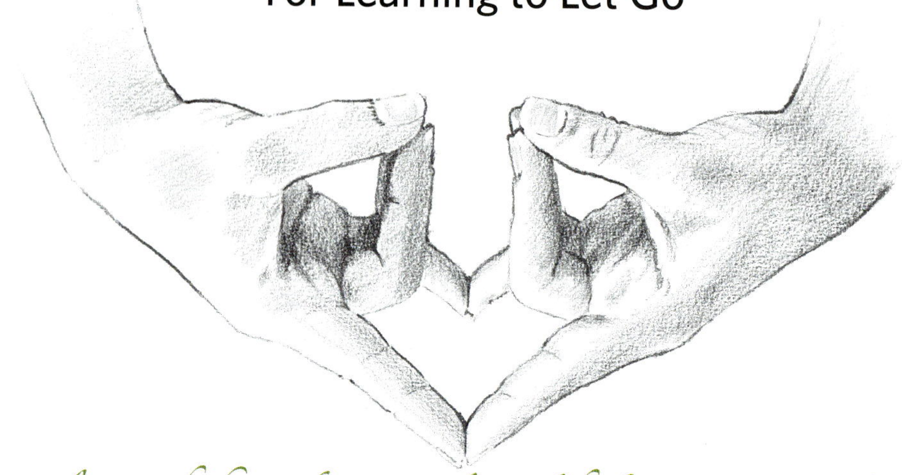

As I let go of the need to control, my life becomes an effortless flow.

CORE QUALITY

Letting Go

ESPECIALLY HELPFUL FOR

- Letting go of attachments.
- Releasing tension from the body.
- Supporting the health of the eliminatory, urinary and reproductive systems.
- Reducing stress and blood pressure.

MUDRAS WITH SIMILAR EFFECTS

Apana, Apanayana, Prajna Prana Kriya

CAUTIONS

The deeply relaxing effects of this gesture may lower blood pressure; those with low blood pressure should proceed cautiously.

INSTRUCTIONS

1. Touch the tips of the thumbs to the tips of the middle and ring fingers of the same hand.
2. Extend the index and little fingers.
3. Bring the tips of the extended little and index fingers together.
4. Hold the gesture below the navel or rest the wrists onto the thighs.
5. Relax the shoulders back and down, with the elbows held slightly away from the body and the spine naturally aligned.

Pranidhana means "surrender," and refers to letting go of all the binding attachments and beliefs that keep us from living with lightness and ease. Surrender is a process that occurs gradually, beginning by learning to recognize and release tension from the physical body. As we sense greater lightness and ease within our bodies, we naturally begin to let go of all we no longer need within the more subtle dimensions of our being, including our thoughts, feelings and beliefs. Through this gradual process of release, we eventually come to see that by letting go we are not actually losing anything, but rather gaining inner peace and the ability to appreciate life more completely. With greater inner peace, we naturally attune to our essential being, inherently whole and complete, with no need to possess or control anything.

Pranidhana mudra directs breath, awareness and energy into the pelvis and the base of the body, dramatically slowing the breath and lengthening the exhalation, cultivating a sense of deep release and relaxation. As we relax more deeply, this gesture naturally enhances our sensitivity to both our physical and subtle bodies, allowing us to perceive the very first seeds of imbalance before they manifest as dis-ease. Pranidhana mudra creates a massaging effect in the pelvis and the base of the body, supporting the health of the eliminatory, urinary and reproductive systems. This gesture also instills a sense of letting go within the mind and emotions, allowing us to release concerns and worries more easily and to appreciate each moment of life more completely.

SYSTEMS BALANCED:

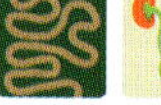  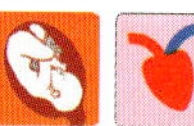

ELEMENTS ACTIVATED:

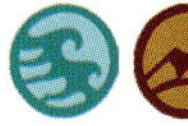 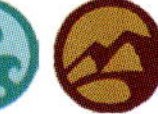

DOSHAS BALANCED:

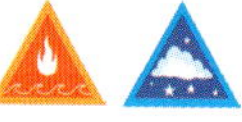

PRANA VAYUS NOURISHED:

CHAKRAS BALANCED:

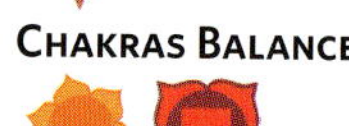

SCALE FROM CALMING TO ENERGIZING:

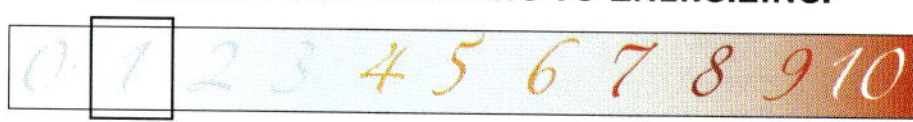

Guided Meditation: Learning to Let Go

- As you hold Pranidhana mudra, take several natural breaths to attune to all the feelings and sensations evoked by this gesture.
- Notice how your exhaling breath is naturally lengthened and directed down toward the base of your body, cultivating a sense of release that allows you to relax more deeply.
- Take several breaths to attune to this growing sense of release, a feeling that you can let go more easily of all that no longer supports your journey.
- In order to deepen your sense of release, begin by experiencing tension in your physical being, gently contracting all of your muscles from your head down to your feet.
- Now, slowly begin to release, starting with your legs and feet and continuing part by part, allowing you to experience greater relaxation and ease throughout your entire being.
- With greater relaxation and ease, take some time to sense how your breath naturally flows more smoothly and freely.
- With body and breath more at ease, you envision greater relaxation and release in all of your activities.
- Begin by envisioning yourself releasing the need to be constantly doing and achieving, especially in the moments you have set aside for relaxing.
- In the space created by this release, take several breaths to sense yourself appreciating the simple things, welcoming each moment as an opportunity to live fully and joyfully.
- Living with greater ease, you naturally let go of the need to judge yourself so harshly, softening self-criticism, allowing all aspects of your being to coexist in greater harmony.
- Embracing yourself more easily, you release the need to control others or judge them so critically, allowing each being to travel their own journey while you focus on your own process of transformation and learning.
- With greater acceptance of yourself and others, you naturally attune more deeply to your own inner being, surrendering to life, allowing its inherent wisdom to guide your journey.
- Guided by life's own inner stream, its changing cycles and seasons no longer affect your essential equanimity, allowing you to live with greater harmony.
- Affirm your ability to release by repeating the following three times, aloud or silently: **"As I learn to let go more easily, I naturally live with greater ease and harmony."**
- Slowly release the gesture, taking several breaths to sense the lightness and ease that come from complete release.
- When you are ready, open your eyes, returning slowly and gently, with a greater sense of release in all dimensions of your being.

Annamaya kosha (physical body)

- **Directs breath and awareness into the pelvis and base of the body, creating a massaging effect that enhances circulation to the eliminatory, urinary and reproductive systems.**
- **Cultivates slow abdominal breathing while lengthening the exhaling breath, reducing stress and blood pressure.**
- **The deep calm cultivated by this gesture may be helpful for anxiety.**
- **The centering effects of this gesture are generally helpful for Vata imbalance.**
- **The calming effects are generally helpful for Pitta imbalance.**

Pranamaya kosha (energy body)

- **Activates Apana vayu, the downward moving current of energy.**
- **Opens and balances the first and second chakras, centers of safety and self-nourishment.**

Manomaya kosha (psycho-emotional body)

- **Cultivates deep calm and a sense of letting go.**

Vijnanamaya kosha (wisdom body)

- **As we learn to let go more easily, we naturally release limiting beliefs, attuning to our inner wisdom, rather than the conditioned patterns of the personality.**

Anandamaya kosha (bliss body)

- **With a greater sense of release, sensations of apprecia-tion, wholeness and deep inner peace arise naturally.**

73

Ushas Mudra

Gesture of the Dawn

For Opening to New Possibilities

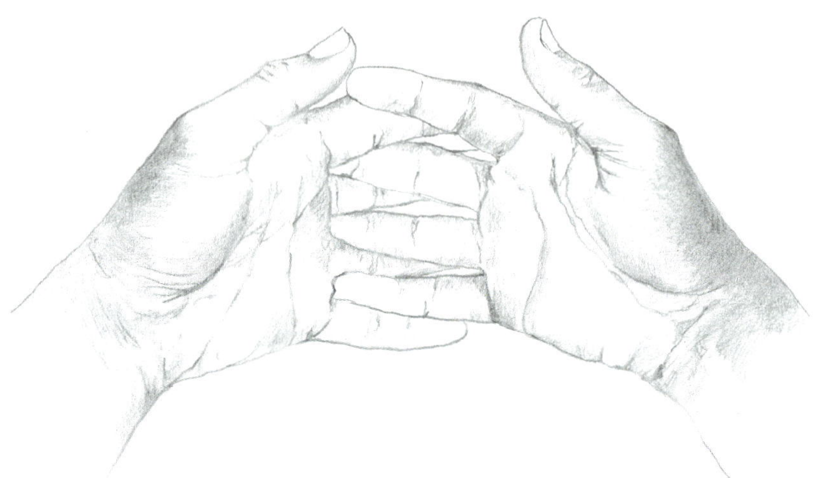

I greet each new day as a mystery
To be lived fully and joyfully.

Core Quality

Opening to New Possibilities

Especially helpful for

- Cultivating more positive attitudes that allow us to manifest all of our possibilities.
- Supporting us in living in the present moment with curiosity and a sense of mystery.

Mudras with similar effects

Padma, Hansi, Vajrapradama, Vajra, Garuda

Cautions

None

Instructions

1. Interlace the fingers loosely and rest the hands on the lap, with the palms upward.
2. The tips of the thumbs may lightly touch each other.
3. Relax the shoulders back and down, with the elbows held slightly away from the body and the spine naturally aligned.

Ushas means "dawn," and Ushas mudra supports us in welcoming each day enthusiastically as a field of infinite possibilities. As we embrace each day more openly with fewer expectations of how things should be, stress and tension are reduced naturally. By welcoming each day more positively, we release the judgments we hold about ourselves and others, allowing us to celebrate life as it is, rather than complaining about how you would like it to be. When we embrace each new day as a field of appreciation and learning, we are able to live in the present moment more completely. With greater presence and appreciation, all of our talents and possibilities unfold naturally, creating a cycle of well-being, vitality and creativity.

Ushas mudra directs breath, awareness and energy to the entire torso, facilitating Full Yogic Breathing, which naturally instills a sense of harmony. This gesture balances the inhalation and exhalation and activates the flow of breath through both nostrils evenly, cultivating greater equanimity, supporting us in welcoming life more positively. The combination of harmonious breathing and a greater sense of equanimity helps to establish a balance of will and surrender in all of our activities. This balance allows us to engage life completely while recognizing that the final results of our actions are often beyond our personal control. Ushas mudra helps to clear the mind, reducing negative thinking, allowing us to meet new projects and activities with a sense of openness and curiosity. With greater harmony, enthusiasm and clarity, we naturally unfold all of our possibilities while experiencing deep appreciation for each moment of living.

Systems Balanced:

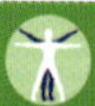

Elements Activated:

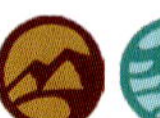
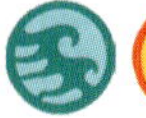

Doshas Balanced:

Prana Vayus Nourished:

Chakras Balanced:

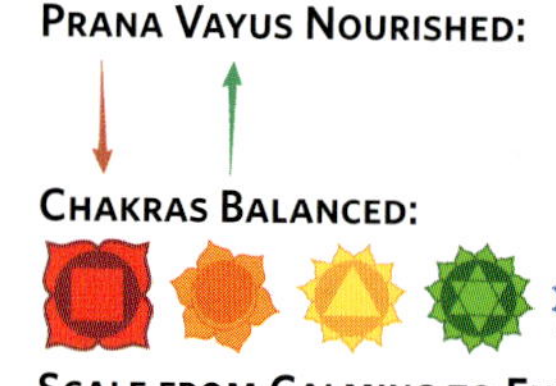

Scale from Calming to Energizing:

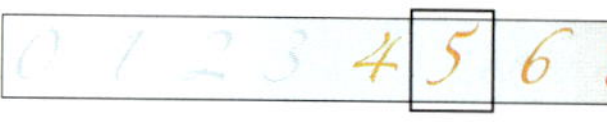

Guided Meditation: Dawn of a New Day

- As you hold Ushas mudra, take several natural breaths to attune to all the feelings and sensations awakened by this gesture.
- Notice how your breath flows smoothly throughout your entire torso, from the base of your body all the way up to the top of your chest.
- Sense how each inhalation cultivates a sense of enthusiasm and uplifting energy, while each exhalation instills a sense of serenity, allowing you to relax completely.
- This balance of enthusiasm and serenity allows you to greet each day as a unique opportunity to unfold all of your talents and possibilities.
- To cultivate this more open way of seeing, visualize yourself in the predawn, ready to embrace the new day with fresh eyes, as if seeing life for the very first time.
- With the sun's first rays, take several breaths to visualize the sky, transformed into a watercolor of orange and gold, a canvas upon which all of your possibilities naturally unfold.
- The background of this watercolor is a clear blue sky, a reflection of your own openness and receptivity, inspiring you to paint your life canvas creatively.
- As the sun rises slowly, its soft light bathes each part of your body progressively, allowing you to absorb the brilliance of this new dawning day.
- Begin by taking several breaths to sense the sun's rays softly illuminating your face, allowing you to see life in fresh, new ways.
- Now, the rising sun gently warms your throat and neck, as you take some time to sense a growing clarity in which you communicate positively and authentically.
- Infused with clarity, sense the dawning rays bathing your shoulders and chest, taking several breaths to fill your heart with uplifting energy and your lungs with vitality.
- Your arms and hands now receive the dawn's growing light, enhancing your sensitivity, allowing you to touch and be touched by other beings in a natural balance of giving and receiving.
- As the sun rises higher, its rays gently warm your solar plexus, awakening the inherent self-esteem that allows you to overcome all challenges along your journey.
- As the sun's full strength illuminates your pelvis, legs and feet, you take several breaths to sense the support of the earth beneath, allowing you to step forward in life confidently.
- Now, the sun's full rays burn the early morning mist away, reflecting your openness and clarity, allowing you to fully appreciate the miracle of this new day.
- With openness and clarity, repeat the following three times, aloud or silently: **"I receive each new day openly and enthusiastically as a field of infinite possibilities."**
- Slowly release the gesture, taking several breaths to sense your infinite possibilities.
- When you are ready, open your eyes, returning slowly and gently, welcoming each new day as a marvelous mystery.

Annamaya kosha (physical body)

• Directs breath and awareness to the entire front of the torso, creating a massaging effect that enhances circulation to all body systems.
• Cultivates a balance of relaxation and alertness, which supports the optimal functioning of the nervous system.
• The harmonizing effects of this gesture are generally helpful for Vata imbalance.
• The soothing effects are generally helpful for Pitta imbalance.
• The cultivation of new ways of seeing is generally helpful for Kapha imbalance.

Pranamaya kosha (energy body)

• Balances Prana and Apana vayus, the upward and downward moving currents of energy.
• Opens and balances the first through fifth chakras.

Manomaya kosha (psycho-emotional body)

• Cultivates calm, mental clarity and centering, which support us in viewing life more positively.

Vijnanamaya kosha (wisdom body)

• As the mind becomes calm and clear, we rest more easily in our true being, opening to life as a field of possibilities.

Anandamaya kosha (bliss body)

• As we welcome each day more openly, we naturally experience the freedom of our true being.

Chapter Fourteen

Invoking Timeless Wisdom

MUDRAS FOR THE EIGHT LIMBS

The *Yoga Sutras of Patanjali,* which is approximately two thousand years old, codifies the essential principles of Yoga in 196 short aphorisms, called *sutras*. The Yoga Sutras outlines the vision of Yoga, its practices and techniques, as well as the experiences that arise along our journey, culminating in an experience of spiritual freedom, called *kaivalya*. The Eight Limbs of Yoga, *Ashtanga Yoga*, are often considered to be the heart of the Yoga Sutras, forming the foundation for the study and practice of Yoga. The Eight Limbs outline a complete path of spiritual transformation, beginning with ethical values; followed by the integration of body and breath; preparing us for progressively deeper states of meditation, leading to an experience of unity, called *Samadhi*.

The Eight Limbs can be described as the "Tree of Yoga." The ethical precepts, the *Yamas*, form the roots; the *Niyamas*, the inner values, form the trunk, providing support. *Asana*, steady and comfortable posture, represents the strong supporting branches. *Pranayama*, breathing techniques, represents the leaves, opening to receive life force energy. *Pratyahara*, turning the senses inward, represents the buds, safeguarding the tree's vital energy so that it eventually blossoms fully. *Dharana*, concentration, is all of the tree's energy focused one-pointedly to prepare for blossoming. *Dhyana*, meditation, is the tree's fragrant flowering while *Samadhi* represents the fruit of Yoga as unity.

The Yamas - Ethical Precepts

Mudra	Yamas
Kapota	Ahimsa Non-violence
Samputa	Satya Truthfulness
Hastaphula	Asteya Non-stealing
Kubera	Brahmacharya Conservation of Energy
Pushpanjali	Aparigraha Non-grasping

The Niyamas - Spiritual Observances

Mudra	Niyamas
Vishuddha	Shaucha Purity
Chaturmukham	Santosha Contentment
Mushtikam	Tapas Spiritual Discipline
Sakshi	Svadhyaya Self-study
Chin	Ishvara Pranidhana Surrender to the Divine

The Other Limbs Culminating in Samadhi

Mudra	Limbs
Murti	Asana Steady & Comfortable Posture
Dirgha Svara	Pranayama Expansion of the Life Force
Ishvara	Pratyahara Withdrawal of the Senses
Abhisheka	Dharana One-pointed Concentration
Dharmadhatu	Dhyana Meditation
Mandala	Samadhi Spiritual Union

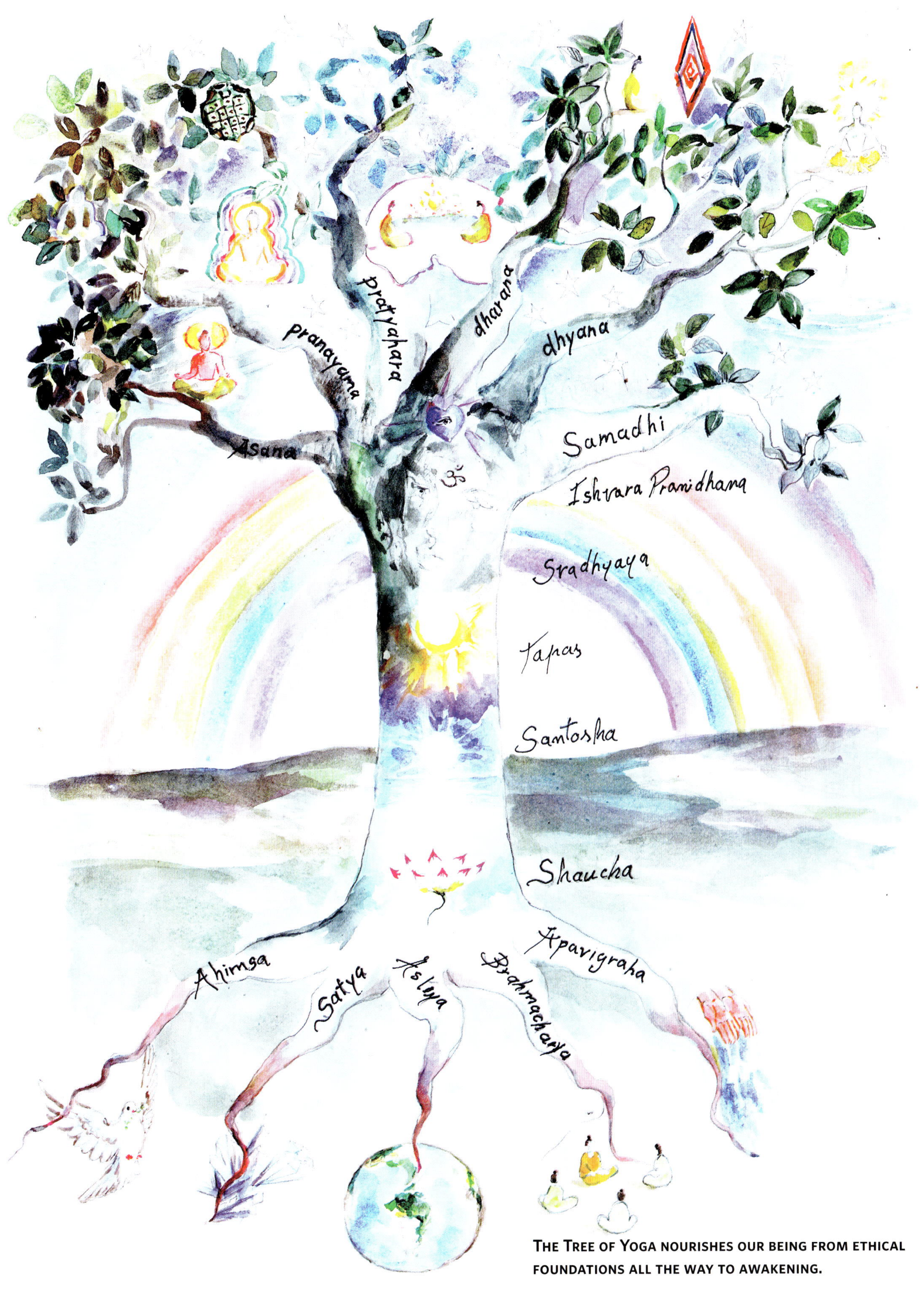

The Tree of Yoga nourishes our being from ethical foundations all the way to awakening.

74

Kapota Mudra

Gesture of the Dove

For Cultivating Non-Violence - Ahimsa

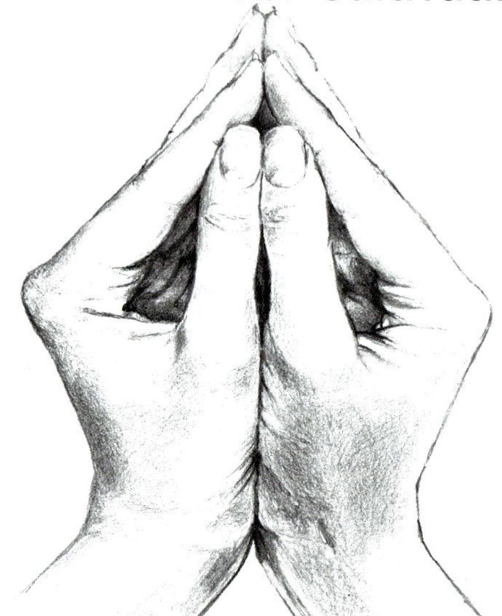

Practicing non-violence at all levels of being, I experience complete inner peace.

Core Quality
Non-violence

Especially helpful for
- Cultivating non-violence and inner peace at all levels of being.
- Supporting the health of the immune system.
- Cultivating self-care and self-healing.
- Facilitating introspection and inner listening.

Mudras with similar effects
Hridaya, Padma, Purna Hridaya, Karuna

Cautions
None

Instructions:
1. Hold the hands in prayer position, in front of the heart, with the hands slightly away from the body.
2. Keep the fingers and the base of the palms together while opening the knuckles away from each other, creating an open space between the palms, resembling a dove's open breast.
3. Relax the shoulders back and down, with the elbows held slightly away from the body and the spine naturally aligned.

Ahimsa, which means "non-violence," is the foundation of the five *Yamas*, the universal ethical values. The practice of Ahimsa encompasses all levels of our being, beginning with our own bodies by adopting a healthy diet and lifestyle, along with adequate rest and stress management. As we embrace our own bodies with greater care and kindness, we naturally expand Ahimsa to include our thoughts and feelings by welcoming them without judging ourselves so harshly. As we practice non-violence toward our bodies and minds, we experience a greater sense of wholeness and inner peace, reducing the need to control and compete, thereby supporting us in practicing non-violence toward other beings. As we expand our vow of Ahimsa to all beings, we recognize our essential unity with all of creation, allowing peacefulness to infuse all of our interactions and activities.

Kapota means "dove," the symbol of peace, and Kapota mudra awakens us to the inherent peace of our own inner being. This gesture directs breath, awareness and energy to the center of the chest, instilling a feeling that we are entering an inner sanctuary of complete comfort and safety. Within this sanctuary, we can embrace and honor our feelings more easily, processing them internally with compassion, rather than acting them out unconsciously. Kapota mudra also cultivates a sense of connectedness, enhancing our experience of unity, allowing acceptance and communion to unfold as the foundation of non-violence. This gesture also directs awareness and breath to the area of the thymus gland, located in the upper chest, supporting the health of the immune system.

Systems Balanced:

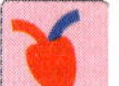 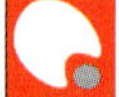

Elements Activated:

Doshas Balanced:

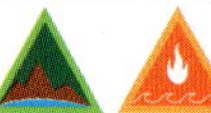 

Prana Vayus Nourished:

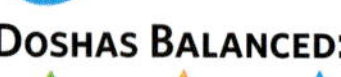

Chakras Balanced:

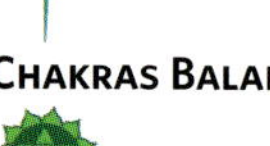

Scale from Calming to Energizing:

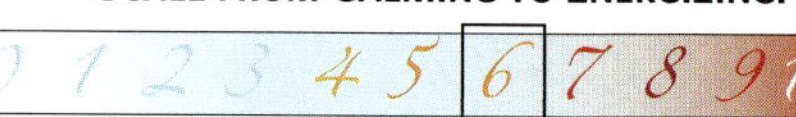

Guided Meditation: A Vow of Peace

- As you hold Kapota mudra, take several natural breaths to attune to all the feelings and sensations evoked by this gesture.
- Notice how your breath is gently directed into your heart center, instilling a sense of inner peace that allows you to rest deeply.
- Take several breaths to rest within your heart, visualizing there a white dove with open wings as a symbol of complete non-violence at all levels of your being.
- Begin by invoking peace at the level of your body, creating an intention to listen to its messages sensitively, naturally guiding you toward greater self-care and self-healing.
- Attune to the white dove within your heart as you make a vow of peace toward your own physical being, chanting silently: "Om Shantih, Shantih, Shantih; Peace, Peace, Peace."
- Now, expand your vow of peace to encompass your own thoughts and feelings, creating an intention to embrace them, without judging yourself so harshly.
- Through heartfelt welcoming, challenging thoughts and feelings are gradually softened and released, allowing you to live with greater self-acceptance and inner peace.
- Attune to the white dove within your heart as you expand your vow of peace to include your psycho-emotional being, chanting silently: "Om Shantih, Shantih, Shantih."
- As your mind and body are immersed in peace, expand your vow of Ahimsa to include your family, friends and community, creating an intention to practice loving kindness and generosity.
- Envision yourself in a circle of cooperation and harmony, joining hands in recognition of the essential unity that allows all to live more peacefully.
- Attune to the white dove within your heart as you expand your vow of peace to include all who share your journey, chanting silently: "Om Shantih, Shantih, Shantih."
- Now, allow your vow of peace to include all of humanity, embracing all cultures, religions and creeds in the spirit of harmony.
- Take several breaths to envision yourself in an ever-expanding circle of peace that encompasses all human beings, joining hands in recognition of our essential unity.
- Attune to the white dove within your heart as you expand your vow of peace to all of humanity, chanting silently: "Om Shantih, Shantih, Shantih."
- With your vow of peace firmly established in relation to yourself and all humanity, you now expand your vow of Ahimsa to include the entire natural world and all living beings.
- Sense the entire web of life as a seamless unity, inspiring you to act consciously, honoring and caring for the natural environment as one with your own being.
- Attune to the white dove within your heart, expanding your vow of peace to encompass all beings as you chant silently: "Om Shantih, Shantih, Shantih."
- Now, take several breaths to rest in the peace of your essential being, a reflection of the oneness and unity that encompasses everything.
- Affirm the light of peace as you repeat the following three times, aloud or silently: **"My vow of complete peace allows me to live in inner and outer harmony."**
- Now, slowly release the gesture, taking several breaths to rest in complete peacefulness.
- When you are ready, open your eyes, returning slowly and gently, affirming your vow of Ahimsa at all levels of your being.

Annamaya kosha (physical body)

• Directs breath and awareness to the center of the chest, creating a massaging effect that optimizes circulation to the area of the thymus gland.
• Directs breath to the middle and upper back, massaging the area of the kidneys and adrenal glands while creating space between the thoracic vertebrae.
• The heart-opening cultivated by this gesture is generally helpful for Pitta imbalance.
• The mildly energizing effects are generally helpful for Kapha imbalance.
• The inner peace cultivated is generally helpful for Vata imbalance.

Pranamaya kosha (energy body)

• Gently activates Prana vayu, the upward moving current of energy.
• Opens and balances the fourth chakra, center of unconditional love.

Manomaya kosha (psycho-emotional body)

• Cultivates compassion and acceptance.
• Instills a sense of serenity, a feeling that the dove of peace is resting within our hearts.

Vijnanamaya kosha (wisdom body)

• Cultivates an experience of empathy that reduces the sense of separation, opening us to our essential unity.

Anandamaya kosha (bliss body)

• Awakens feelings of wholeness and compassion from within the heart center.

75

Samputa Mudra

Gesture of the Treasure Chest

For Cultivating Truthfulness - Satya

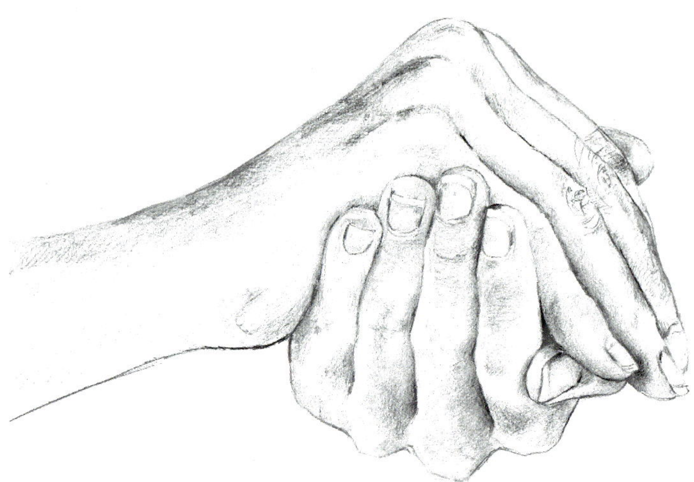

Aligned with my true being,
My thoughts, words and deeds
Reflect complete integrity.

Core Quality

Truthfulness

Especially helpful for

- Connecting to our inner voice of truth in order to communicate clearly and with integrity.
- Supporting the health of the throat and vocal cords.
- Optimizing the health of the thyroid gland, supporting balanced metabolism.
- Receiving guidance for the life journey.

Mudras with similar effects

Garuda, Vishuddha, Shunya, Uttarabodhi

Cautions

None

Instructions

1. Hold the left hand slightly cupped, facing upward, at the level of the navel.
2. Place the right hand, also slightly cupped, over the left so that the right fingers rest on the outer border of the left thumb, creating a hollow space within the hands.
3. Relax the shoulders back and down, with the forearms resting against the sides of the abdomen with the spine naturally aligned.

Satya means "truth," and refers to truthfulness in all of our communications. In order to practice truthfulness, we must first develop the ability to discern what "truth" is. This involves attuning to our authentic being beyond the conditioning of the personality. Until we are able to listen to the voice of our true being, our words may reflect what we believe, but our beliefs are usually just a reflection of our lens of conditioning. As we align with our authentic being, less identified with the subjective likes and dislikes of the personality, we are able to communicate more clearly and authentically. Our communication should also respect *Ahimsa*, non-violence, by speaking not only that which is true, but also that which will cause no harm or suffering to ourselves or others.

Samputa means "a treasure chest," and Samputa mudra awakens us to the treasure of our true inner being, instilling a natural sense of integrity, allowing us to communicate our truth more clearly. This gesture directs breath, awareness and energy to the throat, our center of spiritual purification and clear communication. It relaxes the muscles of the throat and vocal cords, supporting us in communicating easily. This mudra also invites us to turn inward to align with our authentic being, allowing us to receive wisdom and guidance beyond the conditioning of the personality. Samputa mudra cultivates a sense of inner security that supports us in communicating our inner truth clearly, even in the face of challenges and difficulties. This gesture directs breath and energy to the area of the thyroid gland, balancing metabolism.

Systems Balanced:

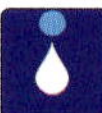

Elements Activated:

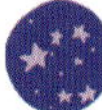

Doshas Balanced:

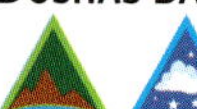

Prana Vayus Nourished:

Chakras Balanced:

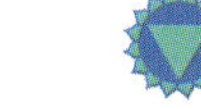

Scale from Calming to Energizing:

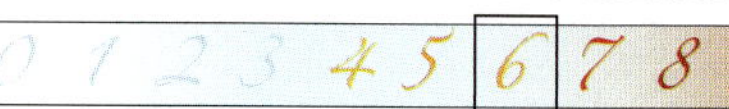

Guided Meditation: Attuning to Your Inner Truth

- As you hold Samputa mudra, take several natural breaths to attune to all the feelings and sensations evoked by this gesture.
- Notice how your breath flows gently upward into your throat center, allowing you to breathe more freely within this area of your being.
- As your breath flows more freely, take some time to attune to the subtle sound of the breath within your air pathways.
- Sense how your inhalation naturally makes the sound "SO" within your throat, and how your exhalation resonates with the sound "HAM."
- Take several breaths to listen to the sacred sound of "SO HAM," reverberating within your throat center.
- As you attune to the sound of "SO HAM," reflect on its deeper meaning, "I AM," referring to your authentic being beyond the limitations of your personality.
- As you align with your true being, you naturally hear your inner voice of truth speaking clearly, guiding your journey of transformation and awakening.
- To attune more deeply to the voice of your authentic being, take some time to reflect on a challenge that you are currently facing.
- Allow this issue to rest within your throat center, taking several breaths to reflect on how it would normally be addressed at the level of your personality.
- Now, focus on the sound of "SO HAM" within your throat center, creating a space of deep inner listening that allows wisdom to arise from within your being.
- Take several breaths to listen clearly and carefully to the messages you are receiving from the voice of your true being, allowing you to see this issue with greater clarity.
- Now, envision the wisdom you have received being integrated into all of your activities and your entire life journey.
- Attuned to your true being, repeat the following three times, aloud or silently: **"Aligned with the voice of my inner being, I communicate clearly and truthfully."**
- Slowly release the gesture, taking several breaths to rest in your essence as truthfulness.
- When you are ready, open your eyes, returning slowly and gently, aligned with your authentic being.

Annamaya kosha (physical body)

• Directs breath and awareness to the throat and neck, creating a massaging effect for the area of the thyroid gland.
• Brings breath and awareness to the vocal cords, cultivating a massaging effect that releases tension and enhances circulation to this area.
• The mildly energizing effects of this gesture are generally helpful for Kapha imbalance.
• The inner security cultivated is generally helpful for Vata imbalance.
• The ability to communicate from our true being is generally helpful for Pitta imbalance.

Pranamaya kosha (energy body)

• Gently activates Udana vayu, the uppermost current of energy.
• Opens and balances the fifth chakra, center of spiritual purification.

Manomaya kosha (psycho-emotional body)

• Draws our awareness inward, inviting self-listening and self-exploration.

Vijnanamaya kosha (wisdom body)

• As we learn to listen to our inner voice, we access the wisdom beyond words that is the language of the true Self.

Anandamaya kosha (bliss body)

• As we become sensitive to the throat area, allowing it to release and relax, feelings of bliss and limitlessness arise naturally.

76

Hastaphula Mudra

Gesture of Open Hands

For Cultivating Non-stealing - Asteya

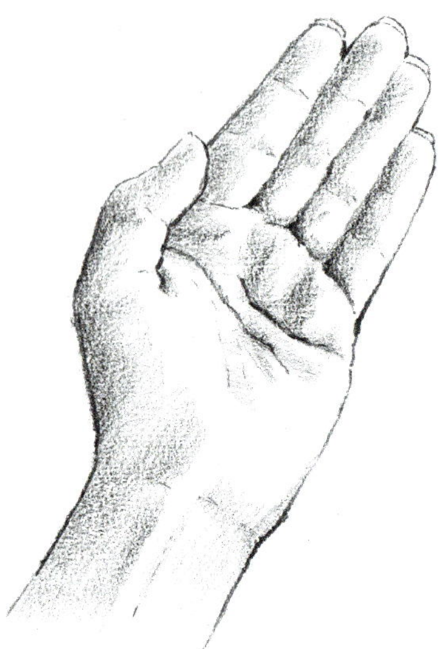

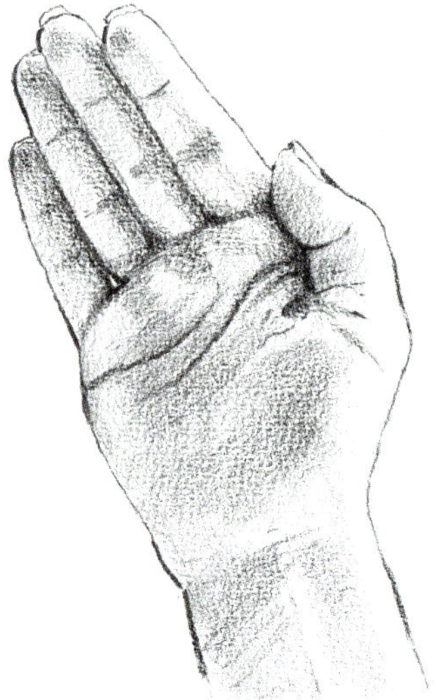

A natural fairness
In all my activities
Allows me to live
In complete harmony.

Core Quality

Non-stealing

Especially helpful for

- Cultivating balanced giving and receiving in all of our activities.
- Optimizing the functioning of the digestive, circulatory and lymphatic systems.
- Deepening our sensitivity to the presence of the life force energy.

Mudras with similar effects

Pushpanjali, Avahana, Dharma Chakra, Purna Jnanam

Cautions

None

Instructions

1. Hold the hands, slightly cupped, in front of the solar plexus, with the palms facing upward.
2. The forearms are parallel to the earth.
3. The hands pulse slightly away from each other with each inhalation, and rest back toward each other on each exhalation.
4. Relax the shoulders back and down, with the spine naturally aligned.

Asteya means "non-stealing," and refers to a natural balance of giving and receiving within all of our interactions and activities. At the most basic level, Asteya involves fairness in our material exchanges. An activity as simple as buying an article of clothing involves awareness of Asteya because goods produced in ways that violate fair exchange may carry a heavy karmic price tag. Asteya is also important within our personal relationships and in our communities, and is practiced by cultivating balanced giving and receiving in relation to material goods, affection and energy. Non-stealing also encompasses our ecological "footprint" on the planet, reminding us to use natural resources consciously in order to maintain global balance and harmony. In the deepest sense, Asteya is the recognition of the value of the life we have received by using all of our talents and possibilities for our own good, for our families and communities and for awakening to our life's deeper meaning.

Hastaphula means "open hands," and Hastaphula mudra lengthens the inhalation and exhalation evenly, evoking a natural balance of giving and receiving in all of our activities. This gesture directs the breath into the solar plexus, enhancing circulation to the digestive system. The enhanced breath in the solar plexus also creates a rhythmic movement of the diaphragm that supports the return of venous blood and lymphatic circulation. At a subtle level, Hastaphula mudra enhances our sensitivity to the life force energy, experienced as a pulsation in the hands. As we attune to our energetic being, we are able to see beyond the limitations of the personality with its likes, dislikes and perceived needs, supporting us in cultivating a balance of giving and receiving.

Systems Balanced:

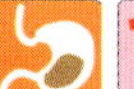 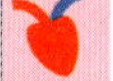 

Elements Activated:

Doshas Balanced:

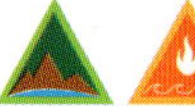  

Prana Vayus Nourished:

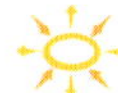

Chakras Balanced:

Scale from Calming to Energizing:

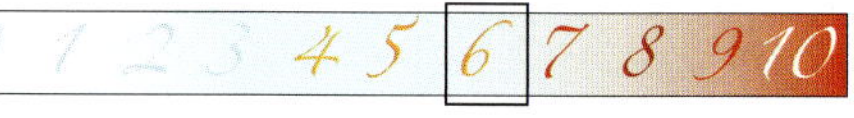

Guided Meditation: Balanced Giving and Receiving

- ॐ As you hold Hastaphula mudra, take several natural breaths to attune to all the feelings and sensations evoked by this gesture.
- ॐ Notice how your breath is gently directed into your solar plexus, allowing you to attune more deeply to your center of personal power and energy.
- ॐ With each inhalation, sense gentle warmth radiating outward from your solar plexus, and with each exhaling breath, allow this area to soften inward and rest.
- ॐ Take several breaths to sense your inhalation and exhalation lengthening evenly, cultivating a sense of balanced giving and receiving at all levels of your being.
- ॐ Begin by reflecting on your balance of giving and receiving within your financial dealings. Ask yourself if there is a natural fairness and integrity between that which you give and that which you receive.
- ॐ With your inhalation, visualize yourself receiving all you need to support your life journey, and as you exhale, sense your natural reciprocity, giving with fairness and generosity.
- ॐ Next, take several breaths to reflect on your level of balance within your relationships. Ask yourself if there is a natural fairness of giving and receiving in terms of your investment of quality time and emotional energy.
- ॐ With your inhalation, visualize the abundant love and support you receive, and as you exhale, affirm your ability to share love and friendship wholeheartedly.
- ॐ Now, take several breaths to reflect on your balance of giving and receiving within your community, sensing your level of natural fairness in relation to all those that contribute to your well-being.
- ॐ With your inhalation, open to receive the support of your community, and as you exhale, affirm your intention to reach out to serve open-heartedly, especially to those that are most in need.
- ॐ Now, sense your level of balanced giving and receiving within the entire web of life, reflecting on your level of gratitude for everything you receive in your interaction with your natural surroundings.
- ॐ With your inhalation, recognize the abundance of nature's bounty and beauty, and as you exhale, envision yourself returning the gift by consciously supporting the natural world's inherent harmony.
- ॐ Now, take some time to sense the even flow of your breathing and your natural balance of giving and receiving within all of your interactions and activities.
- ॐ Affirm your integrity, repeating the following three times, aloud or silently: **"Through balanced giving and receiving, I live in complete integrity."**
- ॐ Slowly release the gesture, taking several breaths to affirm your natural fairness.
- ॐ When you are ready, open your eyes, returning slowly and gently, affirming your ability to balance giving and receiving.

Annamaya kosha (physical body)

• Directs breath and awareness into the solar plexus, creating a massaging effect that optimizes circulation to the digestive system.
• The enhanced movement of the diaphragm assists in the return of venous blood and the circulation of fluid within the lymphatic system.
• The balancing effects of this gesture are generally helpful for Vata, Pitta and Kapha imbalances.

Pranamaya kosha (energy body)

• Gently activates the flow of Samana vayu, the horizontal current of energy.
• Softly massages and opens the third chakra, center of personal power.

Manomaya kosha (psycho-emotional body)

• Cultivates a natural balance of giving and receiving in all of our interactions and activities.

Vijnanamaya kosha (wisdom body)

• With greater awareness of the balance of giving and receiving, we naturally align with the integrity of our true being.

Anandamaya kosha (bliss body)

• As we sense greater balance, feelings of centering and equanimity arise naturally.

77

Kubera Mudra

Gesture of the Lord of Wealth

For Cultivating Conservation of Energy - Brahmacharya

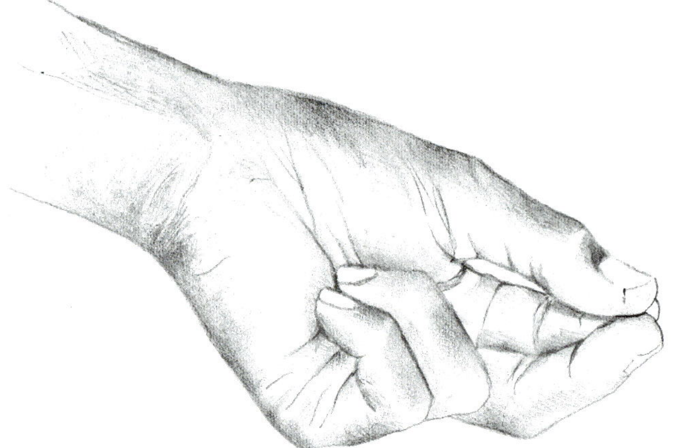

Through conscious conservation of energy,
I experience abundant vitality
Along my spiritual journey.

Core Quality

Conservation of Energy

Especially helpful for

- Cultivating conservation of energy within all dimensions of being.
- Optimizing physical digestion.
- Enhancing circulation to the mid back, kidneys and adrenal glands.
- Digesting life experiences easily with less resentment and worry.

Mudras with similar effects

Pushan, Surya, Vajra

Cautions

None

Instructions

1. Close the hands into fists, with the nails tucked into the crease of the palms and the thumbs outside.
2. Extend the index and middle fingers.
3. Touch the tips of the index and middle fingers to the tips of the thumbs of the same hand.
4. Rest the backs of the hands on the thighs or knees or hold them at the level of the solar plexus, with the forearms parallel to the earth.
5. Relax the shoulders back and down, with the spine naturally aligned.

Brahmacharya is the "conservation of our life force energy," allowing us to unfold all of our possibilities, especially those related to spiritual awakening. Conservation of energy is cultivated at the level of the body by balancing rest and activity and by caring for ourselves optimally. Conservation of energy is also essential at the level of our thoughts and feelings because constant stress, worry and negativity drain us mentally and emotionally, limiting our ability to unfold our possibilities. Brahmacharya is especially important in intimate relationships, which can consume large amounts of energy with doubt, worry, guilt, jealousy or imbalanced sexual activity. As we practice conservation of energy at all levels of being, we experience abundant vitality for supporting our spiritual journey.

Kubera is the "deity of wealth," and Kubera mudra directs breath, awareness and energy into the solar plexus, our center of personal power, increasing circulation to the digestive system and enhancing vitality. This gesture also directs breath to the mid back, kidneys and adrenal glands, cultivating a massaging effect that releases tension from these areas. This mudra also supports psycho-emotional digestion, allowing us to receive life's lessons, process them completely and release any accumulated emotions and memories. With our psycho-emotional digestion more complete, we journey with greater energy and vitality. Kubera mudra also cultivates the self-esteem, courage and determination to overcome obstacles along the spiritual journey, supporting us in releasing habits and beliefs that drain our energy.

Systems Balanced:

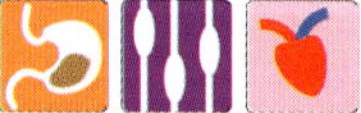

Elements Activated:

Doshas Balanced:

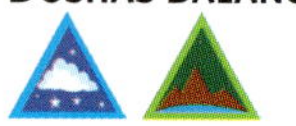

Prana Vayus Nourished:

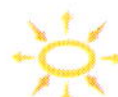

Chakras Balanced:

Scale from Calming to Energizing:

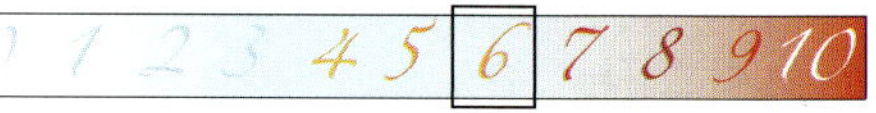

Guided Meditation: Conserving Life Force Energy

ॐ As you hold Kubera mudra, take several natural breaths to attune to all the feelings and sensations evoked by this gesture.

ॐ Notice how your breath is gently directed into your solar plexus, allowing you to attune more deeply with your center of vital energy.

ॐ As you exhale, sense vital energy concentrated in this area, and as you inhale, sense the life force naturally radiating outward.

ॐ As you become more sensitive to your center of vitality, take some time to reflect on the importance of conserving vital energy within all dimensions of your being.

ॐ Begin by reflecting on your use of energy in your daily routine, asking yourself if there is a healthy balance of rest and activity from the time you wake until you sleep.

ॐ With your next exhalation, connect to your solar plexus, and as you inhale, allow balanced energy to radiate outward, providing vitality for all of your daily activities.

ॐ Next, reflect on your use of energy in relation to your career, asking yourself if your needs for success and achievement are producing a level of stress that drains your vitality.

ॐ With your next exhalation, attune to your source of vitality, and as you inhale, sense inherent self-esteem radiating throughout your being, allowing you to unfold all of your talents and possibilities while conserving your life force energy.

ॐ Now, bring awareness to your thoughts and feelings, taking some time to reflect on how much of your energy is consumed by judgment, doubt, resentment or worry.

ॐ With your next exhalation, attune to your solar plexus, and as you inhale, the light of clarity radiates throughout your being, allowing you to see the limiting thoughts, emotions and beliefs that drain your energy.

ॐ Next, reflect on your relationships, exploring whether these are a source of nourishment and vitality or if you allow them to consume your precious energy with conflict, guilt or jealousy.

ॐ With your next exhalation, attune to the center of your being, and as you inhale, affirm your conservation of energy by cultivating healthy relationships that are a source of healing and vitality.

ॐ As you deepen your ability to conserve precious life force energy at all levels of being, take several breaths to envision how you could channel this enhanced vitality toward awakening your life's deeper meaning.

ॐ Affirm conservation of energy, repeating the following three times, aloud or silently: **"As I conserve my precious energy, I naturally awaken my life's deeper meaning."**

ॐ Slowly release the gesture, taking several breaths to sense your balanced energy.

ॐ When you are ready, open your eyes, returning slowly and gently, with a greater commitment to conscious conservation of energy.

Annamaya kosha (physical body)

- **Directs breath and awareness into the solar plexus, creating a massaging effect that increases circulation to the digestive system.**
- **The enhanced movement of the diaphragm assists in the return of venous blood and circulation of lymphatic fluid.**
- **This enhanced movement cultivates a massaging effect for the mid back while supporting the health of the kidneys and adrenal glands.**
- **The energizing effects of this gesture are generally helpful for Kapha imbalance.**
- **The gently warming and centering effects are generally helpful for Vata imbalance.**

Pranamaya kosha (energy body)

- **Activates the flow of Samana vayu, the horizontal current of energy.**
- **Opens and balances the third chakra, center of personal power.**

Manomaya kosha (psycho-emotional body)

- **Builds self-confidence and self-esteem.**
- **Cultivates focused attention.**

Vijnanamaya kosha (wisdom body)

- **This gesture connects us to our true inner wealth, our life force energy to be conserved consciously for spiritual awakening.**

Anandamaya kosha (bliss body)

- **As we attune to our center of energy, sensations of warmth, radiance and self-esteem awaken naturally.**

78 Pushpanjali Mudra

Gesture of Offering Flowers

For Cultivating Non-grasping - Aparigraha

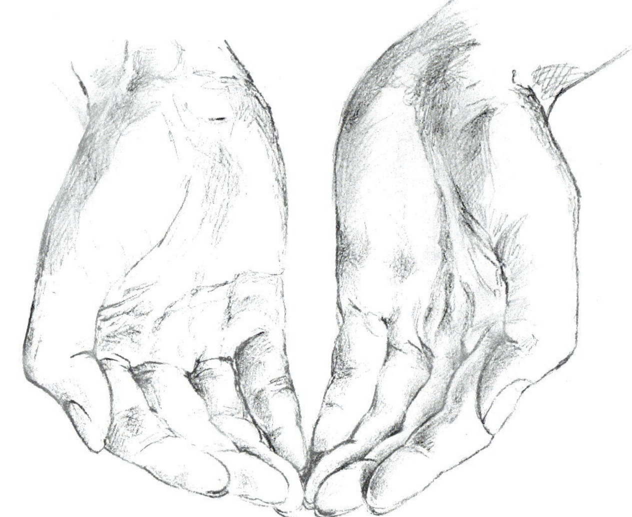

Attuned to the wholeness of my inner being, I naturally hold life more lightly.

Core Quality

Non-grasping

Especially Helpful for

- Releasing attachments at all levels of being.
- Reducing stress and lowering blood pressure.
- Balancing digestion and elimination.
- Instilling appreciation and fluidity.
- Cultivating generosity.

Mudras with similar effects

Apana, Pranidhana, Dvimukham, Chin

Cautions

None

Instructions

1. Gently cup the hands, with the palms facing upward in front of the navel.
2. Touch the outer borders of the little and ring fingers together forming a loose bowl.
3. Allow the wrists to be comfortably separated.
4. The hands extend slightly forward, away from the body, symbolizing an offering.
5. Relax the shoulders back and down, with the spine naturally aligned.

Aparigraha means "non-grasping," and refers to absence of attachment and greed, especially in relation to material possessions beyond our basic needs. Non-grasping also refers to excessive attachment within our relationships and to our own personal history. Through the practice of Aparigraha, we also deepen our ability to release attachment to our beliefs, including spiritual beliefs which, when held too rigidly, become obstacles to awakening. In order to hold life more lightly, it is essential to recognize the inherent wholeness of our true being. As we perceive that we already have everything we need, we no longer reach out to life so desperately for that which we believe will make us complete. As grasping is released, we become co-creators rather than owners, recognizing that life is an ever flowing stream of appreciation and learning, whose beauty is only revealed to those who hold it lightly.

Pushpa means "flower," and *anjali* means "hands joined together in reverence." *Pushpanjali* is therefore an offering of flowers. Pushpanjali mudra lengthens the exhalation, directing the breath into the abdomen, cultivating a sense of relaxation and ease that supports us in releasing attachments more easily. This gesture also instills a sense of openness that allows us to appreciate life exactly as it is in the present moment, without reaching out to fulfil perceived needs endlessly. Pushpanjali mudra also instills a sense of generosity, which is the antidote to grasping. This gesture facilitates both physical and subtle digestion, instilling a sense of natural abundance, a knowing that we have all that we need, making it easier to release neediness and grasping.

Systems Balanced:

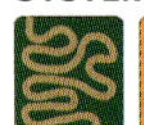
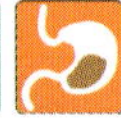

Prana Vayus Nourished:

Elements Activated:

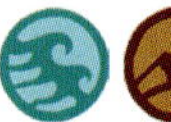
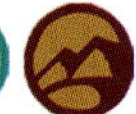

Chakras Balanced:

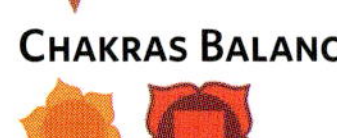

Doshas Balanced:

Scale from Calming to Energizing:

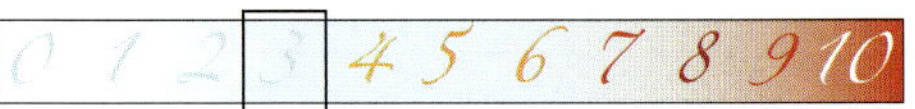

Guided Meditation: **Holding Life Lightly**

ॐ As you hold Pushpanjali mudra, take several natural breaths to attune to all the feelings and sensations evoked by this gesture.

ॐ Notice how your breath is gently directed into your pelvis and abdomen, becoming slow and serene, instilling a sense of contentment and ease.

ॐ With greater contentment and ease, you naturally deepen your ability to hold life more lightly and lovingly, releasing all that no longer supports your journey.

ॐ To deepen your sense of lightness and ease, visualize yourself seated by the edge of a clear flowing stream, your hands filled with flowers, as a symbol of all you have received along your life journey.

ॐ Begin by sensing these flowers as symbols of your material possessions. Take several breaths to hold them lightly and lovingly, honoring them as vehicles, but never the destination of your journey.

ॐ With your next exhaling breath, release into the stream any excessive attachment to your material possessions, naturally allowing you to see that you are always provided for abundantly.

ॐ Now, visualize the flowers within your hands as symbols of your friends and family, recognizing that their love must be held lightly and sensitively, as it only shares its full fragrance when allowed to blossom naturally.

ॐ With your next exhaling breath, release into the stream any excessive attachment to your relationships, allowing them to breathe so that their fragrance and beauty can be experienced completely.

ॐ Next, visualize the flowers in your hands as symbols of your entire history, everything you have done and been along your life journey.

ॐ Within this journey, each chapter has its own unique meaning, but when you hold onto the past too tightly, you are unable to receive the present moment's infinite possibilities.

ॐ With your next exhaling breath, visualize yourself releasing into the stream any attachment to your history that keeps you from moving forward along your journey.

ॐ Finally, sense the flowers in your hands as symbols of all you have received, including your own mind and body, entrusted into your care, but only temporarily.

ॐ As you exhale, release into the stream all excessive attachment to everything you have received, allowing you to live in the present moment lightly and joyfully.

ॐ Holding life more lightly, repeat the following three times, aloud or silently: **"Holding life's gifts more lightly, I journey with greater freedom and ease."**

ॐ Slowly release the gesture, taking several breaths to sense your ability to release all that no longer supports your journey.

ॐ When you are ready, open your eyes, returning slowly and gently, holding life's gifts more lightly and lovingly.

Annamaya kosha (physical body)

• Directs breath and awareness into the pelvis and abdomen, creating a massaging effect that enhances circulation to the digestive and eliminatory systems.
• The enhanced sense of letting go may be helpful for constipation and cramping.
• The enhanced abdominal breathing, together with the lengthened exhalation, helps to reduce stress and lower blood pressure.
• The release of attachment cultivated by this gesture is generally helpful for Kapha imbalance.
• The relaxation cultivated is generally helpful for Pitta imbalance.
• The centering cultivated is generally helpful for Vata imbalance.

Pranamaya kosha (energy body)

• Activates the flow of Apana vayu, the downward moving current of energy.
• Opens and balances the first and second chakras, centers of safety and self-nourishment.

Manomaya kosha (psycho-emotional body)

• Cultivates calm, relaxation, lightness and ease.

Vijnanamaya kosha (wisdom body)

• The open hands represent our recognition that everything is a gift from the Divine, who provides for all our needs, naturally releasing the tendency toward grasping.

Anandamaya kosha (bliss body)

• As we hold life more lightly, we naturally experience gratitude and equanimity.

79 VISHUDDHA MUDRA

Gesture of Purification

For Cultivating Purity - Shaucha

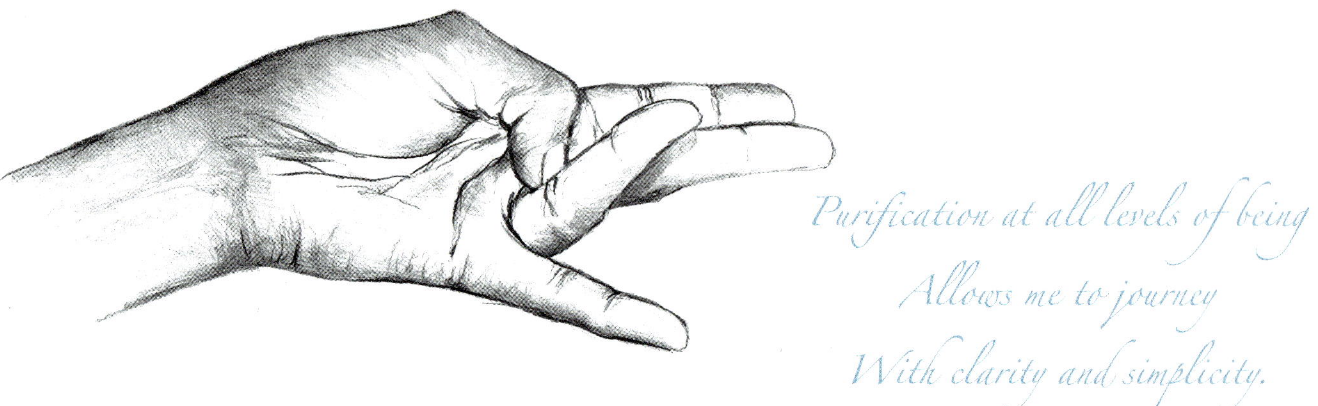

CORE QUALITY

Purity

ESPECIALLY HELPFUL FOR

- Cultivating purity at all levels of being.
- Releasing tension from the neck, throat and vocal cords.
- Aligning the cervical spine.
- Enhancing circulation to the area of the thyroid gland.
- Instilling mental clarity.
- Awakening intuition.

MUDRAS WITH SIMILAR EFFECTS

Garuda, Angushtha, Shunya, Kali

CAUTIONS

Those with hypertension or hyperthyroid conditions should monitor the effects. Shunya, which is less energizing, can be used as a substitute.

INSTRUCTIONS

1. Press the tips of the thumbs into the inner borders of the lowest digit of the ring fingers.
2. Leave the ring fingers extended.
3. The little, middle and index fingers are extended straight out comfortably.
4. Rest the backs of the hands onto the thighs or knees.
5. Relax the shoulders back and down, with the spine naturally aligned.

Shaucha means "purity," and refers to purification at all levels of our being. At the physical level, Shaucha is the purification of our bodies through appropriate diet and lifestyle. Shaucha also refers to purity in our surroundings by creating a clear, open space, inspiring us to live with simplicity, naturally allowing us to focus on our spiritual journey. At the level of the mind, Shaucha is the spaciousness that allows us to meet each new experience openly as a field of appreciation, learning and awakening. When we meet life with fewer judgments and preconceived attitudes, negative thought patterns, emotional reactions and limiting beliefs come to the surface to be seen, witnessed and gradually released. As we meet life with greater openness and simplicity, the purity of our essential being is revealed naturally.

Vishuddha means "purification," and Vishuddha mudra directs breath, awareness and energy into the throat, our center of spiritual purification. This gesture enhances circulation to the vocal cords, releasing tension which cultivates greater ease in speaking and singing. This mudra also increases circulation to the thyroid gland, balancing metabolism and instilling a sense of equanimity that supports our spiritual journey. At a subtle level, this gesture opens and balances *Vishuddha chakra*, supporting the release of limiting beliefs, thereby revealing the inherent purity of our true being. Vishuddha mudra creates space between thoughts, cultivating greater clarity and objectivity, allowing intuition to awaken naturally.

SYSTEMS BALANCED:

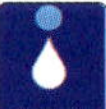

ELEMENTS ACTIVATED:

DOSHAS BALANCED:

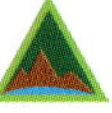

PRANA VAYUS NOURISHED:

CHAKRAS BALANCED:

SCALE FROM CALMING TO ENERGIZING:

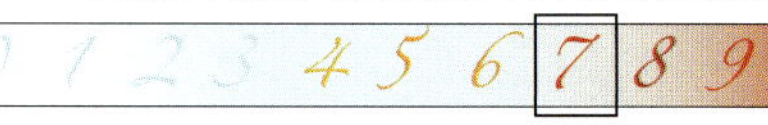

Guided Meditation: Purity at All Levels of Being

- As you hold Vishuddha mudra, take several natural breaths to attune to all the feelings and sensations awakened by this gesture.
- Notice how your breath is gently directed upward into your throat and neck, instilling a sense of spaciousness.
- With each inhalation, your sense of spaciousness expands naturally, and with each exhaling breath, tension from your throat and neck is gradually released.
- As space is created and tension is released, a process of purification naturally occurs within all dimensions of your being.
- Begin by sensing the process of purification within your physical body. Reflect on the extent to which you eat consciously, and only in the quantities you need to support your optimal health and vitality.
- Take several breaths to envision a dietary routine that purifies your body and nourishes it completely.
- Next, explore the level of purity within your surroundings. To what extent does your environment reflect both cleanliness and simplicity, maintaining only what you need to support your journey of transformation and awakening?
- Take several breaths to envision the changes you can make in your surroundings that would allow energy to flow more freely, naturally inspiring your spiritual journey.
- Now, reflect on the level of purity in your use of time and energy. To what extent do you create a clear and open space for spiritual practice, a time to simply be, free from the roles you play in your other activities?
- Take several breaths to envision yourself creating a sacred space of silence and peace where you can attune more deeply to the voice of your authentic being.
- Finally, reflect on purity at the level of your spiritual beliefs. To what extent are you able to release excessive identification with teachers, philosophies and techniques, which are important vehicles, but never the destination of your journey?
- Take several breaths to attune to the simplicity of your true being that is already present beyond all spiritual paths, beliefs, teachings and techniques, waiting to be revealed.
- Affirm your essential purity as you repeat the following three times, aloud or silently: **"By cultivating simplicity, the purity of my essential being is revealed naturally."**
- Slowly release the gesture, taking several breaths to rest in your own pure essence.
- When you are ready, open your eyes, returning slowly and gently, more aligned with the purity of your essential being.

Annamaya kosha (physical body)

• Directs breath and awareness into the neck and throat, creating a massaging effect that improves circulation to the thyroid gland and vocal cords.
• Helps release tension from the neck while supporting the alignment of the cervical spine.
• The energizing effects of this gesture are generally helpful for Kapha imbalance.

Pranamaya kosha (energy body)

• Gently activates Udana vayu, the uppermost current of energy.
• Opens and balances the fifth chakra, center of spiritual purification.

Manomaya kosha (psycho-emotional body)

• Creates space between thoughts.
• Cultivates clarity, supporting psycho-emotional purification.

Vijnanamaya kosha (wisdom body)

• The ability to see with openness and clarity allows us to align more easily with our true being whose very essence is purity.

Anandamaya kosha (bliss body)

• As we release tension from the throat center, an experience of openness and limitlessness arises naturally.

Chaturmukham Mudra

Gesture of Four Faces

For Cultivating Contentment - Santosha

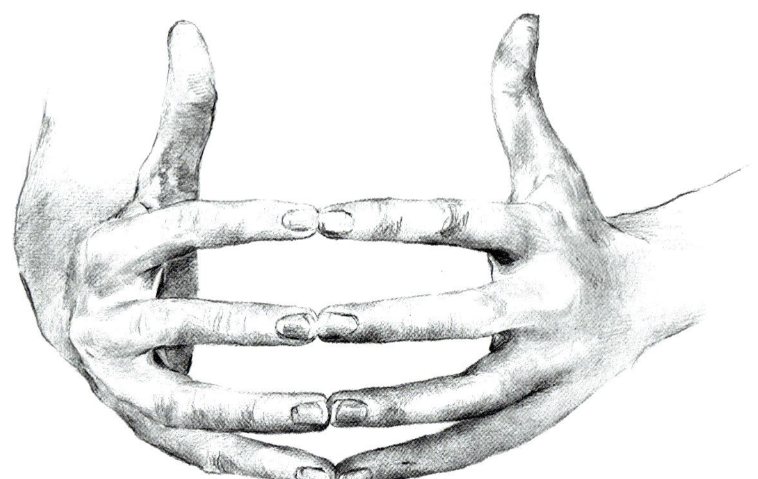

Attuned to the contentment
Of my inner being,
I experience complete serenity.

Core Quality

Contentment

Especially helpful for

- Awakening the essential contentment of our true being.
- Optimizing digestion.
- Instilling optimism and a positive attitude.
- Supporting treatment of depression.

Mudras with similar effects

Dharma Chakra, Ushas, Svadhisthana, Hansi

Cautions

None

Instructions

1. Touch the tips of all the fingers of each hand to the same fingers on the opposite hand.
2. Extend the thumbs straight up.
3. The fingers are separated and rounded as if holding a globe, with the wrists comfortably apart.
4. The gesture can be held slightly away from the body or with the wrists resting comfortably against the abdomen.
5. Relax the shoulders back and down, with the elbows held slightly away from the body and the spine naturally aligned.

Santosha means "contentment," and refers to the ability to remain centered and at peace within our own being no matter what is happening in our surroundings. By cultivating Santosha, we learn to remain balanced in the midst of life's ever present challenges and opportunities, never getting too low when things don't go as planned or too elated when things go well. Contentment is important both at the relative and absolute levels. At the relative level, Santosha is a practice in which we welcome experiences in the most positive way possible, accepting all life brings as a learning and a blessing. At the absolute level, Santosha is a reflection of our true being, inherently whole and complete, and therefore unaffected by life's constant changes. As we rest in our essential contentment, life's challenges may disturb the surface of the sea, but we don't give them the power to affect the calm depths of our inner being.

Chaturmukham means "four faces," and refers to the four joined pairs of fingers in Chaturmukham mudra, as well as the four faces of *Brahma*, the deity of creation. His four faces represent the four cardinal directions, symbolizing his omnipresence. Chaturmukham mudra supports the practice of Santosha by cultivating a sense of calm and ease at all times and in all situations. This gesture directs breath, awareness and energy along the entire front of the body, instilling a sense of comfort and inner security that supports the cultivation of contentment. Chaturmukham mudra further enhances our sense of contentment by facilitating rhythmic breathing that has a balancing effect on our mind and emotions, allowing us to maintain our sense of contentment even in challenging situations.

Systems Balanced:

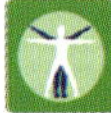

Elements Activated:

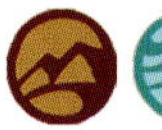
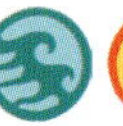

Doshas Balanced:

Prana Vayus Nourished:

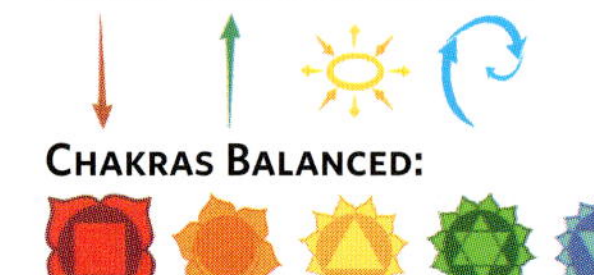

Chakras Balanced:

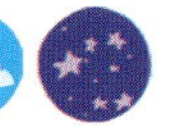

Scale from Calming to Energizing:

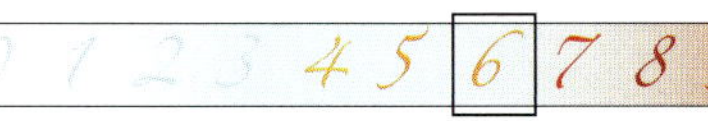

Guided Meditation: Wave of Contentment

- As you hold Chaturmukham mudra, take several natural breaths to attune to all the feelings and sensations awakened by this gesture.
- Notice how your breath flows easily along the front of your body, like a gentle wave of contentment that naturally bathes your entire being.
- Begin by taking several breaths to sense your wave of contentment bathing your physical body, naturally allowing all tension to be released from the crown of your head to the soles of your feet.
- Sensing greater ease within your physical being, your wave of contentment naturally infuses your thoughts and feelings.
- Take several breaths to sense all stress and worry being gradually released, allowing you to experience greater emotional balance at all moments along your journey.
- As your body and mind become calm and serene, waves of contentment support the release of any limiting beliefs that keep you from living joyfully.
- Take several breaths to sense waves of contentment clarifying your ways of seeing, allowing you to live with greater simplicity and harmony.
- As contentment infuses your body, mind and beliefs, take several breaths to rest in the equanimity of your essential being, calm and serene, no matter what storms may be present on the surface of life's sea.
- Affirm your equanimity as you repeat the following three times, aloud or silently: **"Recognizing the contentment of my essential being, I live simply and joyfully."**
- Slowly release the gesture, taking several breaths to rest in complete contentment.
- When you are ready, open your eyes, returning slowly and gently, experiencing greater contentment in all of your activities.

Annamaya kosha (physical body)

• Directs breath and awareness to the entire front of the torso, with a special focus on the abdominal area, enhancing circulation to all the systems of the body, especially the digestive system.
• Lengthens both the inhalation and exhalation, as well as the natural pauses in between, increasing breath capacity.
• The rhythmic movement of the breath releases stress and calms the nervous system.
• The balancing effects of this gesture are generally helpful for all three doshas.

Pranamaya kosha (energy body)

• Balances Prana and Apana vayus while gently activating Samana and Udana.
• Opens and balances the first through fifth chakras.

Manomaya kosha (psycho-emotional body)

• Cultivates emotional balance, contentment and equanimity.
• Instills a sense of optimism.

Vijnanamaya kosha (wisdom body)

• The practice of Santosha gradually reveals contentment to be a natural reflection of our essential being.

Anandamaya kosha (bliss body)

• As we rest in contentment, an experience of wholeness and integration arises naturally.

81

Mushtikam Mudra

Gesture of the Fist

For Cultivating Spiritual Discipline - Tapas

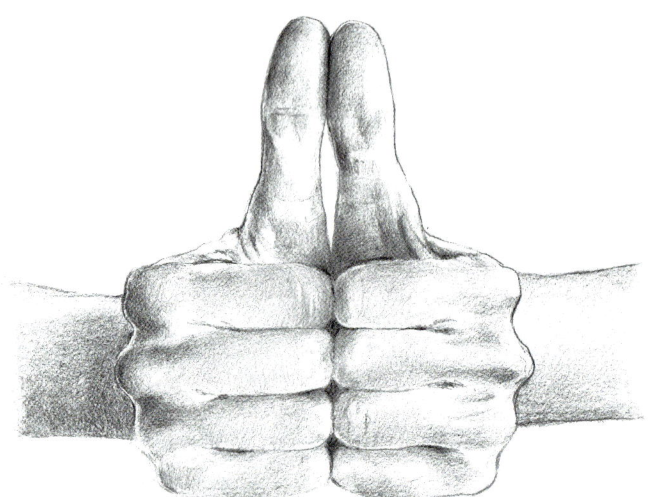

The fire of spiritual discipline
Purifies my being,
Allowing my true Self to
Shine forth radiantly.

Core Quality

Spiritual Discipline

Especially helpful for

- Cultivating spiritual discipline in personal practice and daily life.
- Enhancing the power of digestion and assimilation of nutrients.
- Supporting the health of the kidneys and adrenal glands.
- Cultivating determination and energy.

Mudras with similar effects

Brahma, Merudanda, Shivalingam, Vajra

Cautions

Contraindicated for hypertension and hyperactive digestion. Vajra can be used as a substitute.

Instructions

1. Make the hands into fists, with the thumbs to the outside.
2. Touch the middle digits of the knuckles and the heels of the hands together.
3. Join the thumbs together along their length and extend them upward.
4. Rest the forearms against the abdomen.
5. Relax the shoulders back and down, with the elbows held slightly away from the body and spine naturally aligned.

Tapas means "fire," and refers to the fire of spiritual discipline that burns away impurities at all levels of our being, removing obstacles along our spiritual journey. The practice of Tapas begins by purifying the physical body, strengthening it through regular yogic practices in order to cultivate optimal health as an important foundation for transformation. As the body is strengthened, the practice of Tapas is directed toward our limiting thoughts, feelings and beliefs, cultivating the heat that brings them to the surface where they can be seen and gradually released. As Tapas generates inner heat, there is a tendency to move away from it, and back toward the apparent "safety" of the personality. In the practice of Tapas, however, we consciously embrace this heat, channeling it to hasten the process of transformation. Through this process, the heat of Tapas is gradually transformed into the light of awakening that guides our spiritual journey.

Mushtikam means "fist," and in Mushtikam mudra, both fists come together as a symbol of our determination to attain spiritual freedom through appropriate discipline. In this mudra, the thumbs point straight upward, activating the fire element, cultivating the inner heat that supports the process of transformation. Mushtikam mudra directs breath and awareness into the solar plexus, optimizing our physical digestion and assimilation of nutrients. This gesture also supports the digestion of thoughts, emotions and beliefs that limit our spiritual awakening. Mushtikam mudra supports the opening of the third chakra, our center of personal power, cultivating the willpower that allows us to remain in the heat of spiritual transformation all the way to awakening.

Systems Balanced:

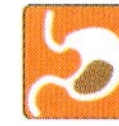

Elements Activated:

Doshas Balanced:

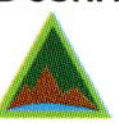

Prana Vayus Nourished:

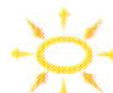

Chakras Balanced:

Scale from Calming to Energizing:

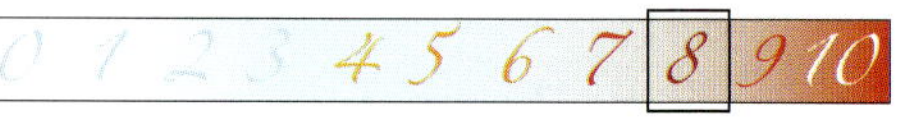

Guided Meditation: Fire of Spiritual Discipline

- As you hold Mushtikam mudra, take several natural breaths to attune to all the feelings and sensations evoked by this gesture.
- Notice how your breath is naturally directed into your solar plexus, your center of personal power and energy.
- Take several breaths to attune to your personal power more deeply, visualizing its source of energy as a flame that burns away all obstacles along your spiritual journey.
- Begin by reflecting on any doubt, resistance, distraction or lethargy that keeps you from practicing with discipline and consistency.
- With your inhaling breath, sense your inner flame glowing brightly, and as you exhale, sense all that keeps you from practicing diligently burned away completely.
- Next, reflect on your level of discipline in relation to dealing with challenging thoughts and feelings, acknowledging how they drain your energy and distract you from the path of awakening.
- With your inhaling breath, your inner flame glows brilliantly, and as you exhale, affirm your commitment to welcome your emotions completely, feeling their heat while simply witnessing, allowing them to be gradually transformed into the light of clarity.
- With greater clarity, you now reflect on your level of discipline in relation to your limiting beliefs. To what extent do you still fall back into old ways of being that no longer support your spiritual journey?
- With your inhaling breath, your inner flame glows brightly, and as you exhale, affirm your intention to release your identification with your limiting beliefs.
- With greater spiritual discipline at all levels of your being, your inner flame of transformation naturally illuminates your path toward awakening.
- Affirm your spiritual discipline, repeating the following three times, aloud or silently: **"Discipline at all levels of being provides a firm foundation for my spiritual journey."**
- Slowly release the gesture, taking several breaths to sense the effects of greater discipline.
- When you are ready, open your eyes, returning slowly and gently, with a deeper commitment to your spiritual journey.

Annamaya kosha (physical body)

- **Directs breath and awareness into the solar plexus, creating a massaging effect that improves circulation to the digestive system.**
- **The increased movement of the diaphragm expands breath capacity, especially at the base of the lungs.**
- **The increased movement of the breath in the mid back creates a massaging effect that enhances circulation to the kidneys and adrenal glands.**
- **The energizing effects of this gesture are generally helpful for Kapha imbalance.**

Pranamaya kosha (energy body)

- **Activates Samana vayu, the horizontal current of energy.**
- **Opens and balances the third chakra, center of personal power.**

Manomaya kosha (psycho-emotional body)

- **Cultivates inner strength, determination, commitment and discipline.**

Vijnanamaya kosha (wisdom body)

- **As the fire of Tapas burns away impurities at all levels of being, wisdom and clarity arise naturally to guide our spiritual journey.**

Anandamaya kosha (bliss body)

- **As the fire of Tapas purifies our being, a sense of inner radiance arises from within the solar plexus.**

82

Sakshi Mudra

Gesture of Witness Consciousness
For Cultivating Self-study - Svadhyaya

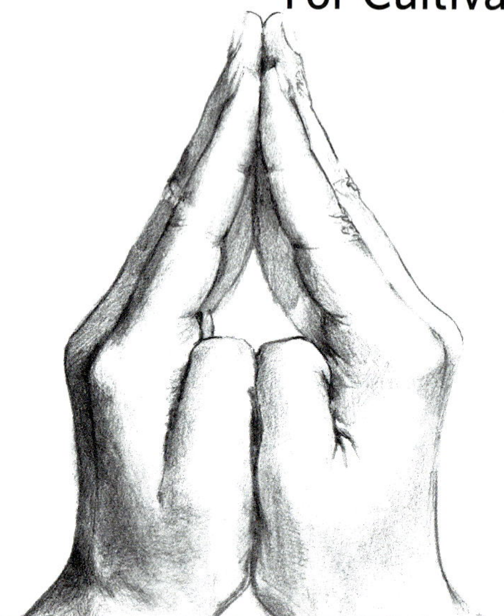

Through exploring limiting beliefs,
Clarity and Self-knowledge arise naturally.

Core Quality
Self-study

Especially helpful for
- Supporting the process of self-study in order to release limiting beliefs, naturally revealing our true being.
- Cultivating equanimity and clarity.
- Relaxing the muscles of the face, especially the jaw, which may be helpful for TMJ dysfunction.

Mudras with similar effects
Jnana, Trishula, Dhyana, Citta

Cautions
Become comfortable with the other gestures in this family before beginning the process of self-study.

Instructions
1. Join the hands in front of the chest, with the fingers pointing upward.
2. Spread the knuckles wide apart while keeping the tips of the fingers and the base of the palms together.
3. Bend the thumbs at the middle digit to touch or come near to the base of the little fingers, forming a triangle as you look through the opening in the hands.
4. Relax the shoulders back and down, with the spine naturally aligned.

Svadhyaya means "self-study," and refers to the recognition of our true being that arises through the exploration and release of our limiting beliefs. The process of self-study is mediated by our "inner witness," called *Sakshi*, the faculty that allows us to observe our body, thoughts, emotions and beliefs without identifying with them so completely. As we explore all that arises within our being without judging or reacting, we gradually release our identification with our conditioning. Through the process of self-study, we also develop compassion, allowing us to see that our limiting beliefs were adopted to fulfill basic needs, such as love, trust or security. As we recognize clearly that these beliefs no longer support our journey, they are gradually released. In the space of clarity created by this release, our inherent positive qualities unfold naturally. The practice of Svadhyaya is supported by the regular study of spiritual texts, including the *Bhagavad Gita* and the *Yoga Sutras of Patanjali*.

Sakshi mudra creates a pattern of triangular breathing that begins outside the nostrils and rises up to merge at the third eye point. This triangular movement of the breath is symbolized by the triangle formed by this gesture. As breath is directed into the third eye, a space of clarity is cultivated, supporting the process of self-study. This gesture also lengthens the inhalation and exhalation evenly while opening both nostrils simultaneously, cultivating a sense of equanimity that facilitates the process of self-study. Sakshi mudra cultivates stability in the seated meditation posture and alignment of the spine, creating a stable foundation for the process of personal investigation.

Systems Balanced:

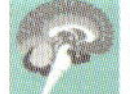
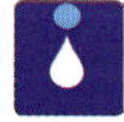
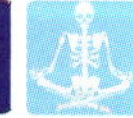
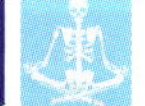

Elements Activated:

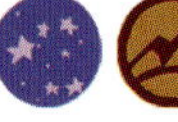
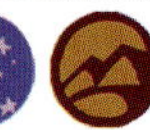

Doshas Balanced:

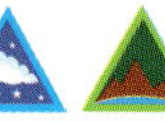

Prana Vayus Nourished:

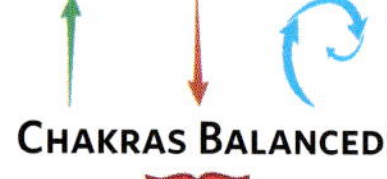

Chakras Balanced:

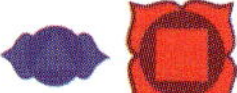

Scale from Calming to Energizing:

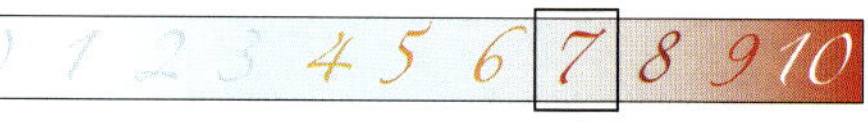

Guided Meditation: The Journey of Self-study

ॐ As you hold Sakshi mudra, take several natural breaths to attune to all the feelings and sensations awakened by this gesture.

ॐ Notice how your breath flows through both nostrils evenly, instilling a greater sense of balance and harmony.

ॐ Take some time to attune to your smooth and even breathing, noticing how it naturally cultivates a space of clarity that supports your practice of self-study.

ॐ Begin your practice of self-study by exploring the sensations within your physical body. Take several breaths to scan your body from your head to your feet, becoming aware of all that is present within your physical being.

ॐ As you embrace sensations more consciously, any resistance is released naturally, allowing you to inhabit your body more fully.

ॐ More at home in your body, take some time to explore your psycho-emotional being, allowing thoughts and feelings to arise and pass away freely, simply witnessing them without identifying, judging or resisting.

ॐ Now, deepen your process of self-study by focusing on a particular feeling that you would normally experience as difficult or challenging.

ॐ Notice how your harmonious breathing allows you to welcome this feeling more easily, taking several breaths to sense its location, color, shape and size within your body.

ॐ As you explore this feeling, allowing it to simply be, notice how resistance is gradually released, naturally cultivating greater ease within your psycho-emotional being.

ॐ Embracing this feeling more openly, your process of self-study can proceed even more deeply.

ॐ As you remain attuned to your challenging feeling, take several breaths to allow any limiting belief related to this feeling to arise within your awareness naturally.

ॐ Explore this belief openly, noticing if it has been repeated along your life journey, perhaps with different characters and scenes, but always with the same central theme.

ॐ Take all the time you need to identify this repeated theme, giving it a name, and also noticing that you adopted it as a way to satisfy a basic need for love, trust or security.

ॐ As you gain clarity around this belief, witnessing it without identifying with it so closely, feelings of heaviness and density naturally begin to release.

ॐ With a greater sense of release, you naturally reconnect with your harmonious breathing, taking some time to allow greater lightness and ease to permeate your entire being.

ॐ As you explore more easily all that arises in your body, thoughts, feelings and beliefs, space is created in which your essential being, beyond all conditioning, is revealed naturally.

ॐ Affirm the process of self-study, repeating the following three times, aloud or silently: **"Through self-study and clear seeing, I naturally align with my true inner being."**

ॐ Slowly release the gesture, taking several breaths to sense your true being with greater clarity.

ॐ When you are ready, open your eyes, returning slowly and gently, with a greater sense of freedom and ease that arises through self-study.

Annamaya kosha (physical body)

• Directs breath and awareness into the neck and head, creating a massaging effect that improves circulation to the area of the pituitary gland.
• Supports correct alignment of the cervical spine.
• Relaxes the muscles of the face, especially the jaw, which may be helpful for TMJ dysfunction.
• The process of self-study is essential for all three doshas, but major imbalances should be addressed before practicing this gesture.

Pranamaya kosha (energy body)

• Balances Prana and Apana vayus, the upward and downward moving currents of energy.
• Gently activates Udana vayu, the uppermost current of energy.
• Opens and balances the first and sixth chakras, centers of safety and wisdom.

Manomaya kosha (psycho-emotional body)

• Creates space between thoughts in which feelings and beliefs can come to the surface to be witnessed more easily.
• Cultivates the centering and equanimity needed for self-study.

Vijnanamaya kosha (wisdom body)

• The release of limiting beliefs through self-study creates a space in which our limitless true being is naturally revealed.

Anandamaya kosha (bliss body)

• As limiting beliefs are released through self-study, an experience of lightness and freedom arises naturally.

83 CHIN MUDRA

Gesture of Consciousness

For Cultivating Surrender to the Divine - Ishvara Pranidhana

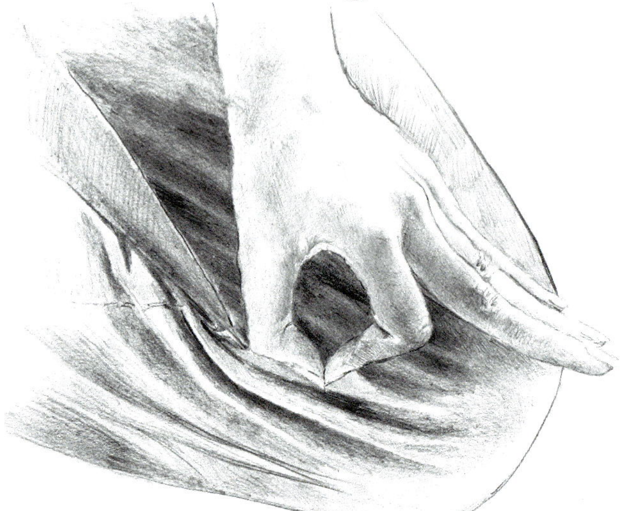

Recognizing the Divine in all of creation, I live with a sense of deep appreciation.

CORE QUALITY
Surrender to the Divine

ESPECIALLY HELPFUL FOR
- Recognizing and honoring the Divine order within all of creation.
- Cultivating silence in the mind.

MUDRAS WITH SIMILAR EFFECTS
Pushpanjali, Avahana, Pranidhana

CAUTIONS
None

INSTRUCTIONS
1. Join the tips of the thumbs to the tips of the index fingers of each hand, forming a circle.
2. Extend the other three fingers straight out comfortably.
3. Turn the palms downward, resting the hands onto the thighs or knees.
4. Relax the shoulders back and down, with the spine naturally aligned.

Ishvara is the "Lord of Creation," and *Pranidhana* means "surrender." In order to understand "surrender to the Lord," we first need to clarify the nature of Ishvara, who is not a creator deity separate from creation, but is the intelligence that pervades all of creation. Ishvara is the universal order, encompassing the physical, psychological and spiritual laws that create, sustain and transform the universe. Because of the all-pervading nature of Ishvara, "surrender to the Lord" is the ability to embrace all of creation with deep reverence and appreciation. As we honor creation deeply, we naturally recognize the Divine in everything, including our own bodies, thoughts and feelings. This recognition of the Divine order within everything allows us to surrender to each moment of life as a gift and a blessing, even when times are difficult or challenging.

Chin means "consciousness," and Chin mudra supports the continual conscious awareness of the Divine presence within all of creation. This gesture facilitates Full Yogic Breathing, expanding breath, awareness and energy along the entire front of the torso. This mudra gently lengthens the exhalation, cultivating a feeling of balance and harmony that allows us to move inward more easily. As we rest within our inner being, a space of silence is created in which we can experience the Divine presence more profoundly. As the Divine presence fills our being, we naturally bow down in reverence to the all-pervading intelligence within everything. Chin mudra balances the first six energy centers, with a special focus on *Ajna chakra*, awakening the clarity that allows us to recognize the Divine presence at each step of our journey.

SYSTEMS BALANCED:

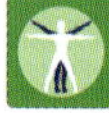

ELEMENTS ACTIVATED:

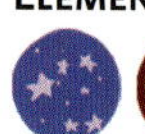
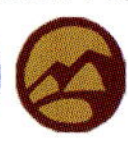

DOSHAS BALANCED:

PRANA VAYUS NOURISHED:

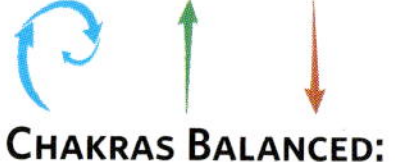

CHAKRAS BALANCED:

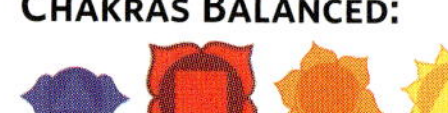
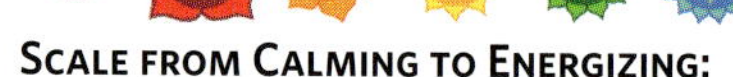

SCALE FROM CALMING TO ENERGIZING:

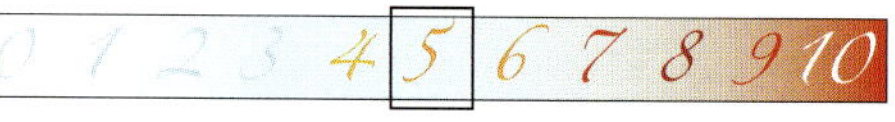

Guided Meditation: **Seeing the Divine in Everything**

- As you hold Chin mudra, take several natural breaths to attune to all the feelings and sensations awakened by this gesture.
- Notice how your breath flows smoothly and evenly throughout your entire body, allowing you to relax more deeply.
- With a greater sense of relaxation, you become more sensitive to the presence of Divine intelligence and energy permeating all of creation, including your own being.
- Take several breaths to attune to this all-pervading Divine energy, sensing it as the source and essence of everything.
- Begin by sensing Divine energy within the natural laws that maintain dynamic balance and harmony, from the farthest stars to the smallest seeds, holding within them the potential to bring forth majestic trees.
- Take several breaths to affirm your deep reverence and gratitude for all of creation's mystery, as a reflection of the Divine light within all things.
- Now, sense the Divine essence within your own body, infusing your physical being with life force energy, orchestrating your entire physiology with miraculous efficiency.
- Take several breaths to sense your deep reverence and gratitude for every system, organ, tissue and cell of your being, given as a precious vehicle for your life journey.
- Next, recognize the Divine light within your senses, acknowledging hearing, touch, sight, taste and smell as essential instruments for meeting your basic needs and exploring creation's infinite beauty.
- Take several breaths to affirm your deep reverence and gratitude for all of your senses, allowing you to perceive the Divine source within everything.
- Now, acknowledge your mind as a reflection of the Divine, appreciating its capacity to process thoughts and feelings in past, present and future time, weaving a tapestry that unfolds all of your possibilities, naturally guiding you toward spiritual awakening.
- Take several breaths to affirm your deep reverence and gratitude for your thoughts and feelings, especially those that are challenging, for they provide the learning that ultimately allows you to see the Divine in everything.
- Recognizing the Divine within everything, you realize your life's deepest meaning - to become one with creation's unfolding mystery.
- Affirm the one source energy, repeating the following three times, aloud or silently: **"Seeing the Divine in everything, I experience all of life as a gift and a blessing."**
- Slowly release the gesture, taking several breaths to rest in gratitude and reverence.
- When you are ready, open your eyes, returning slowly and gently, recognizing the Divine essence that permeates all of creation.

Annamaya kosha
(physical body)

- **Facilitating Full Yogic Breathing along the entire front of the body, supporting the health of all body systems.**
- **Gently lengthens the exhaling breath, helping to calm the nervous system.**
- **Supports optimal spinal alignment, facilitating seated meditation.**
- **The complete breath cultivated by this gesture is generally helpful for Kapha imbalance.**
- **The enhanced focus and concentration are generally helpful for Vata imbalance.**
- **Surrendering to the spiritual source is generally helpful for Pitta imbalance.**

Pranamaya kosha
(energy body)

- **Balances all prana vayus, with a special focus on Udana vayu, the uppermost current of energy.**
- **Opens and balances the first six energy centers, with a special focus on Ajna chakra, center of wisdom.**

Manomaya kosha
(psycho-emotional body)

- **Calms, centers and focuses the mind.**
- **Creates space between thoughts, releasing obstacles to meditation.**

Vijnanamaya kosha
(wisdom body)

- **The recognition of the Divine order in everything, allows us to align with our own true being as a reflection of Divinity.**

Anandamaya kosha
(bliss body)

- **As we surrender to the Divine intelligence within creation, we experience our own essence as deep stillness and bliss.**

Murti Mudra

Gesture of the Body

For Cultivating Steady and Comfortable Posture - Asana

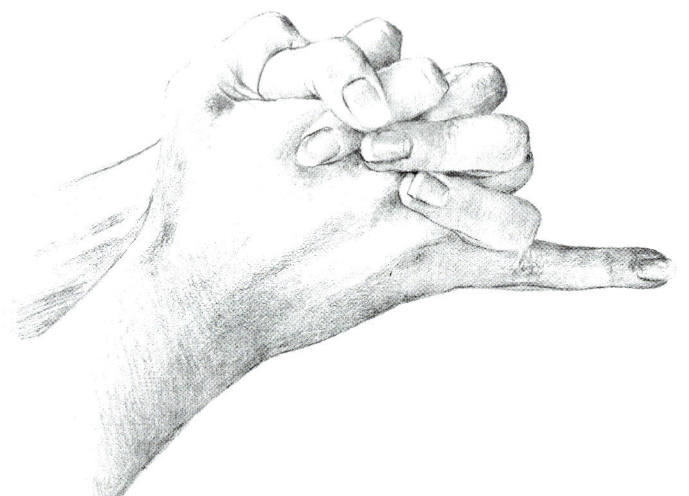

Steadiness and comfort
At all levels of being
Provides a firm foundation for
My spiritual journey.

Core Quality

Steady and Comfortable Posture

Especially helpful for

- Cultivating a balance of steadiness and ease in meditation and daily living.
- Supporting optimal alignment of the spine.
- Releasing stress and lowering blood pressure.
- Supporting the treatment of anxiety.
- Enhancing body awareness.

Mudras with similar effects

Chinmaya, Palli, Prajna Prana Kriya, Rupa

Cautions

None

Instructions

1. Interlace the fingers to the outside, with the right thumb crossed over the left, and the palms pressed lightly together.
2. Extend the little fingers straight out and gently press them together along their length.
3. Rest the hands below the navel or on the lap.
4. Relax the shoulders back and down, with the elbows slightly away from the body and the spine naturally aligned.

Asana means "seat," and in the context of Patanjali's Eight Limbs of Yoga refers to a posture that is both ***sthira***, "steady" and ***sukha***, "comfortable." This balance of steadiness and comfort is the foundation for optimal seated posture in meditation. Finding balanced posture is like tuning a stringed instrument; if the chords are too loose, the sound is dull; if the chords are too tight, the sound is tense and shrill. When the strings are perfectly tuned, the sound is harmonious. As we experience this balance of steadiness and comfort in our posture, the breath naturally becomes smooth and rhythmic. As body and breath are harmonized, the mind and senses naturally become calm and serene, allowing us to enter into meditation more easily. This harmony of body, breath and mind, cultivated in seated meditation, can then be integrated into all of our interactions and activities, allowing us to encounter all situations with an attitude of steadiness and ease.

Murti means "body," "form" or "image." Murti mudra directs breath, awareness and energy into the base of the body, supporting us in developing a balance of stability and comfort within all dimensions of our being, the essence of Asana. This gesture cultivates stability by enhancing our sense of grounding and connection to the earth. It also lengthens and aligns the spine, providing postural support. As our sense of support is increased, we naturally inhabit our bodies more fully. As a counterpart to stability, Murti mudra lengthens the exhalation, facilitating slow, deep abdominal breathing, naturally cultivating comfort and relaxation. This balance of steadiness and comfort allows us to remain fully present and completely at ease in the seated meditation posture and in daily living.

Systems Balanced:

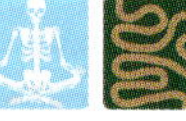
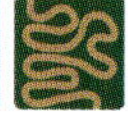

Elements Activated:

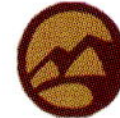

Doshas Balanced:

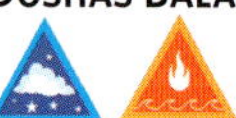

Prana Vayus Nourished:

Chakras Balanced:

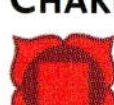

Scale from Calming to Energizing:

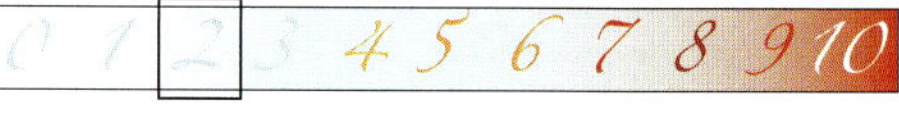

Guided Meditation: Balancing Steadiness and Ease

- As you hold Murti mudra, take several natural breaths to attune to all the feelings and sensations evoked by this gesture.
- Notice how your breath is gently directed downward toward the base of your body, instilling a sense of steadiness and grounding.
- Sense how your exhaling breath is lengthened naturally, becoming slow and serene, cultivating comfort and ease.
- As this combination of steadiness and ease infuses each area of your body, it naturally cultivates effortless seated posture.
- Begin by experiencing the balance of steadiness and ease within the base of your body, legs and feet, sensing these areas deeply rooted to the earth beneath and, at the same time, relaxed comfortably.
- The balance of steadiness and ease now naturally encompasses your pelvis, sacrum and hips, allowing you to be firmly centered while resting in complete comfort.
- Now, allow the balance of steadiness and ease to permeate your abdomen, solar plexus, low and mid back, experiencing the entire middle region of your body both supported and relaxed.
- Your balance of steadiness and ease now encompasses your chest and upper back, allowing you to sense your entire rib cage steady and comfortable.
- As your torso is infused with steadiness and ease, now take several breaths to sense this equilibrium permeating your spinal column completely.
- With each inhalation, your spine lengthens naturally, cultivating alignment and stability, while each exhaling breath allows the natural curves of your spine to soften and release, instilling suppleness and flexibility.
- With your torso and spinal column balanced, your shoulders, arms and hands naturally reflect this harmony, resting with both stability and ease along your body.
- The balance of steadiness and ease now encompass your neck and head, lengthening your cervical spine while drawing your chin back and in, allowing your head to rest evenly over your body.
- Take some time to sense how this perfect balance of steadiness and ease in your physical being is naturally reflected in your steady and easeful breathing.
- With body and breath in perfect harmony, the balance of steadiness and ease naturally permeates your thoughts and feelings, allowing you to be completely focused and, at the same time, relaxed completely.
- Now, take several breaths to experience the perfect balance of steadiness and ease throughout your entire being, allowing you to rest in perfect harmony.
- Affirm your balanced posture as you repeat the following three times, aloud or silently: **"The balance of steadiness and ease allows me to rest in complete harmony."**
- Now, slowly release the gesture, taking several breaths to rest in perfect balance.
- When you are ready, open your eyes, returning slowly and gently, integrating the balance of steadiness and ease into all of your activities.

Annamaya kosha (physical body)

• Directs breath and awareness to the base of the body, creating a massaging effect that improves circulation to the eliminatory system.
• Lengthens the exhalation, activating the relaxation response, which reduces stress and blood pressure.
• The enhanced body awareness supports the health of the musculo-skeletal system.
• The grounding effects of this gesture are generally helpful for Vata imbalance.
• The calming effects are generally helpful for Pitta imbalance.

Pranamaya kosha (energy body)

• Activates Apana vayu, the downward moving current of energy.
• Opens and balances the first chakra, center of safety.

Manomaya kosha (psycho-emotional body)

• Cultivates deep calm and serenity while enhancing concentration, making this an excellent gesture for anxiety.

Vijnanamaya kosha (wisdom body)

• The balance of steadiness and comfort helps us to recognize the equanimity of our essential being.

Anandamaya kosha (bliss body)

• As our posture becomes steady and comfortable, sensations of deep inner peace arise naturally.

85 Dirgha Svara Mudra

Gesture of Expanded Breath

For Expanding Life Force Energy - Pranayama

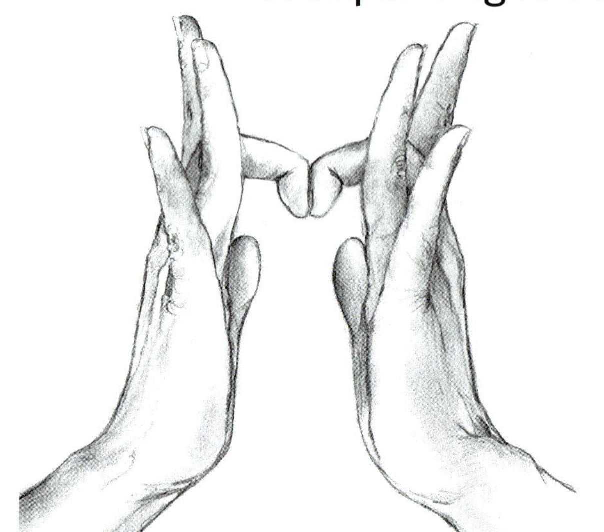

Attuned more deeply to my breathing,
The life force vitalizes my entire being.

Core Quality

Expansion of Life Force Energy

Especially helpful for

- Increasing breath capacity and expanding the free flow of life force energy.
- Releasing constriction from the rib cage.
- Supporting alignment of the spine.
- Cultivating enthusiasm and vitality.

Mudras with similar effects

Madhyama Sharira, Urdhvam Merudanda, Medha Prana Kriya

Cautions

Contraindicated for asthma when in crisis.

Instructions

1. Hold the hands facing each other in front of the chest, with the fingers pointing upward.
2. Bend the middle fingers downward and press the nails of the middle fingers against each other.
3. Extend the other fingers straight up, with the palms parallel to each other.
4. Relax the shoulders back and down, with the elbows slightly away from the body and the spine naturally aligned.

Pranayama is composed of two Sanskrit roots: *prana* is "life force energy," and *ayama* is "expansion." Pranayama is the expansion of the life force energy through yogic breathing techniques. The breath is the primary vehicle for expanding and channeling prana. The various techniques of Pranayama regulate the location of the breath in the body, the length of inhalation and exhalation, and the duration of the pauses. Pranayama techniques range from very calming to energizing. At the physical level, breathing techniques optimize lung capacity, harmonizing all the systems of the body. At the psycho-emotional level, Pranayama cultivates harmony and equanimity, allowing us to enter and remain in meditation more easily. At the spiritual level, breathing techniques create a sense of spaciousness that allows us to move beyond the limitations of the personality, supporting our journey of spiritual awakening.

Dirgha means "lengthened," and *svara* means "breath." Dirgha Svara mudra expands the entire rib cage, increasing breath capacity while enhancing our awareness of all four phases of breathing: the inhalation, the natural pause, the exhalation and the natural rest. The rhythmic movement of the rib cage facilitated by this gesture helps to release chronic contraction from the muscles of respiration. Dirgha Svara mudra is energizing, cultivating enthusiasm and vitality. As this gesture expands the life force energy, it also supports us in channeling it into all the areas of our body, supporting optimal health and healing while creating a sense of spaciousness in which awakening occurs naturally.

Systems Balanced:

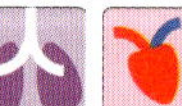
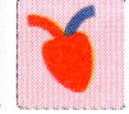

Elements Activated:

Doshas Balanced:

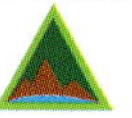

Prana Vayus Nourished:

Chakras Balanced:

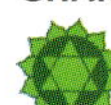

Scale from Calming to Energizing:

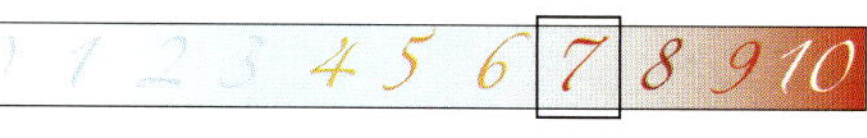

Guided Meditation: **Expanding Life Force Energy**

- As you hold Dirgha Svara mudra, take several natural breaths to attune to all the feelings and sensations awakened by this gesture.
- Notice how your breath flows smoothly through your chest, side ribs and upper back, naturally deepening your sensitivity to your own breathing process.
- As you attune more deeply to your wavelike breathing, your awareness of its four phases expands naturally.
- With each inhalation, your rib cage expands fully to receive vital energy, followed by a pause in which your lungs absorb the life force completely.
- With each exhalation, you experience a sense of release, followed by a pause, allowing you to rest deeply.
- Sense this wavelike movement naturally lengthening each of the phases of breathing, expanding breath capacity and your ability to absorb the life force more efficiently.
- As you attune more deeply to the expansion of vital energy, you are able to channel it to each part of your body, enhancing your overall level of vitality.
- Begin by inhaling vital energy, expanding your lungs completely, and as you exhale, direct the life force down into your pelvis, legs and feet.
- Take several breaths to sense these areas expanding and releasing energetically in synchrony with your wavelike breathing.
- As your lower body breathes more completely, sense this area nourished and vitalized by the life force energy.
- Now, fill your lungs with vital energy, and as you exhale, direct the life force into your abdomen, solar plexus, low and mid back.
- Take several breaths to sense these areas expanding and relaxing energetically in synchrony with your wavelike breathing.
- As your breath flows more freely, allow your wave of breathing to bathe the entire middle region of your body with vital energy.
- With your next inhalation, expand your lungs with vital energy, and with your exhaling breath, direct the life force into your chest, upper back, shoulders, arms and hands.
- Take several breaths to sense these areas expanding and releasing in synchrony with your wavelike breathing.
- As your wave of breathing nourishes your chest and upper extremities, sense these areas infused with vital energy.
- With your next inhalation, your lungs expand completely, and as you exhale, your wave of breath gently rises up into your neck and head, nourishing your brain and senses with clarity and vitality, as your facial expression reflects a growing serenity.
- Now, sense your entire body expanding and relaxing energetically in synchrony with your wavelike breathing, allowing the life force energy to vitalize your entire being.
- Affirm greater vitality, as you repeat the following three times, aloud or silently: **"As the life force permeates my entire being, I am filled with radiant vitality."**
- Slowly release the gesture, taking several breaths to sense your expanded vitality.
- When you are ready, open your eyes, returning slowly and gently, sensing enhanced energy to support your spiritual journey.

Annamaya Kosha (Physical Body)

• Directs breath and awareness to the entire rib cage, expanding breath capacity.
• The enhanced movement of the rib cage helps to release muscular contraction from the thoracic area.
• Facilitates optimal alignment of the spine.
• The expanded breath may be helpful for some respiratory conditions, such as asthma when not in crisis.
• The clearing and energizing effects of this gesture, together with the expansion of the rib cage, are generally helpful for Kapha imbalance.

Pranamaya Kosha (Energy Body)

• Activates Prana vayu, the upward moving current of energy.
• Opens and balances the fourth chakra, center of unconditional love.

Manomaya Kosha (Psycho-Emotional Body)

• Cultivates a sense of confidence in relation to the breathing process.
• Cultivates a sense of balanced giving and receiving.

Vijnanamaya Kosha (Wisdom Body)

• As we attune to the life force energy, we deepen our sensitivity to the more subtle realms of our being.

Anandamaya Kosha (Bliss Body)

• With the life force flowing freely, feelings of expansiveness, limitlessness and freedom arise naturally.

86

Ishvara Mudra

Gesture of the Lord of Creation
For Drawing the Senses Inward - Pratyahara

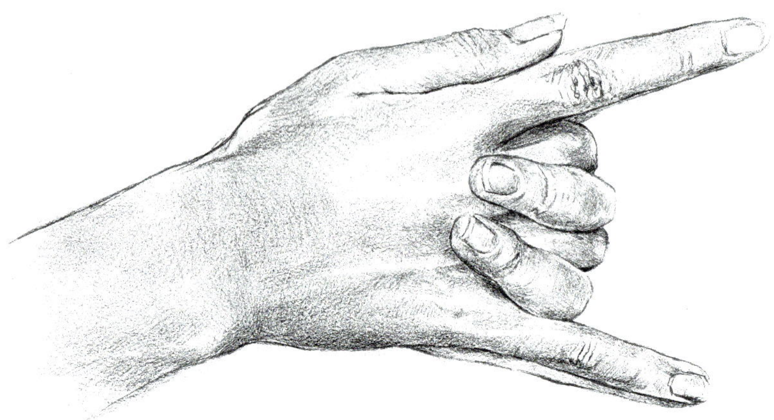

As my senses rest deeply,
I experience greater peace and clarity.

Core Quality
Withdrawal of the Senses

Especially helpful for
- Reducing excessive sensory stimulation and processing accumulated sensory impressions.
- Supporting the health of the eliminatory and digestive systems.
- Cultivating abdominal breathing, reducing stress and instilling a sense of deep relaxation and restoration.

Mudras with similar effects
Gupta, Kurma, Shankha, Samputa

Cautions
None

Instructions
1. Interlace the fingers to the outside with the base of the palms touching.
2. Extend the little and index fingers.
3. Place the thumbs alongside each other, resting them onto the index fingers.
4. Rest the forearms onto the abdomen, with the extended fingers facing forward.
5. Relax the shoulders back and down, with the elbows slightly away from the body and the spine naturally aligned.

Pratyahara is derived from two Sanskrit words: ***ahara*** meaning "food," and ***prati*** meaning "away from." Pratyahara refers to "turning away from all that is ingested." In the context of Yoga, Pratyahara means withdrawing the senses from excessive sensory stimuli in order to allow the mind to rest and regain its inherent clarity. As the senses move inward, the mind does not become silent immediately and, in fact, it may even become more agitated. This is due to the accumulated thoughts, feelings and memories, whose release require time, patience and the ability to witness them without identifying. As these accumulated sensory impressions are "digested," the stress and tension that accompany them are released, allowing the senses to be restored naturally. As the senses and mind become more calm, clear and serene, inner silence arises naturally, allowing us to remain in the steady stream of meditation more easily.

Ishvara is "the Lord of creation," the universal order and harmony that pervades everything. Ishvara mudra cultivates this harmony within our own being, instilling a sense of deep calm, which allows the senses to turn inward naturally. This gesture directs breath, awareness and energy to the abdomen and base of the body, supporting the functioning of the digestive and eliminatory systems. Ishvara mudra slows the breath and lengthens the exhalation, cultivating a sense of calm and inner peace that supports the subtle digestion of sensory impressions, thoughts, feelings and memories. This gesture also helps to create space between thoughts, cultivating inner silence.

Systems Balanced:

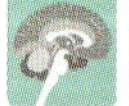
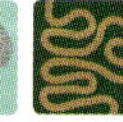
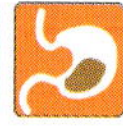
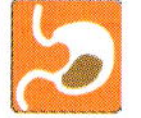

Elements Activated:

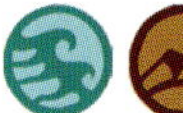
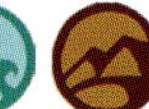

Doshas Balanced:

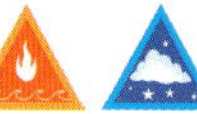

Prana Vayus Nourished:

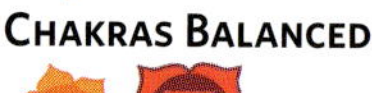

Chakras Balanced:

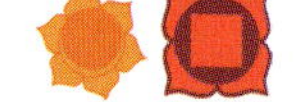

Scale from Calming to Energizing:

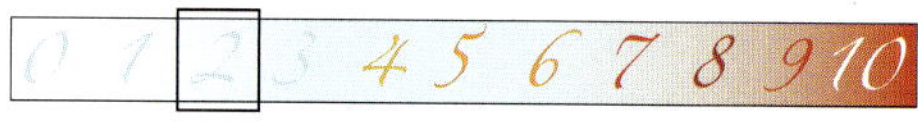

Guided Meditation: Turning the Senses Inward

- As you hold Ishvara mudra, take several natural breaths to attune to all the feelings and sensations evoked by this gesture.
- Notice how your breath is gently directed into your abdomen and the base of your body, cultivating a sense of comfort and ease that allows you to relax completely.
- As you relax more deeply, your senses turn inward naturally, allowing you to align with your essential being.
- Begin by attuning to your sense of hearing, listening to the most distant sounds you can perceive, then gradually bringing your awareness closer and closer to the sounds that are most near.
- Now, allow your sense of hearing to turn inward, taking several breaths to explore the subtle sounds within your being, including the sound of your breathing and your own heart beating.
- Next, attune to your sense of touch, feeling the contact between your body and the place you sit, the sensation of your clothing against your skin, and the plane of contact between your eyelids.
- Now, allow your sense of touch to turn inward, feeling the stream of air entering your nostrils, and flowing down to gently caress your air passages.
- As hearing and touch turn inward, your sense of sight follows naturally, visualizing in your mind's eye the landscape of your surroundings, beginning far away and gradually moving closer until you come to the image of your own body.
- Now, allow your sense of sight to turn inward, visualizing your internal world, allowing any colors, shapes or images to naturally appear.
- Next, bring awareness to your sense of taste, imagining a flavor that reminds you of a time when you felt completely at peace, deeply savoring this taste together with the accompanying feeling.
- Now, your sense of taste turns inward, allowing this sense of comfort and peace to encompass your entire being, infusing you with absolute tranquility.
- As hearing, touch, sight and taste turn inward, you attune to your sense of smell, perceiving any fragrances in the air you breathe, such as the scent of flowers carried on the breeze.
- Now, allow your sense of smell to turn inward, imagining a pleasant aroma that you can recall easily, allowing its fragrance to spread throughout your being.
- As all of your senses turn inward, your mind naturally becomes calm and serene, allowing you to rest in the silence of your essential being.
- With your senses resting deeply, repeat the following three times, aloud or silently: **"As my senses turn inward naturally, I rest in the silence of my essential being."**
- Now, slowly release the gesture, taking several breaths to experience your senses completely at rest.
- When you are ready, return slowly and gently, turning your senses outward gradually, while remaining aligned with your essential being.

Annamaya kosha (physical body)

• Directs breath and awareness into the abdomen and base of the body, creating a massaging effect that increases circulation to the digestive and eliminatory systems.
• Calms the nervous system and senses, supporting their optimal functioning.
• The calming effects of this gesture are generally helpful for Pitta imbalance.
• The reduction of sensory stimuli is generally helpful for Vata imbalance.

Pranamaya kosha (energy body)

• Gently stimulates Apana vayu, the downward moving current of energy.
• Opens and balances the first and second chakras, centers of safety and self-nourishment.

Manomaya kosha (psycho-emotional body)

• Instills a sense of deep calm, which naturally facilitates the practice of Pratyahara.
• Supports the subtle "digestion" of accumulated thoughts and feelings.

Vijnanamaya kosha (wisdom body)

• The inner silence experienced by the withdrawal of the senses serves as a doorway to the clarity of our essential being.

Anandamaya kosha (bliss body)

• As the senses are fully restored, sensations of joy, peace and well-being awaken naturally.

87

Abhisheka Mudra

Gesture of Anointing

For One-Pointed Concentration - Dharana

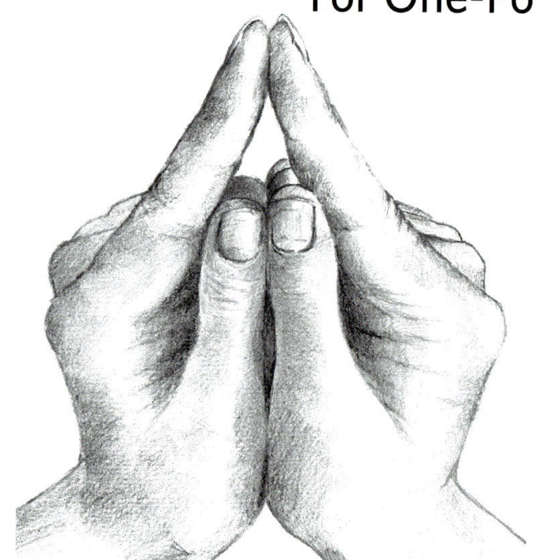

Deepening my one-pointed concentration,
I enter smoothly and easily into meditation.

Core Quality

One-pointed Concentration

Especially helpful for

- Improving concentration by focusing on a chosen object as a preparation for meditation.
- Enhancing digestion.
- Clarifying our life purpose and vision.

Mudras with similar effects

Vajra, Anushasana, Jnana, Trishula

Cautions

None

Instructions

1. Hold the hands in front of the solar plexus, with the palms facing each other.
2. Make the hands into loose fists, with the thumbs to the outside.
3. Bring the base of the palms and fists together.
4. Extend the index fingers and join their pads together.
5. Join the sides of the thumbs and rest them in the space between the index fingers.
6. Relax the shoulders back and down, with the elbows held slightly away from the body and the spine naturally aligned.

Dharana, which means "concentration," is the ability to focus the mind steadily and comfortably on a chosen object. This object may be external, such as a *Yantra*, a geometric symbol used for meditation, or internal, such as the symbol Om visualized at the third eye. As we develop the ability to focus the mind for longer periods, it becomes more stable and serene, allowing us to enter into meditation more easily. Developing one-pointed concentration is a gradual process because the very nature of our everyday mind is movement, scanning our environment constantly for opportunities and threats. This state of vigilance is necessary for survival and for meeting our basic needs, but as we embrace the spiritual path, the mind must be trained to focus inwardly and to release its attachment to the external environment. As we begin the practice of Dharana, it is natural for the mind to drift away from its object. By continually and gently bringing the mind back, it gradually becomes more still and serene, allowing us to remain focused more easily.

Abhisheka means "anointing," and refers to consecrating a sacred image by pouring milk, yogurt, ghee or honey onto it. The shape of the hands in Abhisheka mudra resembles the instrument used in anointing. This gesture brings breath, awareness and energy to the solar plexus, activating the power of digestion while enhancing energy and mental clarity, which support our ability to focus one-pointedly. Abhisheka mudra further enhances one-pointed concentration by awakening *Ajna chakra*, our center of wisdom and clear seeing, thereby allowing us to focus the mind more easily and to develop greater clarity.

Systems Balanced:

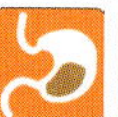 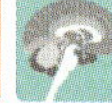

Elements Activated:

Doshas Balanced:

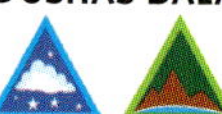

Prana Vayus Nourished:

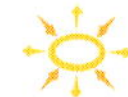

Chakras Balanced:

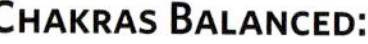

Scale from Calming to Energizing:

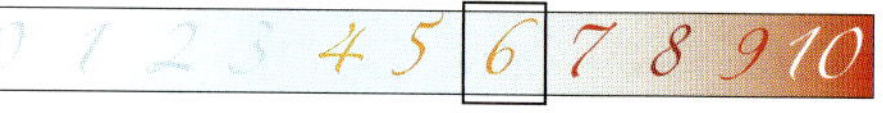

Guided Meditation: Inner Flame of Concentration

- As you hold Abhisheka mudra, take several natural breaths to attune to all the feelings and sensations evoked by this gesture.
- Notice how your breath is naturally directed into your solar plexus, instilling a sense of warmth and radiance.
- Take several breaths to sense this radiance more deeply, visualizing its source as a small flame at the center of the solar plexus, providing a natural point of concentration on which your mind can rest completely.
- Take some time to notice all the details of this flame, visualizing the gold and orange at its base, its luminous blue tip, and its gently curving shape.
- At first your flame may waiver and your attention may drift away. If so, calmly invite your mind back to rest on your flame without judging yourself in any way.
- Take several breaths to continue this process, noticing that each time your mind wanders and you bring it back gently, your level of concentration deepens naturally.
- As your concentration deepens, your breath becomes slower and more serene, allowing your mind to rest on your flame effortlessly.
- Thoughts may still arise, but you simply allow them to come and go naturally while inviting your awareness back to your flame, gently but steadily.
- As your awareness rests on your flame more easily, your mind gradually becomes centered and serene, allowing you to experience greater harmony.
- With greater harmony, you enter into the stream of meditation effortlessly.
- With your mind calm and serene, repeat the following three times, aloud or silently: **"As my mind rests one-pointedly, I experience deep inner peace and harmony."**
- Slowly release the gesture, taking several breaths to sense your enhanced concentration.
- When you are ready, open your eyes, returning slowly and gently, with a greater ability to focus one-pointedly.

Annamaya kosha (physical body)

• Directs breath and awareness to the solar plexus, creating a massaging effect that enhances circulation to the digestive system.
• Expands the breath at the back of the rib cage, creating space between the vertebrae.
• The expansion of the breath in the mid back increases circulation to the kidneys and adrenal glands.
• The enhanced focus is helpful for stress reduction.
• The one-pointed concentration cultivated by this gesture is generally helpful for Vata imbalance.
• The mildly energizing effects are generally helpful for Kapha imbalance.

Pranamaya kosha (energy body)

• Activates Samana vayu, the horizontal current of energy.
• Opens and balances the third and sixth chakras, centers of personal power and wisdom.

Manomaya kosha (psycho-emotional body)

• Cultivates calm in the mind and emotions.
• Creates space between thoughts as a support for one-pointed concentration.

Vijnanamaya kosha (wisdom body)

• Concentration develops the clarity that allows us to align with our true Self more easily.

Anandamaya kosha (bliss body)

• As concentration deepens, serenity, equanimity and clear seeing arise naturally.

88

Dharmadhatu Mudra

Gesture of Tranquility

For Meditation - Dhyana

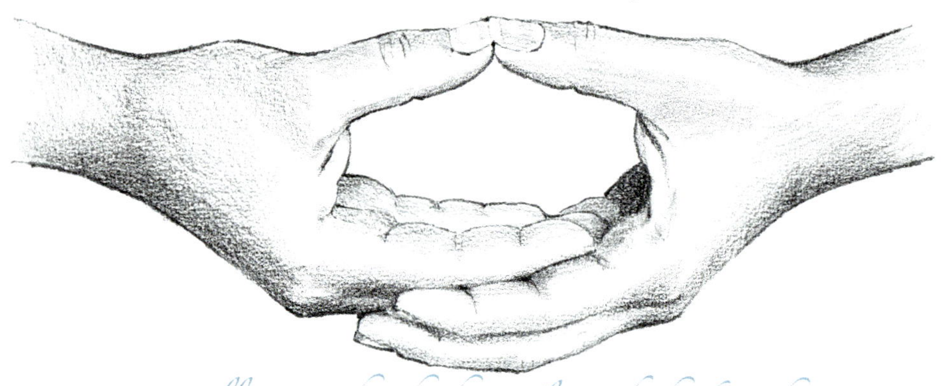

Following the rhythmic flow of the breath,
The mind finds a natural place of rest.

Core Quality

Meditation

Especially helpful for

- Supporting us in welcoming and witnessing thoughts and feelings in meditation.
- Reducing stress and calming the nervous system.
- Integrating body, breath, senses and mind.
- Experiencing the silent space between thoughts.

Mudras with similar effects

Jnana, Dhyana, Bhairava

Cautions

None

Instructions

1. Rest the left hand onto the lap, with the palm facing upward.
2. Rest the back of the right hand onto the palm of the left hand.
3. Touch the tips of the thumbs gently together, forming an oval shape.
4. Relax the shoulders back and down, with the elbows held slightly away from the body and the spine naturally aligned.

Dhyana, which means "meditation," is a steady stream of pure awareness that we gradually come to recognize as our natural state of being. Each of the limbs of Yoga plays an important role in preparing us for meditation. The *Yamas* and *Niyamas*, the ethical foundation, reduce inner and outer conflict. *Asana* cultivates a balance of steadiness and ease in our physical seat. *Pranayama* expands our life force energy, providing the vitality that allows us to remain in meditation more easily. *Pratyahara*, drawing the senses inward, reduces external distractions. *Dharana* cultivates one-pointed concentration, allowing the mind to become more calm and serene. Dhyana, meditation, is a natural extension of Dharana in which all effort is released. In meditation, body, breath, senses and mind are integrated naturally into a single harmonious stream of awareness. A key to meditating with greater ease is the ability to welcome all that arises at all levels of our being without identifying so completely. By welcoming and witnessing, resistance is released, allowing us to remain in meditation effortlessly.

Dharmadhatu refers to the "purified mind," free of conditioning. It is the essential nature of the mind that has been purified along the spiritual journey. Dharmadhatu mudra is also called the Cosmic mudra and is commonly used in Zen Buddhist meditation. This gesture allows breath, awareness and energy to flow naturally along the entire front of the body, instilling a steady and calm rhythm in the breath, which serves as a natural point of focus on which the mind can rest. This mudra cultivates an experience of serenity, which supports the process of welcoming and witnessing. With greater serenity, we naturally experience the inherent silence of our true being.

Systems Balanced:

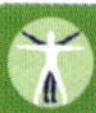

Elements Activated:

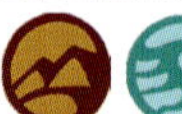
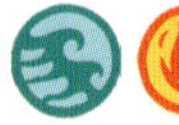

Doshas Balanced:

Prana Vayus Nourished:

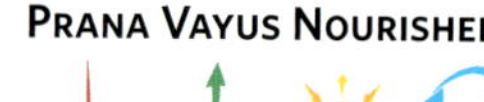

Chakras Balanced:

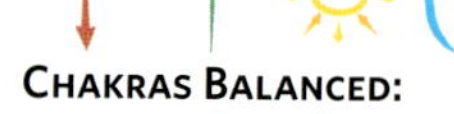
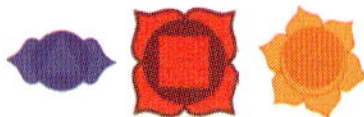

Scale from Calming to Energizing:

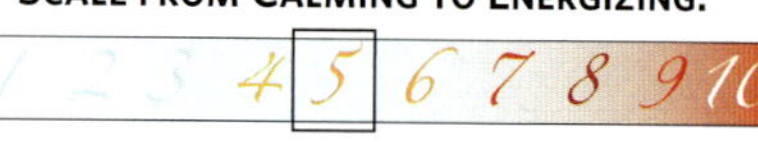

Guided Meditation: Welcoming and Witnessing

ॐ As you hold Dharmadhatu mudra, take several natural breaths to attune to all the feelings and sensations awakened by this gesture.

ॐ Notice how your breath flows smoothly and easily up and down along the entire front of your body, naturally calming your mind and instilling a sense of serenity.

ॐ With greater calm and serenity, you are able to welcome all that arises within your being while simply witnessing, allowing you to enter into meditation more easily.

ॐ Begin by welcoming all that arises within your physical body. Take several breaths to scan from the crown of your head to the soles of your feet, exploring all sensations and embracing them openly.

ॐ Now, expand your welcoming to encompass your breathing. Take some time to follow the natural flow of your breath from the base of your body to the crown of your head.

ॐ Allow your breath to flow freely throughout your entire being, sensing your breathing as a natural balance of giving and receiving.

ॐ Next, attune to your senses, allowing any sounds, fragrances, tastes or images from outside or within your being to arise naturally.

ॐ Take several breaths to embrace all sensory stimuli as pure energy, allowing them to be naturally integrated with the sensations in your body and the flow of your breathing.

ॐ As body, breath and senses are welcomed and integrated completely, you embrace your thoughts and feelings more easily.

ॐ Take several breaths to allow any thoughts or feelings to arise naturally, experiencing them as waves of pure energy that arise and pass away freely.

ॐ Now, welcome all that arises within your being, allowing body, breath, senses, and mind to be integrated naturally.

ॐ Through this integration of all that arises within your being, you enter into the stream of meditation effortlessly.

ॐ As you rest in the meditation stream, you sense the harmony and clarity that are the essence of your true being.

ॐ Resting in meditation's stream, repeat the following three times, aloud or silently: **"Welcoming all that arises within my being, I rest in meditation effortlessly."**

ॐ Now, slowly release the gesture, taking several breaths to rest in effortless meditation.

ॐ When you are ready, open your eyes, returning slowly and gently, integrating the essence of meditation into all of your activities.

Annamaya kosha (physical body)

• Directs breath, awareness and energy to the entire front of the body, cultivating a balance of alertness and relaxation, which supports the optimal functioning of all the systems of the body.
• The balancing effects of this gesture are generally helpful for all three doshas.

Pranamaya kosha (energy body)

• Balances all prana vayus.
• Opens and balances the first through sixth chakras with a focus on Ajna chakra, center of wisdom.

Manomaya kosha (psycho-emotional body)

• Instills calm and serenity.
• Cultivates centering, allowing us to remain present in meditation while maintaining sufficient energy to dispel lethargy.

Vijnanamaya kosha (wisdom body)

• Through welcoming and witnessing, we reduce the tendency to identify with thoughts and feelings so completely.

Anandamaya kosha (bliss body)

• As we rest in conscious presence, feelings of equanimity, wholeness and contentment arise naturally.

89 Mandala Mudra

Gesture of the Circle

For Attaining Spiritual Union - Samadhi

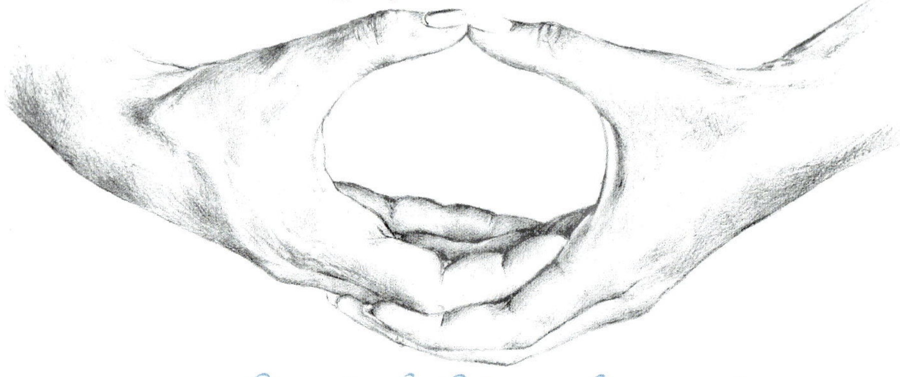

In the circle of wholeness of my true being,
I experience my essence as freedom and unity.

Core Quality

Spiritual Union

Especially Helpful For

- Glimpsing deeper states of meditation beyond the personality, allowing us to experience our essence as unity.
- Supporting all the systems of the physical body in functioning optimally.

Mudras with Similar Effects

Bhairava

Cautions

None

Instructions

1. Rest the left hand onto the lap, with the palm facing upward.
2. Rest the back of the right hand onto the palm of the left hand.
3. Touch the tips of the thumbs gently together, forming a wide open circle shape.
4. Relax the shoulders back and down, with the elbows held slightly away from the body and the spine naturally aligned.

The word *Samadhi* is made up of three Sanskrit roots: ***sam*** means "united with," ***a***, in this context, means "toward," and ***dha*** means "to hold." Samadhi refers to the mind resting in its natural state of unity. The experience of Samadhi has been described as immersion in an ocean of infinite bliss, as complete union with the Divine and as a sense of oneness with all of creation. In Samadhi, all sense of separation is released, allowing the meditator and the object of meditation to naturally merge as a seamless unity. Within this unified state, we experience our essential essence as pure Consciousness beyond all conditioning. The Yoga Sutras describes several levels of Samadhi, and each level refers to the degree to which the movements of the mind have been mastered, allowing the meditator to rest in progressively deeper states of unity in meditation.

Mandala means "circle," and Mandala mudra directs breath, awareness and energy throughout our entire body, cultivating an experience of wholeness in which all dimensions of our being are integrated naturally. This growing sense of wholeness allows us to glimpse more easily our true nature as unity. As we experience integration and unity, the systems of our body naturally reflect this harmony. At a symbolic level, the circular shape of Mandala mudra represents the unity of all creation, instilling a sense of our oneness with the entire web of life. As this sense of oneness becomes more complete, any remaining sense of separation is released, allowing us to experience all of life as a circle of unity. As we deepen our sense of oneness, *Sahasrara chakra*, at the crown of the head, opens naturally, allowing us to glimpse our essential nature as freedom and unity.

Systems Balanced:

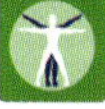

Elements Activated:

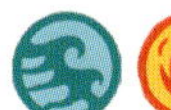

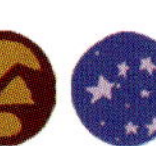
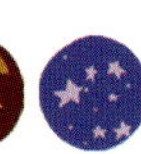

Doshas Balanced:

Prana Vayus Nourished:

Chakras Balanced:

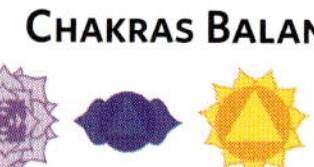
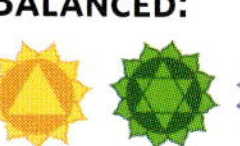
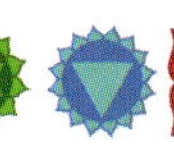
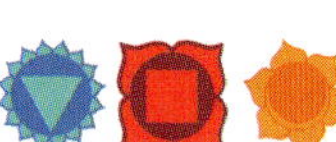

Scale from Calming to Energizing:

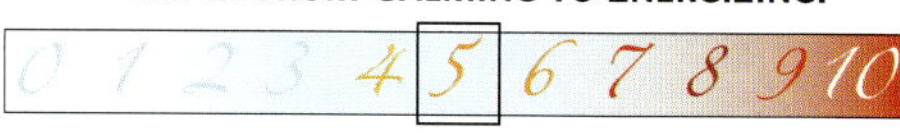

Guided Meditation: The Journey of Unity

- Begin with your hands resting comfortably on your thighs or knees as you prepare to embark on a journey to glimpse Samadhi, an experience of complete unity.
- Begin by placing your hands in Murti mudra. Take several natural breaths to scan through your body from your feet to the crown of your head, making subtle adjustments to find a posture that is steady and comfortable, the essence of Asana.
- As you inhabit your body with steadiness and ease, all areas of your being are integrated naturally, forming the foundation for your meditation journey.
- Firmly supported in your physical seat, place your hands in Dirgha Svara mudra. Sense your breath flowing out from the center of your chest to infuse every area of your being with life force energy, the essence of Pranayama.
- Sense the contours of your body expanding and releasing energetically in synchrony with your breathing, experiencing your entire being as a field of radiant energy.
- With body and breath integrated, place your hands in Ishvara mudra. Allow your senses to turn inward naturally, beginning with smell, followed by taste, touch, sight and hearing, guiding you toward the silence of your inner being.
- As your senses rest inward, you naturally enter an inner sanctuary, experiencing the silence of your true being, the essence of Pratyahara.
- As body, breath and senses are integrated naturally, you place your hands in Abhisheka mudra. Rest your awareness on a small flame at the center of your solar plexus, cultivating one-pointed concentration, the essence of Dharana.
- Maintain your concentration gently but steadily, bringing your awareness back to your flame when necessary, allowing your mind to rest upon its point of focus more easily.
- With one-pointed concentration, place your hands in Dharmadhatu mudra. Notice how all effort is gradually released, allowing body, breath, senses and mind to merge as a single stream, entering into meditation, Dhyana, naturally.
- Maintain this flowing stream through welcoming and witnessing all that arises within your being, allowing you to rest in meditation effortlessly.
- As you rest in meditation, place your hands in Mandala mudra. Now, take several breaths to allow the meditator and the experience of meditation to merge as a seamless unity.
- Take several breaths to rest in this experience of absolute unity, the essence of Samadhi, the culmination of your Yoga journey.
- Affirm your experience of unity, repeating the following three times, aloud or silently: **"Integrating all limbs of the Yoga journey, I experience my essential unity."**
- Slowly release the gesture, beginning your return journey by focusing on your solar plexus. Now, gradually allow your senses to turn outward.
- Next, focus on the steady flow of your breath and, finally, become fully present and grounded in your physical body.
- When you are ready, open your eyes, returning slowly and gently, fully integrating the limbs of Yoga.

Annamaya kosha
(physical body)

- **Promotes whole body breathing which supports the optimal functioning of all body systems.**
- **Promotes optimal breathing in all parts of the lungs.**
- **The balancing effects of this gesture are generally helpful for all three doshas.**

Pranamaya kosha
(energy body)

- **Balances all prana vayus.**
- **Balances and integrates all seven chakras, with a special focus on the sixth and seventh, centers of wisdom and unity.**
- **Balances the three main nadis.**

Manomaya kosha
(psycho-emotional body)

- **Cultivates a sense of integration and wholeness.**

Vijnanamaya kosha
(wisdom body)

- **As we gain glimpses of unity, we naturally open a doorway to the recognition of our true being.**

Anandamaya kosha
(bliss body)

- **As we glimpse our essential wholeness and unity, an experience of bliss and limitlessness arises naturally.**

Chapter Fifteen

Ten Steps to Freedom

MUDRAS FOR SPIRITUAL AWAKENING

Along the spiritual path, we move from the identification with the limited personality to an experience of our limitless true being, from fragmentation to wholeness, from doubt to clarity and from suffering to freedom. Most spiritual traditions present the cultivation of positive qualities as an important support for our spiritual journey. We begin by cultivating these qualities consciously and, as conditioning is released, we gradually come to see that these positive qualities are reflections of our own true being.

The following spiritual qualities have been especially helpful in our own journey toward healing and awakening. Each of these qualities is supported by a specific mudra along with its accompanying inspiration, meditation and affirmation.

1. **Commitment**, **Sthirata** - Making the spiritual journey our first priority.

2. **Openness**, **Vipulachetana** - Gaining a wider, more open perspective of ourselves, life and other people.

3. **Faith**, **Shraddha** - Developing confidence in our true inner being, allowing it to guide our spiritual journey.

4. **Acceptance**, **Kshanti** - Welcoming all that happens in our lives wholeheartedly as a learning and a blessing.

5. **Compassion**, **Karuna** - Recognizing our essential unity with all beings.

6. **Discernment**, **Viveka** - Distinguishing clearly between our limited personality and our limitless true being.

7. **Equanimity**, **Samatva** - Resting in our center securely so that we are not shaken by life's ups and downs so easily.

8. **Spiritual Energy**, **Shakti** - Cultivating the vitality that supports our spiritual journey.

9. **Self-Mastery**, **Vashitvam** - Releasing identification with our conditioning to become the masters of our own destiny.

10. **Freedom**, **Moksha** - Integrating wisdom and compassion, allowing us to experience the freedom and unity that are the essence of our true being.

Spiritual qualities and the mudras that awaken them

Mudra	Core Qualities
Shivalingam	Commitment Sthirata
Shunya	Openness Vipulachetana
Palli	Faith Shraddha
Avahana	Heartfelt Acceptance Kshanti
Karuna	Compassion Karuna
Purna Jnanam	Spiritual Discernment Viveka
Varahkam	Equanimity Samatva
Shakti	Spiritual Energy Shakti
Uttarabodhi	Self-mastery Vashitvam
Kaleshvara	Spiritual Liberation Moksha

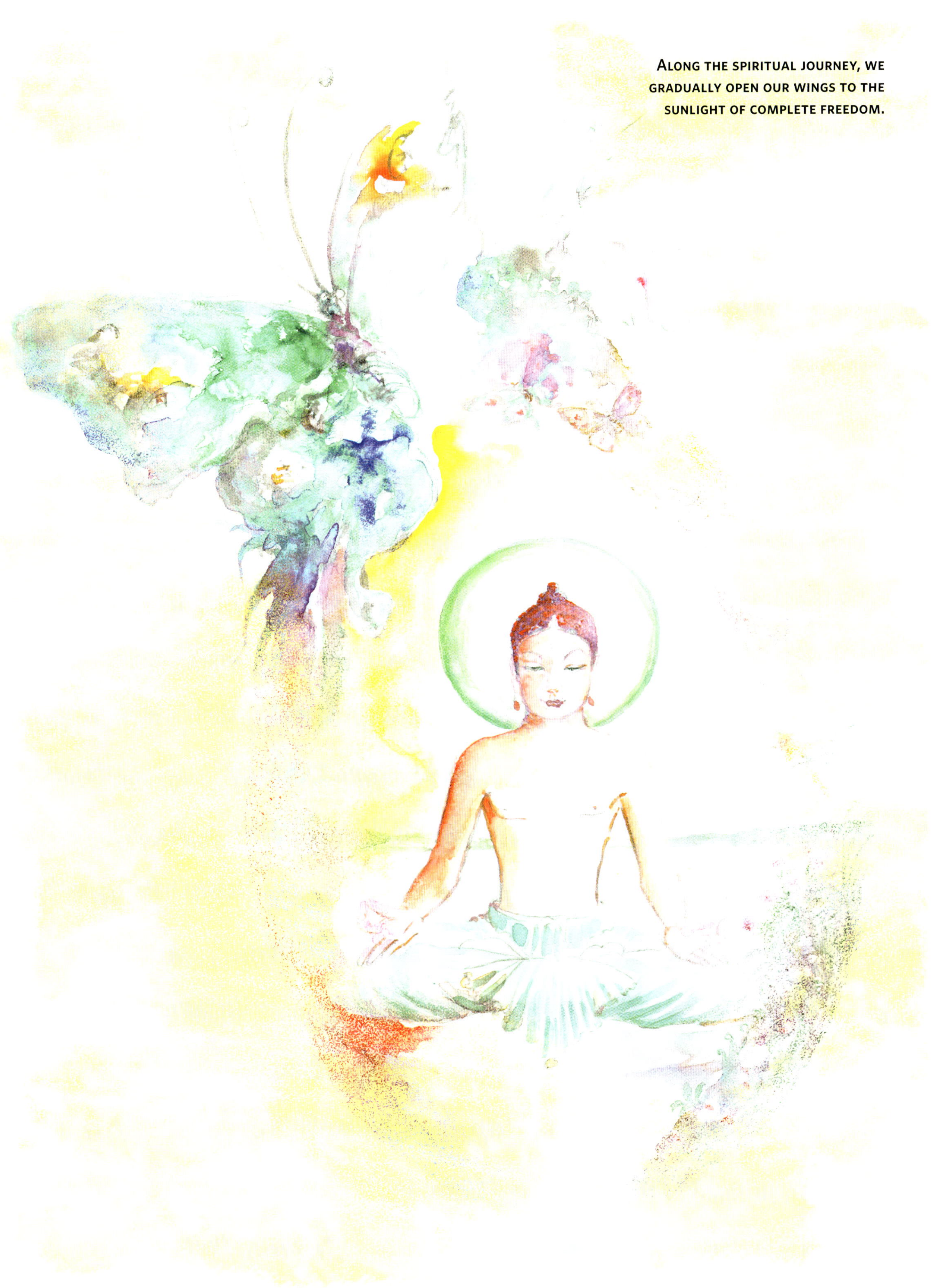

Along the spiritual journey, we gradually open our wings to the sunlight of complete freedom.

90

Shivalingam Mudra

Gesture of the Symbol of Shiva

For Cultivating Spiritual Commitment - Sthirata

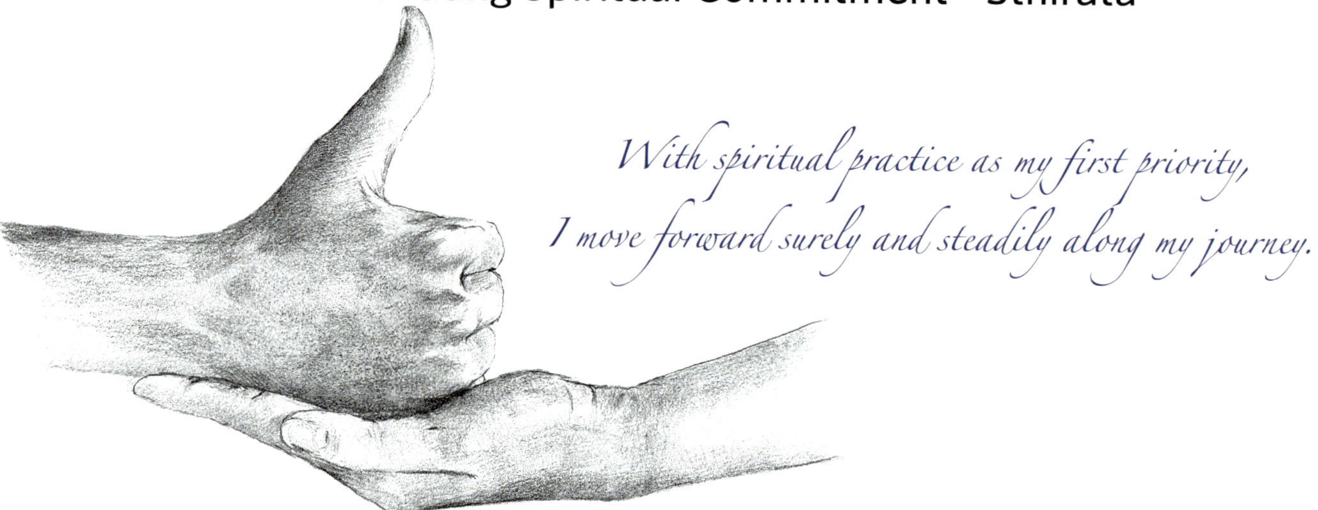

Core Quality

Spiritual Commitment

Especially helpful for

- Strengthening commitment to spiritual practice.
- Supporting optimal postural alignment, which facilitates meditation.
- Enhancing the power of digestion.
- Cultivating determination and one-pointed concentration.

Mudras with similar effects

Merudanda, Mushtikam, Brahma, Matangi, Adhi

Cautions

Contraindicated for hypertension. Adhi, which is less energizing, can be used as a substitute.

Instructions

1. Place the left hand, palm upward, in front of the lower abdomen.
2. Make the right hand into a fist, with the right thumb extended upward.
3. Place the right hand onto the center of the left palm.
4. Relax the shoulders back and down, with the elbows held slightly away from the body and the spine naturally aligned.

Sthirata, which means "commitment," is an important foundation for the spiritual journey. Life offers a wide variety of possibilities and directions that can keep us searching for fulfilment in the outside world endlessly. When we decide to embark on the spiritual journey, focusing on our life's deepest meaning in the form of self-knowledge, it is essential to make spiritual transformation our first priority. At the level of the personality, we often follow our own wants and needs through the accumulation of material possessions, status, success and security. The spiritual path, however, asks us to explore the limitations within these perceived wants and needs in order to awaken to our authentic inner being, which is inherently whole and complete. Identified with the personality, we are guided by the norms of culture and society. For the spiritual journey, however, our motivation arises internally, which requires tremendous determination and commitment in order to proceed all the way to awakening.

Shiva is the deity associated with fervent commitment to spiritual practice. *Linga* is the symbol of Shiva's spiritual power. Shivalingam mudra instills a sense of Shiva's firm commitment to the spiritual path. This gesture directs breath, awareness and energy into the solar plexus, our center of personal power, cultivating the determination to move beyond all obstacles along our spiritual journey. This energy, when awakened and integrated fully, is channeled upward into our higher energy centers of compassion, purification and clarity, cultivating the wisdom that guides us toward awakening. This mudra also cultivates a sense of grounding, creating a firm foundation for our journey by instilling a sense of trust that life will always support us fully.

Systems Balanced:

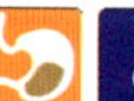 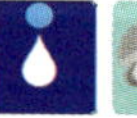 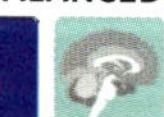 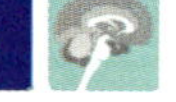

Elements Activated:

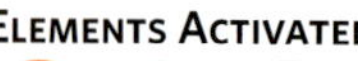

 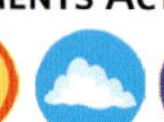 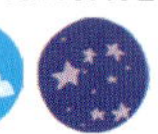

Doshas Balanced:

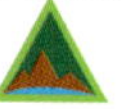

Prana Vayus Nourished: check this

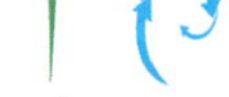

Chakras Balanced:

 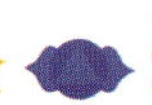 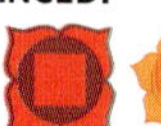 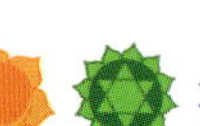

Scale from Calming to Energizing:

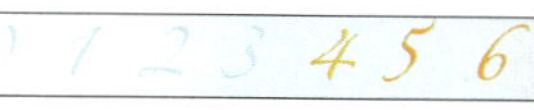 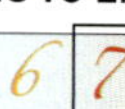 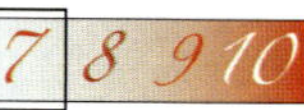

Guided Meditation: **Firm Spiritual Commitment**

- As you hold Shivalingam mudra, take several natural breaths to attune to all the feelings and sensations evoked by this gesture.
- Notice how your breath is naturally directed upward from your solar plexus upward into your chest, neck and head, instilling a sense of uplifting energy that supports your spiritual journey.
- As you embark on this journey, firm commitment is an absolute necessity, allowing you to overcome challenges, moving steadily toward awakening.
- The first aspect of spiritual commitment is developing a consistent practice. Reflect on your ability to maintain a regular spiritual practice in the midst of your daily activities, especially when you encounter challenges and difficulties.
- Take several breaths to envision the changes you could make in your lifestyle and daily routine that would support you in making spiritual practice your first priority.
- The next facet of spiritual commitment is creating a personal practice that meets your unique needs for transformation and awakening within all dimensions of your being.
- Developing a personal practice requires deep commitment, because it asks you to choose methods and techniques that bring to the surface the most challenging aspects of your personality.
- Take several breaths to envision a personal practice that would reveal and transform all the most challenging aspects of your being, allowing them to be gradually seen and released.
- The third facet of spiritual commitment is maintaining continual awareness of your habit patterns and limiting beliefs that drain your energy and keep you from moving forward along your spiritual journey.
- Even with a committed practice and a sincere intention to release your limiting beliefs, you may fall back into old patterns based on perceived needs for security, success, relationships or material possessions.
- Take several breaths to envision new ways of perceiving yourself, the world and other beings that would support you in releasing patterns of conditioning.
- As all the facets of spiritual commitment are integrated within your being, sense your breath flowing more freely toward your higher centers of awakening, providing the clarity for your spiritual journey.
- Affirm your commitment as you repeat the following three times, aloud or silently: **"With firm commitment to my spiritual journey, I move steadily toward awakening."**
- Slowly release the gesture, taking several breaths to affirm your absolute commitment.
- When you are ready, open your eyes, returning slowly and gently, more deeply committed to your spiritual journey.

Annamaya kosha (physical body)

- **Directs breath and awareness into the abdomen and solar plexus, creating a massaging effect that improves circulation to the digestive system.**
- **Directs breath and awareness upward into the throat, neck and head, enhancing circulation to the area of the thyroid and pituitary glands.**
- **Brings breath and awareness to area of the kidneys, adrenal glands and mid back, creating a massaging effect that improves circulation to this area.**
- **Supports optimal alignment of the spine.**
- **The energizing effects of this gesture are generally helpful for Kapha imbalance.**

Pranamaya kosha (energy body)

- **Activates Samana, Prana and Udana vayus, the horizontal, upward moving and uppermost currents of energy.**
- **Opens and balances the first through sixth chakras, with a special focus on the third and sixth, centers of personal power and wisdom.**

Manomaya kosha (psycho-emotional body)

- **Instills commitment and determination.**
- **Enhances trust and self-esteem.**
- **Cultivates one-pointed focus.**

Vijnanamaya kosha (wisdom body)

- **Only with firm commitment can we release our limiting beliefs in order to gradually reveal our true being.**

Anandamaya kosha (bliss body)

- **Cultivates an experience of energy, clarity and vitality.**

91

Shunya Mudra

Gesture of Emptiness

For Cultivating Openness to Transformation - Vipulachetana

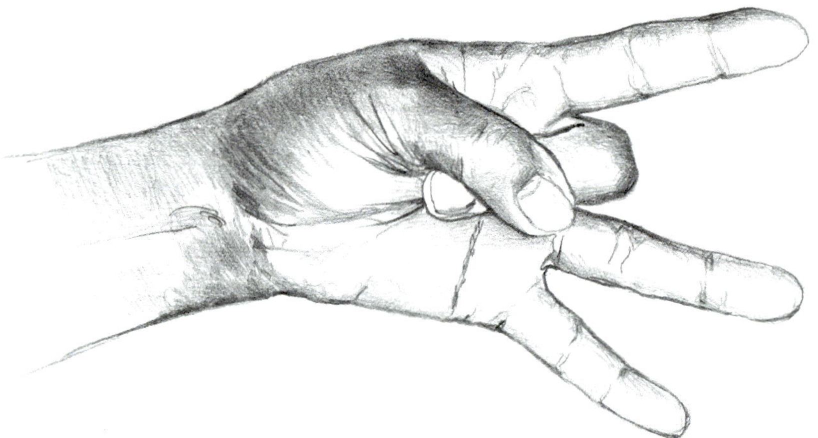

With greater openness
To new ways of seeing,
Space is created for the
Journey of awakening.

Core Quality

Opening to Transformation

Especially Helpful For

- Cultivating a more open way of seeing and being that allows transformation to occur more easily.
- Releasing tension from the area of the shoulders, throat, neck and head.
- Supporting the treatment of auditory problems.
- Supporting the health of the thyroid gland.
- Creating space between thoughts, which helps to release limiting beliefs.
- Opening us to new possibilities.

Mudras With Similar Effects

Akasha, Vishuddha, Garuda

Cautions

None

Instructions

1. Bend the middle fingers down to touch the mounds at the base of the thumbs.
2. Use the thumbs to hold the middle fingers in place.
3. Rest the backs of the hands onto the thighs or knees.
4. Relax the shoulders back and down, with the spine naturally aligned.

With firm commitment to our spiritual journey, we are ready to take the next step, *Vipulachetana*, "opening to transformation." Openness is essential for the spiritual journey because it allows us to see and release the patterns of conditioning that keep us from recognizing the freedom of our true being. A more open way of seeing and being also helps to relax the mind and body, releasing the tension that drains our energy and keeps us from moving forward. The importance of cultivating openness is illustrated by story of the Zen master who received a university professor for tea. The professor talked incessantly about his theoretical knowledge of Zen while the master filled the professor's cup until it overflowed. When the professor saw his cup spilling over, he asked the master what he was doing. The master replied with a smile, "Until your mind is like an empty cup, you will never understand the true essence of Zen."

Shunya means "zero" as well as "empty," and Shunya mudra cultivates a space of openness in which we develop the ability to view ourselves and our lives with greater objectivity and clarity. This gesture directs breath, awareness and energy into the area of the throat and neck, helping to release tension, thereby creating a space of openness in which conditioning can be seen and released more easily. The release of tension cultivated by this gesture enhances circulation to the area of the thyroid gland, supporting balanced metabolism. Shunya mudra creates space between thoughts so that we don't identify with our conditioning so completely. As conditioning is released, this gesture supports the awakening of intuition, allowing us to attune to our inner voice, which guides us along the spiritual journey.

Systems Balanced:

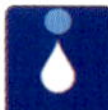

Elements Activated:

Doshas Balanced:

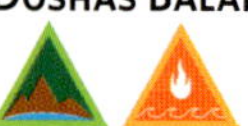

Prana Vayus Nourished:

Chakras Balanced:

Scale from Calming to Energizing:

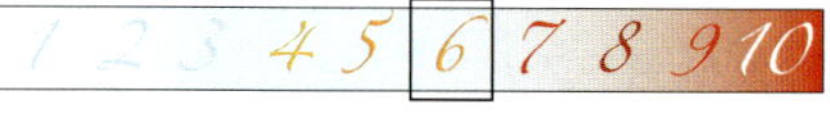

Guided Meditation: Opening to Transformation

ॐ As you hold Shunya mudra, take several natural breaths to attune to all the feelings and sensations awakened by this gesture.

ॐ Notice how your breath is gently directed into your throat and neck, cultivating a greater sense of openness.

ॐ With each inhalation, this sense of openness is naturally increased, and with each exhalation, tension from your throat and neck is gradually released.

ॐ As tension is released, you naturally open to new ways of seeing and being, creating space in which spiritual transformation can occur more easily.

ॐ To deepen your ability to see yourself, others and life more openly, bring to mind an issue or challenge that you are currently facing.

ॐ Supported by your rhythmic breathing, sense this issue gently resting within your throat center, allowing thoughts and feelings to arise naturally.

ॐ Use your breath to enhance your sense of opening, allowing any tensions that accompany this issue to be gradually released, together with your breathing.

ॐ As tension is released, take several breaths to embrace this issue more lightly and spaciously, naturally allowing you to gain greater clarity.

ॐ With greater clarity, intuition awakens naturally, allowing you to expand your horizons in order to perceive new possibilities for the issue you are exploring.

ॐ As you envision these new possibilities, take some time to reflect on more open ways of seeing that will allow you to bring them into being.

ॐ As you integrate new possibilities, you naturally sense greater lightness and ease permeating your entire being, allowing you to continue your spiritual journey with a greater sense of inner freedom.

ॐ Affirm your growing openness, repeating the following three times, aloud or silently: **"Open to new ways of seeing and being, spiritual transformation occurs naturally."**

ॐ Slowly release the gesture, taking several breaths to sense your greater openness to transformation.

ॐ When you are ready, open your eyes, returning slowly and gently, more open to new possibilities along your spiritual journey.

Annamaya kosha (physical body)

- **Directs breath and awareness to the throat and neck, creating a massaging effect that increases circulation to the area of the thyroid gland.**
- **Expands the breath in the upper chest, cultivating energy and vitality.**
- **May be helpful for hearing problems.**
- **The mildly energizing effects of this gesture are generally helpful for Kapha imbalance.**
- **The cultivation of new ways of seeing is generally helpful for Pitta imbalance.**

Pranamaya kosha (energy body)

- **Activates the flow of Udana vayu, the uppermost current of energy.**
- **Opens and balances the fifth chakra, center of spiritual purification.**

Manomaya kosha (psycho-emotional body)

- **Slows the train of thoughts, creating space for transformation.**

Vijnanamaya kosha (wisdom body)

- **Within the space of transformation, conditioning is witnessed and gradually released, opening a doorway to our authentic being.**

Anandamaya kosha (bliss body)

- **As tension is released from the area of the throat and neck, feelings of openness and limitlessness arise naturally.**

92 Palli Mudra

Gesture of the Shelter

For Cultivating Trust in Your Inner Guide - Shraddha

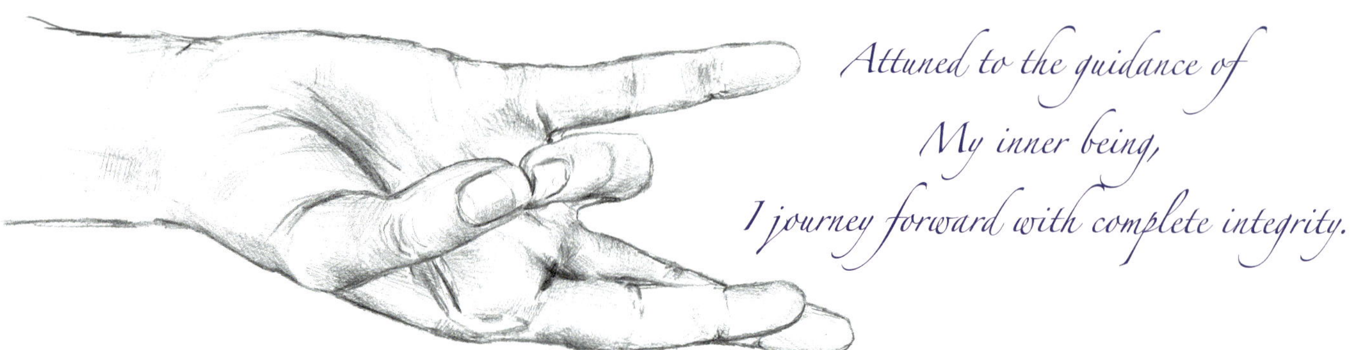

Core Quality

Trusting Inner Guidance

Especially helpful for

- Cultivating self-confidence, optimism and energy for the spiritual journey.
- Supporting optimal alignment of the spine.
- Enhancing our sense of embodiment.
- Balancing digestion.

Mudras with similar effects

Vajra, Vajrapradama, Abhaya Varada

Cautions

None

Instructions

1. Wrap the middle fingers over the index fingers.
2. Touch the tips of the thumbs to the tips of the ring fingers of the same hand.
3. Extend the little fingers straight out.
4. Rest the backs of the hands onto the thighs or knees. Alternatively, this gesture can be held with the hands at shoulder height, with the palms facing forward.
5. Relax the shoulders back and down, with the spine naturally aligned.

Shraddha means "faith," but rather than faith in a religious system or an external deity, it refers to trust in the guidance of our own being as we move forward along our spiritual journey. Teachers, teachings, methodologies and philosophies all support this journey, but it is a deepening sense of inner trust that ultimately guides us toward awakening. The first fruits of our spiritual journey may be experienced as a greater sense of relaxation, mental clarity or reduced neediness or worry. These initial experiences enhance our confidence in the spiritual path and in our own inner guidance. As we see the positive benefits that come from our own process of transformation, we naturally embrace the spiritual path more deeply, releasing the limiting beliefs that keep us from moving toward awakening. Our deepening faith supports us even when the path is challenging, reminding us that all experiences provide important learnings along our journey.

Palli means "shelter," and Palli mudra provides a shelter along our spiritual journey by enhancing our sense of trust, support and centering. This gesture facilitates Full Yogic Breathing, which flows most strongly along the back of the body. The flow of breath and energy throughout the back of the body, naturally lengthens and aligns the spine. At a subtle level, this alignment is experienced as a sense of integrity within our thoughts, words and deeds, which serves as a shelter along our spiritual journey. As this mudra cultivates alignment and centering, it also enhances our sense of embodiment. Palli mudra lengthens both the inhalation and the exhalation, facilitating rhythmic breathing, which instills a sense of equanimity, further supporting us in remaining centered and focused along our journey.

Systems Balanced:

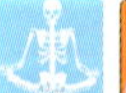 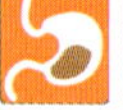 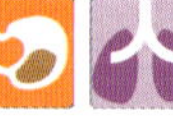 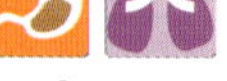

Elements Activated:

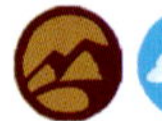 

Doshas Balanced:

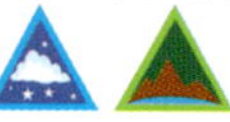

Prana Vayus Nourished:

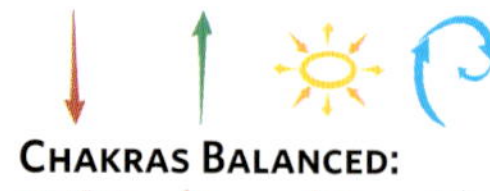

Chakras Balanced:

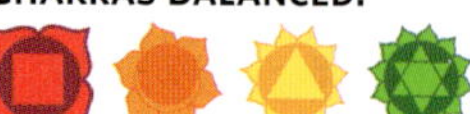

Scale from Calming to Energizing:

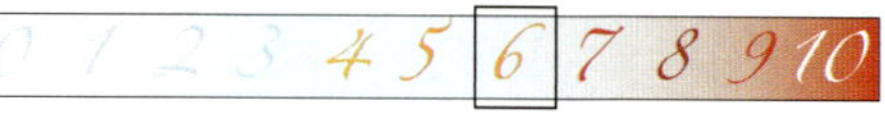

Guided Meditation: Trusting Inner Guidance

- As you hold Palli mudra, take several natural breaths to attune to all the feelings and sensations awakened by this gesture.
- Notice how your breath flows gently along your spinal column. With each inhalation, space is created between each vertebra, and with each exhalation, sense your spine aligned naturally.
- Take several breaths to experience this alignment within the central axis of your body, naturally instilling a sense of centering that allows you to trust more completely in the guidance of your inner being.
- Trust in your inner guide is an essential support for your spiritual journey, allowing you to attune to the wisdom and clarity that illuminate your path toward awakening.
- Begin by reflecting on how your inner guide has illuminated your way to different paths and teachings, noticing how each was absolutely necessary at a certain point in your journey for supporting your process of transformation and learning.
- Take several breaths to affirm the guidance of your inner being, illuminating your steps surely and steadily toward each of the teachings that plays a part in your awakening.
- Now, reflect on how your inner guide has supported your journey, even in times of doubt and uncertainty, ultimately transforming your challenges into opportunities for learning and awakening.
- Take several breaths to affirm the guidance of your inner being, illuminating your steps, especially when your journey is challenging.
- Next, reflect on how your inner guide has served you faithfully in knowing when a change of direction is needed, even if this involves moving beyond paths or practices that you have held as sacred.
- Take several breaths to affirm the guidance of your inner being, illuminating your steps whenever a change of direction is needed.
- Finally, reflect on how your inner guide has always shown the way toward the truth of your being, beyond all techniques and philosophies, teachers and teachings, guiding you toward your life's deeper meaning.
- Take several breaths to affirm the guidance of your inner being, illuminating your steps beyond all teachings and techniques, supporting you completely at each moment of your journey.
- Affirm inner guidance, as you repeat the following three times, aloud or silently: **"Trusting in the guidance of my inner being, I journey forward confidently."**
- Slowly release the gesture, taking several breaths to affirm your trust in your own inner guidance.
- When you are ready, open your eyes, returning slowly and gently, with a sure sense of guidance along your journey.

Annamaya kosha (Physical body)

• Cultivates Full Yogic Breathing, creating a massaging effect throughout the torso, which supports the health of all the body systems.
• Directs breath and awareness up and down the spinal column, creating space between the vertebrae and supporting optimal alignment.
• The grounding and centering cultivated by this gesture are generally helpful for Vata imbalance.
• The uplifting energy cultivated is generally helpful for Kapha imbalance.

Pranamaya kosha (Energy body)

• Balances Prana and Apana vayus, the upward and downward moving currents of energy.
• Gently activates Samana and Udana vayus, the horizontal and uppermost current of energy.
• Opens and balances the first five chakras.

Manomaya kosha (Psycho-emotional body)

• Instills trust and self-confidence.
• Cultivates steadiness and one-pointed concentration.

Vijnanamaya kosha (Wisdom body)

• Instills faith, supporting a willingness to release limiting beliefs, creating space in which guidance toward our true Self awakens naturally.

Anandamaya kosha (Bliss body)

• Cultivates an experience of inner alignment, integrity and equanimity.

93

Avahana Mudra

Gesture of Invocation

For Cultivating Heartfelt Acceptance - Kshanti

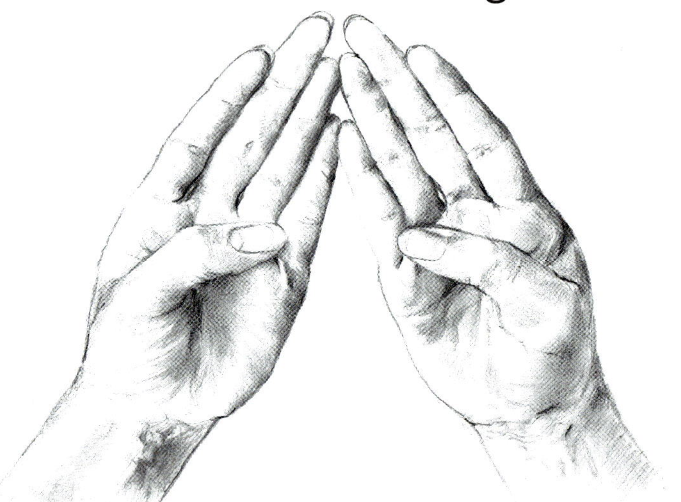

Through heartfelt acceptance,
I open to receive
All of life
As a learning and a blessing.

Core Quality

Heartfelt Acceptance

Especially helpful for

- Opening the frontiers of the heart to welcome all of life as a learning and a blessing.
- Learning to welcome challenges as opportunities.
- Optimizing digestion and assimilation.
- Supporting the healthy functioning of the immune system.
- Instilling optimism and energy.

Mudras with similar effects

Purna Hridaya, Hastaphula, Hridaya, Vajrapradama

Cautions

None

Instructions

1. Hold the palms upward in front of the solar plexus, with the fingers together.
2. Touch the tips of the thumbs to the base of the ring fingers of each hand.
3. Touch the outer borders of the tips of the ring and little fingers together.
4. Keep the wrists comfortably apart, with the forearms resting against the abdomen.
5. Relax the shoulders back and down, with the spine naturally aligned.

Kshanti is wholehearted acceptance of all that life brings as a learning and a blessing. When we embrace life unconditionally, we come to see that even the most challenging experiences are an important part of our learning. These challenges and difficulties reveal the limiting beliefs that need to be released in order to proceed toward awakening. As we practice heartfelt acceptance, we recognize that everything is part of a larger plan whose intention is always to reveal the limitlessness of our true inner being. This larger plan is a reflection of the universal intelligence, which always gives us exactly what we need for awakening at each step of our journey. Through wholehearted acceptance, the frontiers of our hearts expand naturally, cultivating compassion and empathy, allowing us to embrace others' ways of seeing, as well as our own history. Acceptance does not mean living life passively, but rather choosing to embrace all life experiences positively as a doorway to awakening.

Avahana is an "invocation," seeking the blessing of a deity. Avahana mudra directs breath, awareness and energy upward from the solar plexus, our center of personal power, to the chest, our center of unconditional love and compassion. The movement of energy from the center of will to the center of compassion reflects the process of wholehearted acceptance. As we welcome life more completely, we move from a focus on our own personal needs to a wider perspective in which every step of our journey is embraced as a process of learning. Avahana mudra cultivates the equanimity, optimism and energy that allow us to receive challenges more confidently as opportunities for learning in which there are always solutions and possibilities.

Systems Balanced:

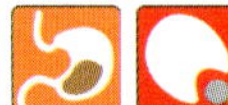
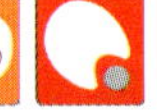

Prana Vayus Nourished:

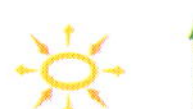

Elements Activated:

Chakras Balanced:

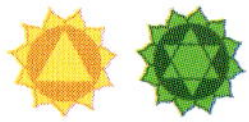

Doshas Balanced:

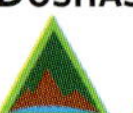

Scale from Calming to Energizing:

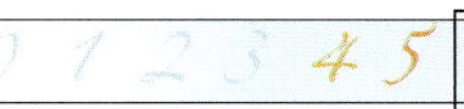
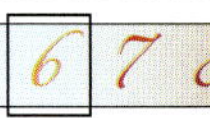
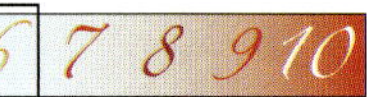

Guided Meditation: Heartfelt Acceptance

- ॐ As you hold Avahana mudra, take several natural breaths to attune to all the feelings and sensations evoked by this gesture.
- ॐ Notice how your breath flows gently upward from your solar plexus into your chest, instilling a sense of ease and openness.
- ॐ With greater openness, the quality of acceptance unfolds naturally, allowing you to embrace all that life offers wholeheartedly.
- ॐ Begin by taking several breaths to welcome everything in your natural surroundings, embracing the seasons with ease, as reflections of life's ever flowing stream.
- ॐ As you learn to accept nature's ever changing scenery, you release resistance and learn to embrace each moment's unique beauty.
- ॐ Now, take several breaths to embrace the different facets of your personality, welcoming your habits and tendencies with humor and empathy, rather than judging yourself harshly or taking yourself too seriously.
- ॐ Take some time to welcome all aspects of your personality, creating space in which they can be transformed gradually and naturally.
- ॐ Next, take several breaths to deepen your ability to embrace others and their points of view more openly, honoring and learning from different ways of seeing and being.
- ॐ As you embrace others more openly, you release any tendency to be critical or demanding, acknowledging that all of your interactions play an important role in your process of learning.
- ॐ Now, open to embrace your own history, seeing that each chapter in your life journey has been an essential part of your process of transformation and awakening.
- ॐ Take several breaths to welcome every chapter of your life wholeheartedly by seeing that even the greatest challenges actually turned out to be blessings.
- ॐ Finally, welcome life as a whole, no matter what is happening, recognizing that everything that occurs has its own meaning within your journey.
- ॐ Take several breaths to expand the frontiers of your heart, receiving all that life offers as a learning and a blessing, guiding you surely toward awakening.
- ॐ Affirm your heartfelt acceptance, repeating the following three times, aloud or silently: **"As I embrace life wholeheartedly, everything becomes a doorway to awakening."**
- ॐ Slowly release the gesture, taking several breaths to experience the lightness and ease that come from heartfelt acceptance of all that life brings.
- ॐ When you are ready, open your eyes, returning slowly and gently, sensing yourself more open and accepting.

Annamaya kosha (physical body)

• Directs breath and awareness into the solar plexus and chest, creating a massaging effect that enhances circulation to the digestive and cardiovascular systems.
• Gently enhances circulation to the area of the thymus gland.
• Directs the breath into the middle and upper back, creating space between the shoulder blades and between the vertebrae of the thoracic spine, supporting optimal alignment.
• The mildly energizing effects of this gesture are generally helpful for Kapha imbalance.
• The heartfelt acceptance cultivated is generally helpful for Pitta imbalance.

Pranamaya kosha (energy body)

• Activates Samana and Prana vayus, the horizontal and upward moving currents of energy.
• Opens and balances the third and fourth chakras, centers of personal power and unconditional love.

Manomaya kosha (psycho-emotional body)

• Cultivates acceptance, gratitude and surrender.
• Develops a willingness to embrace challenges as opportunities.

Vijnanamaya kosha (wisdom body)

• By embracing difficult situations as opportunities for learnings, the limiting beliefs which restrict our freedom are revealed and gradually released.

Anandamaya kosha (bliss body)

• Through heartfelt acceptance, hope and optimism naturally spring from within our own being.

94

Karuna Mudra

Gesture of Compassion

For Cultivating Compassion - Karuna

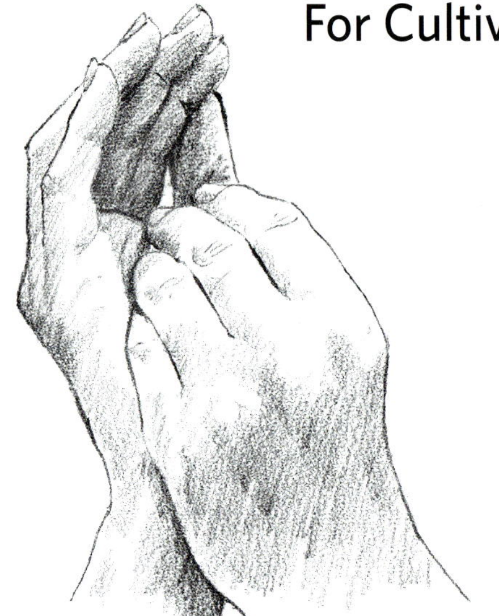

Through the eyes of the heart,
I clearly see that all beings
Seek happiness and freedom from suffering.

Core Quality

Compassion

Especially helpful for

- Cultivating compassion toward ourselves and all beings.
- Supporting the health of the cardio-respiratory and immune systems.
- Relaxing the muscles of the chest, thereby helping to reduce stress.
- Relaxing the muscles of the face and jaw, which may be helpful for TMJ dysfunction.

Mudras with similar effects

Hridaya, Purna Hridaya, Padma, Kapota

Cautions

None

Instructions

1. Gently cup your left hand and hold it with the palm facing your heart.
2. Cup the right hand and place the fingertips of the left hand at the base of the fingers of the right hand.
3. The outer border of the left thumb rests alongside the right thumb, with the upper digit of the left thumb, resting on the middle digit of the right thumb.
4. Relax the shoulders back and down, with the spine naturally aligned.

Karuna, which means "compassion," is the ability to see that all beings, just like ourselves, ultimately seek happiness and release from suffering. We normally see the world through the lens of our own personality, focused on ourselves and our own needs. This narrow perspective tends to create separation from others, who are also focused on their own needs, often resulting in misunderstanding, competition and conflict. Through the eyes of compassion, we learn to focus on the similarities rather than the differences between ourselves and others. The essence of compassion is understanding that all are searching for love and security within the limits of their understanding. As our compassion expands, we also see that our search for love and security is ultimately a quest for the wholeness and unity of our own true being. Compassion begins with ourselves, because it is only when we can embrace all the facets of our own being wholeheartedly that we are able to accept others and life more openly.

In Karuna mudra, the left palm is directed toward our own heart as a symbol of self-compassion while the right palm is turned outward toward others, symbolizing universal compassion. This gesture brings breath, awareness and energy to the center of the chest, gently massaging the physical heart and the thymus gland. Karuna mudra focuses the breath into the left nostril and left side of the chest, making this gesture slightly calming, which supports the opening of the heart and the cultivation of compassion. This gesture naturally expands our ability to live with joy and harmony, traveling the spiritual path lightly and easily in unison with all beings.

Systems Balanced:

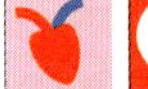 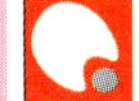

Elements Activated:

Doshas Balanced:

 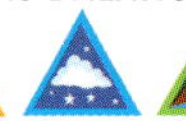

Prana Vayus Nourished:

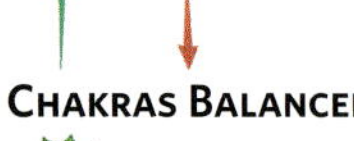

Chakras Balanced:

Scale from Calming to Energizing:

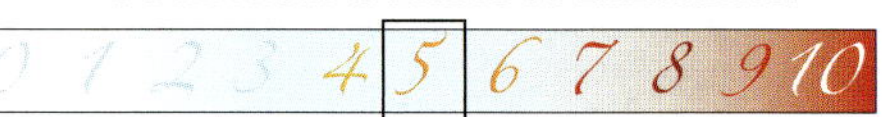

Guided Meditation: **Awakening Compassion**

- As you hold Karuna mudra, take several natural breaths to attune to all the feelings and sensations awakened by this gesture.
- Notice how your breath is gently directed into your chest, instilling calm and serenity that unfolds from deep within your heart center naturally.
- As you attune to your heart, you gradually develop the sensitivity that allows you to embrace yourself, life and all other beings compassionately.
- Take several breaths to reflect on the extent to which you are able to offer compassion to yourself by acknowledging that all of your actions were ultimately an attempt to find the love, support and security that are the essence of your true being.
- Attuning deeply to your heart center, offer compassion to yourself, honoring your journey wholeheartedly, dissolving all self-judgment, shame and guilt naturally.
- As you embrace yourself compassionately, you naturally enhance your ability to offer loving kindness to those you care for deeply, embracing both their positive and challenging qualities.
- Bring into your heart the image of someone you care for deeply, releasing any expectation of how they should be, creating a space of openness in which their transformation, and yours, can occur more easily.
- As you offer compassion to yourself and to those you care for deeply, you gradually develop the ability to offer compassion to those with whom you experience separation or difficulty.
- Bring into your heart the image of someone you find challenging, perceiving their authentic being rather than focusing on their actions and beliefs.
- As you hold this person within your heart of compassion, clearly see that all of their actions are based on a need for love, support and security, even if those needs are expressed inappropriately.
- By seeing this person compassionately, your feelings of judgment, anger and resentment are released more easily, allowing you to see this person and yourself more objectively, while creating safe and appropriate boundaries.
- Now, open your heart of compassion to all beings, honoring each person's journey, recognizing that all of us are moving, within the limits of our understanding, toward a vision of unity.
- Affirm your growing compassion, repeating the following three times, aloud or silently: **"With a heart of compassion, I clearly see that we all share a journey toward unity."**
- Slowly release the gesture, taking several breaths to rest within your heart of compassion.
- When you are ready, open your eyes, returning slowly and gently, sensing your heart of compassion guiding your journey.

Annamaya kosha (physical body)

• Directs breath and awareness into the chest, gently massaging the heart and thymus gland.
• Relaxes the muscles of the chest, thereby helping to reduce stress.
• Releases tension from the face and jaw, which may be helpful for TMJ dysfunction.
• The cultivation of compassion is generally helpful for Vata and Pitta imbalances.
• The enhanced breath in the chest is generally helpful for Kapha imbalances.

Pranamaya kosha (energy body)

• Balances Prana and Apana vayus, the upward and downward moving currents of energy.
• Opens and balances the fourth chakra, center of unconditional love.

Manomaya kosha (psycho-emotional body)

• Cultivates a sense of calm, patience, safety and inner nourishment that support us in releasing judgment toward ourselves and others.

Vijnanamaya kosha (wisdom body)

• As the heart opens, we gradually come to see that compassion is a reflection of our true being.

Anandamaya kosha (bliss body)

• As our subtle heart expands, waves of nourishment and healing flow out from the heart center.

95 Purna Jnanam Mudra

Gesture of Complete Wisdom

For Cultivating Spiritual Discernment - Viveka

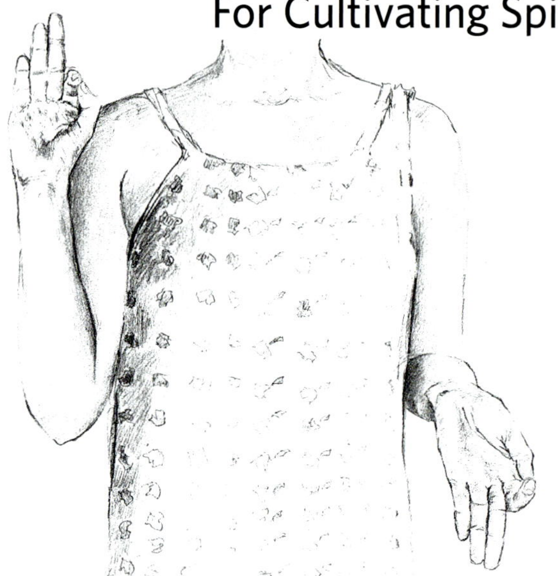

Discernment allows me to recognize clearly
My true Self
Beyond the limited personality.

Core Quality

Spiritual Discernment

Especially helpful for

- Cultivating discernment between our true being and the conditioned personality.
- Integrating all the polarities of our being, cultivating a balance of activity and rest, supporting the health of all the bodily systems.
- Cultivating calm and spaciousness in which we open to receive guidance.

Mudras with similar effects

Dharma Chakra, Jnana, Dhyana

Cautions

None

Instructions

1. Touch the tips of the index fingers to the thumbs of the same hand with the other fingers together and extended.
2. Hold the right hand at the level of the right shoulder, facing forward.
3. Hold the left forearm parallel to the earth, with the left hand bent downward so that the left palm is facing forward at the level of the pelvis.
4. Relax the shoulders back and down, with the spine naturally aligned.

Viveka, which means "spiritual discernment," is the ability to differentiate clearly between the limited personality and our limitless true being. The personality is characterized by change and a sense that there is always something "out there" that we need in order to become happy and complete. On the contrary, spiritual discernment allows us to see that we are inherently whole and complete. As we gradually recognize our inherent wholeness, we experience greater contentment and equanimity, a sense that we are at peace no matter what is happening in our surroundings. The quality of Viveka is cultivated by seeing our psycho-emotional patterns and beliefs more objectively rather than acting them out unconsciously. Every time we catch ourselves beginning to react based on our conditioning and, instead, choose to act consciously, we diminish the power of our beliefs to determine our behavior, thoughts and feelings. As our identification with these beliefs is gradually released, our true Self naturally comes to the forefront of all our activities.

Purna means "full" or "complete," and *Jnanam* means "knowledge." *Purna jnanam* refers to the continual experiential awareness of our true being in all our interactions and activities. In Purna Jnanam mudra, the breath originates at the bottom of the left lung and moves diagonally up to the top of the right lung, integrating the lunar and solar, feminine and masculine facets of our being, allowing us to experience greater integration and harmony. This sense of greater harmony naturally supports the awakening of discernment. This gesture also expands the pauses at the end of the inhalation and exhalation, cultivating a space of inner silence in which clear seeing awakens naturally.

Systems Balanced:

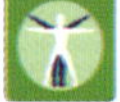

Elements Activated:

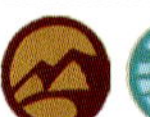
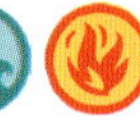

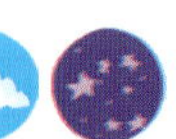
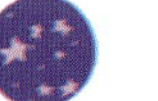

Doshas Balanced:

Prana Vayus Nourished:

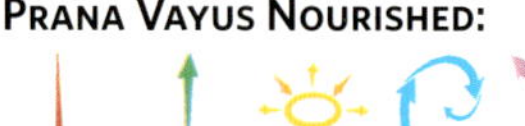

Chakras Balanced:

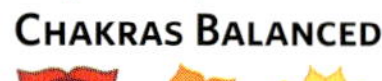
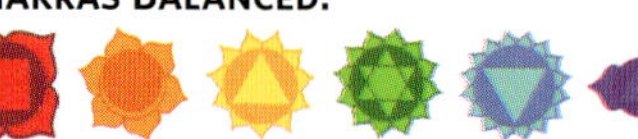

Scale from Calming to Energizing:

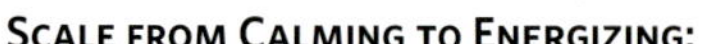
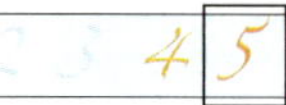

Guided Meditation: Cultivating Spiritual Discernment

- As you hold Purna Jnanam mudra, take several natural breaths to attune to all the feelings and sensations awakened by this gesture.
- Notice how each inhaling breath expands your torso, front, sides and back, and how each exhalation allows your entire rib cage to fully soften and relax.
- Sense how this rhythmic expansion and release supports freer breathing throughout your entire being.
- As you breathe more freely, tension is released, allowing you to rest within your authentic being, naturally loosening your identification with your personality.
- To discern more clearly between your true Self and your limited personality, visualize a shelf on which you place, temporarily, all the various facets of your identity.
- Begin by placing your wallet on the shelf, with all of your personal information, including your name, age, address and description.
- Next, place your possessions on the shelf: money, house, car and bank accounts, everything that gives you a sense of security, recognizing their importance in supporting your journey, but also seeing that they are ultimately temporary.
- Now, place all of your certificates, diplomas and degrees on the shelf, everything that represents your process of learning along your life journey.
- Reflect on how your degrees represent your career and role in society, which you also place on the shelf temporarily.
- Next, place your friends and family on the shelf, separating from them only momentarily, as part of a process that will allow you to honor them more deeply.
- Now, place your likes and dislikes on the shelf, your emotions, thoughts, judgments and beliefs, everything that defines your everyday personality.
- Finally, place your own body on the shelf, including its state of health, honoring it as the vehicle for your life journey while recognizing that it is ultimately temporary.
- Take several breaths to observe everything on the shelf, becoming aware of the one who is left – the simple conscious being who is observing everything.
- Now, try to place this conscious presence on the shelf, noticing that no matter how hard you try, it always remains, because it is your essential Self.
- Take some time to rest within your essential Self, noticing a growing lightness and ease, as if a weight has been taken off your shoulders, allowing you to relax completely.
- With the weight of the personality released, you experience your essential Self as inherently whole and complete, allowing you to rest in deep silence and inner peace.
- Now, with an enhanced ability to discern your true being, return to the shelf and welcome everything back gradually, recognizing that everything on the shelf plays an essential role within your journey of appreciation and awakening.
- Aligned with your true being, repeat the following three times, aloud or silently: **"By placing everything on the shelf temporarily, my true being is revealed clearly."**
- Slowly release the gesture, taking several breaths to rest in your essential Self.
- When you are ready, open your eyes, returning slowly and gently, discerning more clearly between your authentic being and your limited personality.

Annamaya kosha (physical body)

• Lengthens the inhaling and exhaling breaths evenly as well as the pauses, facilitating a balance of alertness and relaxation, which supports the function of all bodily systems.
• The balancing effects of this gesture are generally helpful for Vata, Pitta and Kapha imbalances.

Pranamaya kosha (energy body)

• Balances all prana vayus, with a special focus on Prana and Apana vayus.
• Opens and balances the first six chakras.

Manomaya kosha (psycho-emotional body)

• Improves concentration, which stabilizes the mind, supporting the development of discernment.
• Creates space between thoughts.

Vijnanamaya kosha (wisdom body)

• In an environment of spaciousness and calm, we more easily discern between the conditioned personality and our limitless true being.

Anandamaya kosha (bliss body)

• As we release the stress and tension associated with the conditioning of the personality, the wholeness and bliss of the true Self arise naturally.

96 VARAHKAM MUDRA

Gesture of the Boar

For Cultivating Equanimity - Samatva

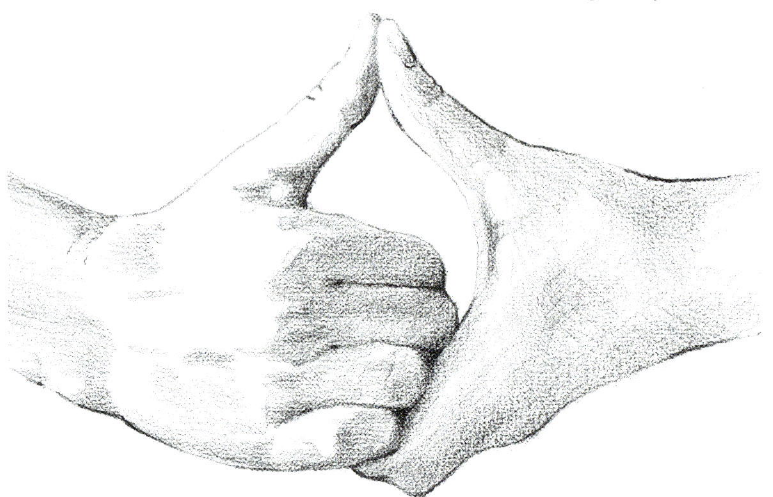

Centered in my authentic being,
I meet life's challenges
With greater equanimity.

CORE QUALITY
Equanimity

ESPECIALLY HELPFUL FOR
- Cultivating equanimity.
- Balancing all the systems of the body.
- Releasing tension from the middle and upper back.
- Bringing circulation to the area of the kidneys and adrenal glands.

MUDRAS WITH SIMILAR EFFECTS
Dharma Chakra, Abhaya Varada, Trimurti, Vajra, Svasti

CAUTIONS
None

INSTRUCTIONS
1. Hold the left hand in front of the solar plexus, palm up, and place the right hand above the left hand, palm down.
2. Clasp the fingers together and draw the hands gently apart.
3. Place the tips of the thumbs together, rotating the hands in opposite directions so that both thumbs are pointing upward.
4. Relax the shoulders back and down, with the elbows held away from the body and the spine naturally aligned.

Samatva, which means "equanimity," is the balance and centering that awakens naturally as we align with our true inner being. At the level of the personality, life can be a "roller coaster" of ups and downs that creates imbalance both in the mind and body. When we ride this "roller coaster" unconsciously, we experience the results in the form of both elation and suffering. As we align with our inner being, we experience a sense of centering and equanimity beyond the constant changes at the level of the personality. As we deepen our equanimity, we tend to return to balance more quickly and easily when we encounter challenges along our journey. With a growing sense of equanimity, challenges are experienced as waves that arise and pass away on the surface of life's sea without disturbing the peace of our essential being.

Varahka means "boar," and Varahkam is one of the incarnations of the deity *Vishnu*, the sustainer of the universe, who maintains balance and harmony within all the rhythms and cycles of creation. Varahkam mudra evokes Vishnu's ability to maintain dynamic balance within the inner universe of our mind and body. In this gesture, the breath flows upward along the front of the body on the inhalation, and then down the back on the exhalation. Within this circle of harmonious breathing, a sense of harmony arises naturally. This harmonious breathing also creates a massaging effect within the torso that supports health and healing within all the systems of the body. The circuit of breath and energy cultivated by this gesture enhances embodiment and a sense of grounding. The combination of grounding and harmony cultivates an experience of deep equanimity.

SYSTEMS BALANCED:

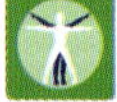

ELEMENTS ACTIVATED:

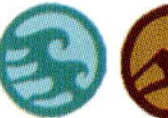
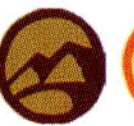

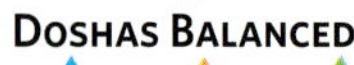

DOSHAS BALANCED:

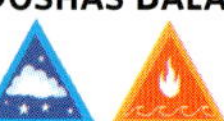

PRANA VAYUS NOURISHED:

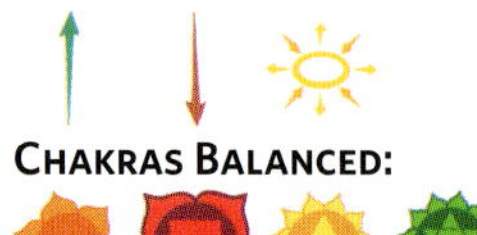

CHAKRAS BALANCED:

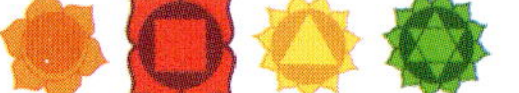

SCALE FROM CALMING TO ENERGIZING:

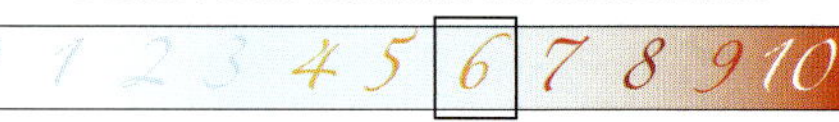

Guided Meditation: Circle of Equanimity

ॐ As you hold Varahkam mudra, take several natural breaths to attune to all the feelings and sensations evoked by this gesture.

ॐ With each inhalation, your breath flows upward along the front of your body, and with each exhalation, it flows smoothly down your back, creating a circle of energy that naturally harmonizes your entire being.

ॐ Take some time to sense this circuit of energy, flowing in synchrony with your breathing, instilling a sense of equanimity that you integrate into all of your activities.

ॐ To sense greater equanimity within your daily routine, visualize yourself at the dawn of a new day, creating an intention to maintain balance at all times, places and in all situations.

ॐ You begin by taking a few moments to sit in peace, welcoming all that this new day might bring by understanding that everything has its own purpose and meaning within your journey.

ॐ Visualize the people and events you may encounter throughout this day. Recognizing that some interactions may be smooth and easy while others may be challenging, you create an intention to meet them all with equanimity.

ॐ You remain aligned more easily with your essential equanimity by constantly remembering that life is a field of learning in which every interaction has its own place within your journey.

ॐ As you prepare for your day, you review your plans and expectations carefully, honoring the importance of sincere effort in achieving your objectives in the best possible way.

ॐ At the same time, you recognize that the results you receive may be very different from what you've envisioned initially.

ॐ By resting within your circle of equanimity, you can allow the results of your actions to unfold naturally, with less attachment and anxiety, knowing that everything that happens has its own meaning within the larger picture of your life journey.

ॐ As you prepare for your day, you also recognize that equanimity does not occur immediately. There may be moments when you begin to lose your balance and ease due to the pressures of daily living.

ॐ With a sincere intention to remain aligned with your true being, you become aware of the first signs of imbalance more easily, and rather than becoming impatient, critical or demanding, you reconnect with your essential equanimity.

ॐ Now, envision your day drawing to a close. Your sense of equanimity may have been challenged and your composure may have risen and fallen, but you have developed the ability to return to your circle of equanimity.

ॐ Resting in equanimity, repeat the following three times, aloud or silently:
"Attuned to my essential equanimity, I embrace all that I meet along my journey."

ॐ Now, slowly release the gesture, taking several breaths to rest completely within your circle of equanimity.

ॐ When you are ready, open your eyes, returning slowly and gently, continuing your journey with greater equanimity.

Annamaya kosha (physical body)

• Creates a circuit of breath within the torso that enhances circulation, nourishing all of the body systems.
• Directs breath into the back, creating a massaging effect that helps to release muscular contraction.
• The enhanced breathing in the mid back increases circulation to the area of the kidneys and adrenal glands.
• The grounding and centering cultivated by this gesture are generally helpful for Vata imbalance.
• The equanimity cultivated is generally helpful for Pitta imbalance.
• The expansion of the breath is generally helpful for Kapha imbalance.

Pranamaya kosha (energy body)

• Balances Prana and Apana vayus, the upward and downward moving currents of energy.
• Gently activates Samana vayu, the horizontal current.
• Opens and balances the first through the fourth chakras, with a special focus on the second, center of self-nourishment.

Manomaya kosha (psycho-emotional body)

• Enhances a sense of body awareness.
• Supports emotional balance.

Vijnanamaya kosha (wisdom body)

• Through deepening equanimity, we come to experience it as a reflection of our true being.

Anandamaya kosha (bliss body)

• As we live with greater equanimity, feelings of joy and unity arise naturally.

97

SHAKTI MUDRA

Gesture of the Goddess

For Awakening Spiritual Energy - Shakti

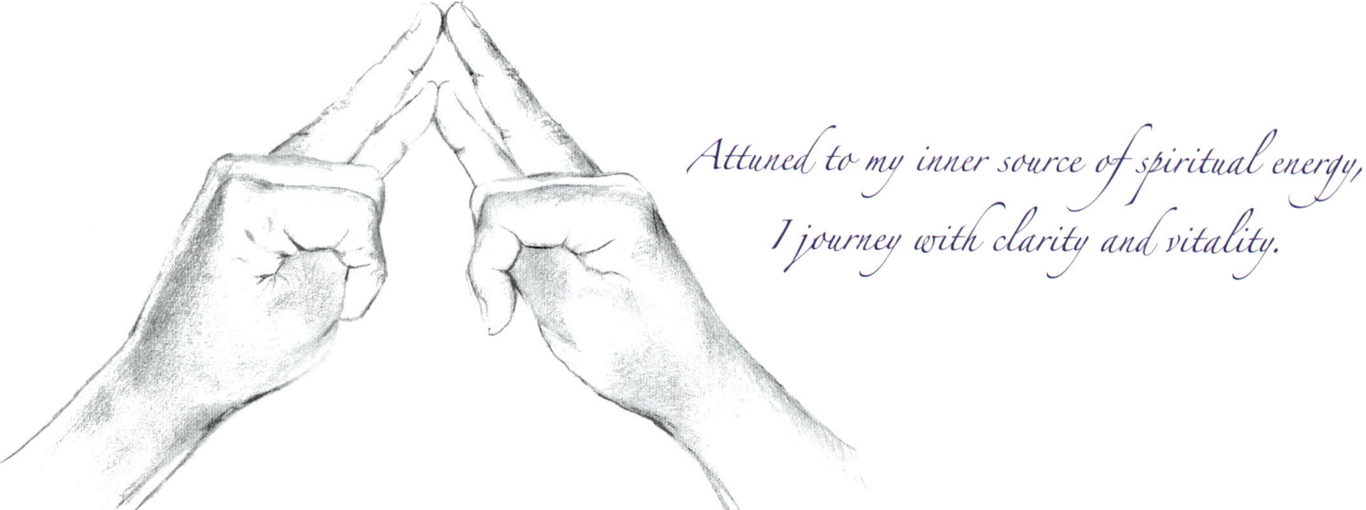

Attuned to my inner source of spiritual energy, I journey with clarity and vitality.

CORE QUALITY

Awakening Spiritual Energy

ESPECIALLY HELPFUL FOR

- Awakening the potential energy that inspires and guides our journey of awakening.
- Supporting the health of the urinary, reproductive and eliminatory systems.
- Cultivating a sense of support and centering as the foundation for our spiritual journey.

MUDRAS WITH SIMILAR EFFECTS

Svadhisthana, Adho Merudanda, Vittam

CAUTIONS

None

INSTRUCTIONS

1. Bring the palms of the hands together below of the navel, with the fingers facing outward.
2. Keep the tips of the little and ring fingers together and separate the base of the palms, thumbs, middle and index fingers.
3. Wrap the index and middle fingers loosely around the thumbs.
4. Rest the wrists against the abdomen.
5. Relax the shoulders back and down, with the spine naturally aligned.

Shakti is the "potential energy of spiritual awakening," personified as a female deity. As limiting conditioning at the level of the personality is released, tremendous amounts of energy are made available for the spiritual journey. As our level of energy increases, it supports and hastens our process of transformation, opening doorways to the subtle realms of our being. At the beginning of our journey, most of our energy is consumed by meeting our perceived needs and avoiding situations that appear to be threatening. As we proceed along the spiritual journey, there is an evolution within our values and priorities that naturally redirects our energy toward spiritual awakening. This evolutionary journey of transformation is symbolized by the upward movement of Shakti through the *chakras*, culminating in spiritual liberation.

Shakti mudra supports us in awakening the energy of transformation within all dimensions of our being. This gesture directs breath, awareness and energy from the base of the body, where Shakti lies dormant, upward to the second chakra, where it expands and is concentrated. Shakti mudra instills a feeling of a vast ocean of potential energy that can be channeled upward through all the energy centers all the way to *Sahasrara* at the crown of the head, where we experience our essential nature as pure Consciousness. The expanded flow of breath and energy throughout the pelvic area cultivated by this gesture supports the eliminatory, urinary and reproductive systems in functioning optimally.

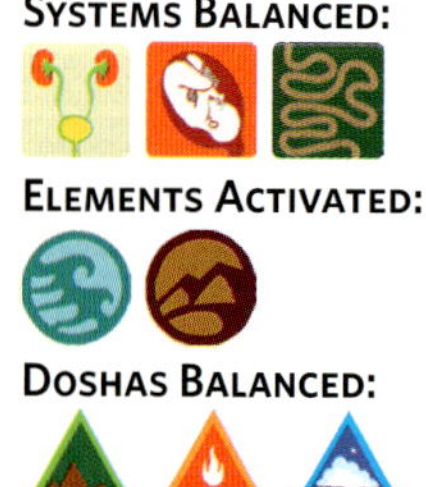

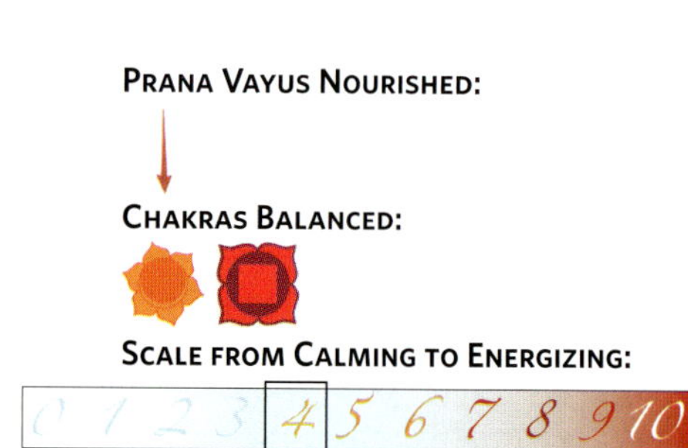

Guided Meditation: Awakening Spiritual Energy

- As you hold Shakti mudra, take several natural breaths to attune to all the feelings and sensations awakened by this gesture.
- Notice how your breath is gently directed into your lower abdomen and pelvis, sensing this area as a vast ocean of potential energy that can be channeled to dissolve all blockages within your chakras, cultivating vitality for your spiritual journey.
- Begin by visualizing four red petals at the base of your body. As you inhale, attune to your ocean of energy, and as you exhale, sense Muladhara Chakra filled with vitality.
- Infused with vital energy, these petals blossom naturally, untying all the knots related to survival needs, allowing you to move forward with a greater sense of security.
- Now, visualize six orange petals within your pelvis. As you inhale, attune to your ocean of energy, and as you exhale, sense Svadhisthana Chakra filled with vitality.
- Infused with vital energy, your orange lotus blossoms naturally, releasing all blockages related to relationships and sexuality, allowing you to continue your journey with greater emotional balance and a sense of centering.
- Now, visualize ten golden petals at your solar plexus. As you inhale, attune to your inner ocean, and as you exhale, sense radiant golden energy infusing your center of self-esteem.
- Filled with vital energy, your third chakra blossoms radiantly, releasing any knots related to self-esteem and your place in society, allowing you to manifest your life purpose confidently.
- Now, visualize twelve emerald petals at your heart center. As you inhale, attune to your inner ocean, and with your exhaling breath, sense these petals infused with vital energy.
- Energized completely, your emerald lotus blossoms naturally, releasing any sense of resentment, guilt or loneliness, allowing you to expand the frontiers of your heart to live with love, compassion and generosity.
- Next, visualize the sixteen sky blue petals of your throat chakra. As you inhale, attune to your ocean of vitality, and as you exhale, Vishuddha Chakra opens naturally.
- Sense this lotus blossoming completely, releasing all limiting beliefs that keep you from recognizing your authentic being and speaking your truth clearly.
- Now, attune to the two violet petals between your eyebrows. As you inhale, connect to your inner ocean, and as you exhale, sense your third eye infused with vitality.
- As this violet lotus blossoms naturally, all knots of confusion and doubt are released completely, allowing you to see your life's deeper meaning with clarity.
- Vital energy now flows up to the crown of your head, allowing the thousand petals of crystal light to blossom infinitely, revealing your true nature as freedom and unity.
- Now, with all of your chakra petals unfolding completely, you experience the abundant spiritual energy that supports you all the way to final awakening.
- Filled with vital energy, affirm the following three times, aloud or silently: **"As all knots are released from my energetic being, I journey easily toward awakening."**
- Slowly release the gesture, taking several breaths to rest in pure energy.
- When you are ready, open your eyes, returning slowly and gently, filled with vitality.

Annamaya kosha (physical body)

• Directs breath and awareness to the base of the body and pelvis, improving circulation to the eliminatory, urinary and reproductive systems.
• The mobilization of energy cultivated by this gesture is generally helpful for Kapha imbalance.
• The enhanced awareness of subtle energy is generally helpful for Pitta imbalance.
• The centering cultivated is generally helpful for Vata imbalance.

Pranamaya kosha (energy body)

• Activates Apana vayu, the downward moving current of energy.
• Opens and balances the first and second chakras, whose energy is channeled upward for awakening the other centers.

Manomaya kosha (psycho-emotional body)

• Cultivates emotional balance and equanimity.

Vijnanamaya kosha (wisdom body)

• As we become more sensitive to our energetic body, we loosen our identification with the personality, thereby aligning with our true being more easily.

Anandamaya kosha (bliss body)

• As spiritual energy rises upward through the chakras, an experience of bliss, freedom and limitlessness is awakened.

98

Uttarabodhi Mudra

Gesture of Highest Wisdom
For Cultivating Self-mastery - Vashitvam

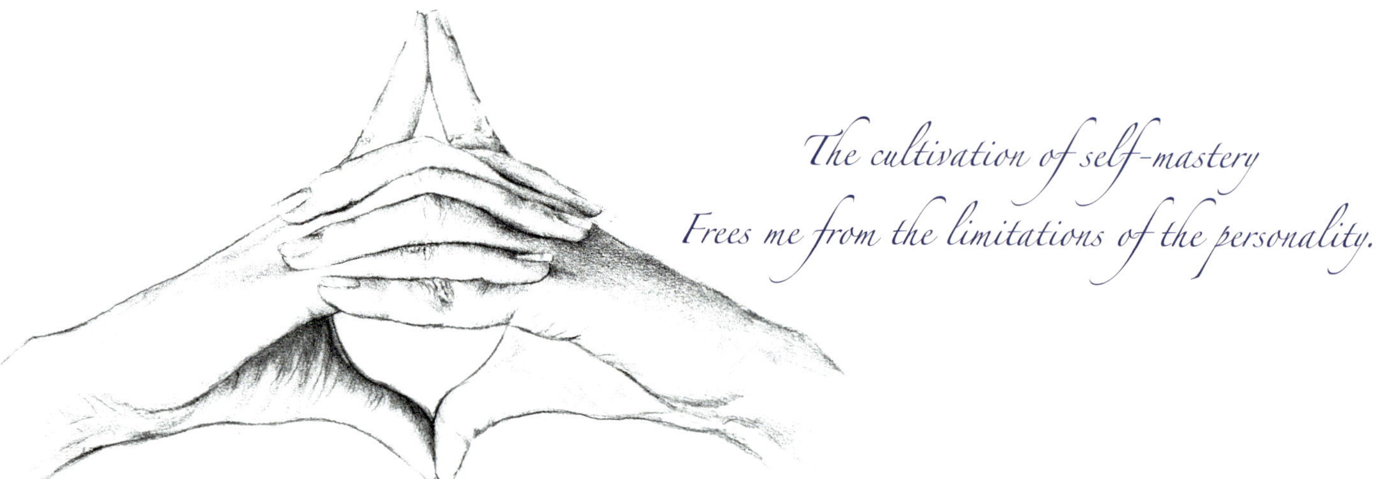

Core Quality
Self-mastery

Especially helpful for
- Developing self-mastery.
- Expanding the breath throughout the rib cage, especially at the sternum and side ribs.
- Enhancing immunity.
- Cultivating a sense of integrity and authenticity.

Mudras with similar effects
Jnana, Citta, Svadhyaya

Cautions
None

Instructions
1. Interlace the fingers to the outside, with the left little finger as the base.
2. Press the tips of the index fingers together and the tips of the thumbs together.
3. Extend the index fingers upward and the thumbs downward.
4. Place the thumbs and index fingers against the sternum, with the index fingers at the sternal notch.
5. Relax the shoulders back and down, with the elbows held away from the body and the spine naturally aligned.

Vashitvam, which means "self-mastery," marks a turning point in the spiritual journey in which we no longer identify with the limiting beliefs at the level of the personality. As we witness these beliefs, the thoughts and feelings associated with them lose the power to control our life journey. As we develop greater self-mastery, our true Self naturally comes to the forefront of all of our activities. In this way, we are able to live in the world, engaged completely, responding objectively and compassionately to every situation that we meet. When challenging thoughts and emotions arise, we witness them as vehicles for seeing and releasing any remaining limiting beliefs.

Uttara means "highest," and *bodhi* means "wisdom." *Uttarabodhi* refers to our ability to remain aligned with our true being in all of our interactions and activities. Uttarabodhi mudra directs breath, awareness and energy to the chest, enhancing circulation to the area of the thymus gland, supporting the health of the immune system. This gesture instills a balance of steadiness and ease in the breath, mind and body, which supports us in remaining aligned with our true Self, especially when we encounter challenges along our journey. Uttarabodhi mudra support a growing sense of self-mastery in which the likes and dislikes of the personality lose their power to draw us into their "stories," allowing us to live with ease within our authentic being.

Systems Balanced:

Elements Activated:

Doshas Balanced:

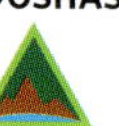

Prana Vayus Nourished:

Chakras Balanced:

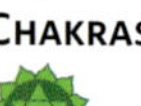

Scale from Calming to Energizing:

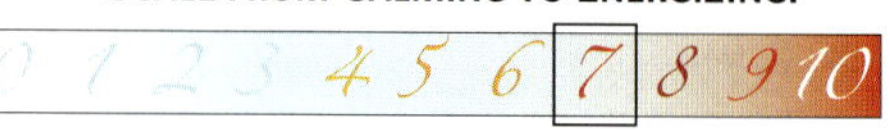

Guided Meditation: Developing Self-mastery

- As you hold Uttarabodhi mudra, take several natural breaths to attune to all the feelings and sensations awakened by this gesture.
- Notice how your breath is naturally directed into your chest, creating a space of inner silence and rest where you can attune to your deeper Self.
- As you attune more deeply to your authentic being, you naturally receive guidance for your journey, allowing you to cultivate self-mastery.
- Your journey of self-mastery begins at the level of your physical body, by caring for it optimally while recognizing that it is not an end in itself, only a vehicle for awakening.
- Take several breaths to reflect on your relationship with your body. To what extent are you ruled by its cravings, and to what extent are you able to witness these, refining your self-mastery?
- Next, explore self-mastery at the level of your psycho-emotional being, your ability to utilize your thoughts and feelings as vehicles for learning and awakening.
- Take several breaths to reflect on your relationship with your thoughts and feelings. Are you ruled by their fluctuations or able to allow them to simply be without identifying so completely, thereby refining your self-mastery?
- Now, take several breaths to reflect on your relationship with your deepest beliefs. To what extent are you ruled by them rigidly and unconsciously, limiting your horizons and possibilities?
- As you deepen your level of self-mastery in relation to your beliefs, you are able to witness them more easily, adhering to them less rigidly, naturally opening to the clarity of your true being.
- With greater self-mastery, you gradually release your identification with your conditioning, allowing you to align with the freedom and unity of your authentic being.
- Affirm your self-mastery as you repeat the following three times, aloud or silently: **"With self-mastery at all levels of being, I live with freedom and authenticity."**
- Now, slowly release the gesture, taking several breaths to rest in your authentic Self.
- When you are ready, open your eyes, returning slowly and gently, with a greater sense of self-mastery.

Annamaya kosha (physical body)

• Directs breath and awareness into the entire rib cage, especially to the sternum and side ribs, creating a massaging effect that improves circulation to the area of the thymus gland.
• The energizing effects of this gesture are generally helpful for Kapha imbalance.

Pranamaya kosha (energy body)

• Activates Prana vayu, the upward moving current of energy.
• Opens and balances the fourth chakra, center of unconditional love.

Manomaya kosha (psycho-emotional body)

• Cultivates stability in the mind and emotions.
• Cultivates a sense of self-confidence and inner trust that supports self-mastery.

Vijnanamaya kosha (wisdom body)

• The stability in the mind that occurs through self-mastery is a reflection of the changeless nature of our true being.

Anandamaya kosha (bliss body)

• With enhanced self-mastery, we engage life fully with a sense of complete freedom.

99

Kaleshvara Mudra

Gesture of the Lord of Time
For Attaining Spiritual Freedom - Moksha

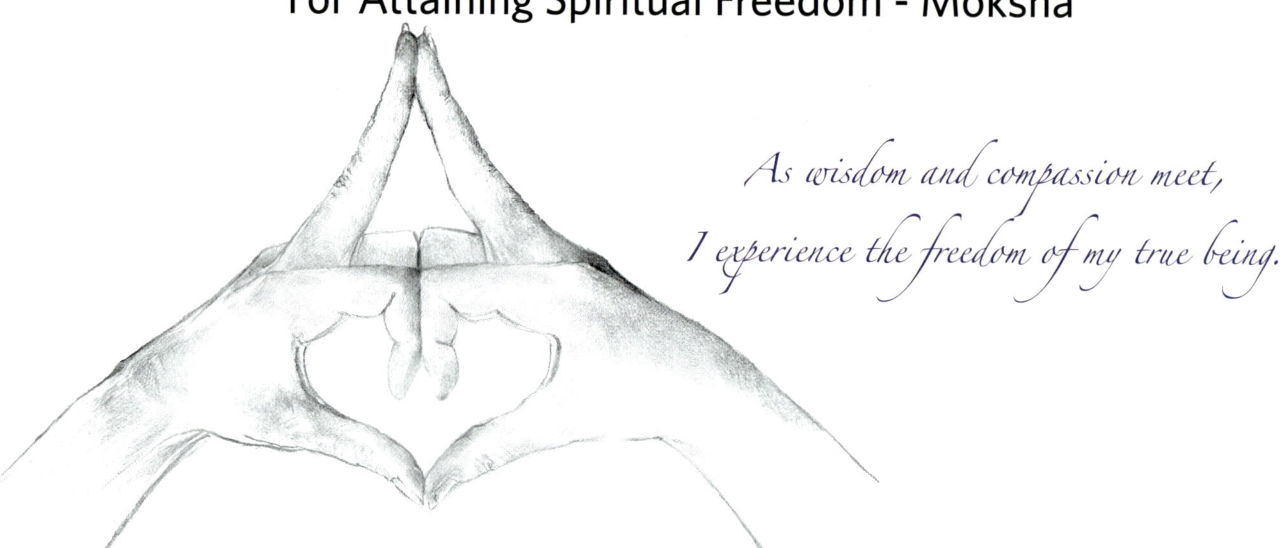

As wisdom and compassion meet,
I experience the freedom of my true being.

Core Quality
Spiritual Freedom

Especially helpful for
- Integrating wisdom and compassion to reveal the essence of our true being as the lived experience of freedom and unity.
- Supporting the health of the neuro-endocrine system.

Mudras with similar effects
Mandala, Tejas, Ananta

Cautions
None

Instructions
1. Hold the palms facing each other in front of the heart, with the pads of the middle fingers touching.
2. Join the backs of the middle digit of the index fingers.
3. Join the pads of the thumbs and press them downward, forming a heart.
4. The little and ring fingers rest naturally inward.
5. Hold the gesture about a hand's width away from the heart.
6. Relax the shoulders back and down, with the elbows held away from the body and the spine naturally aligned.

Moksha, "spiritual liberation," is the culmination of the spiritual journey as the moment to moment experience of freedom and unity. Spiritual liberation requires both wisdom and compassion. Wisdom is absolute clarity in regard to the nature of our true being, free from the limitations of our conditioning. This recognition is experienced as a homecoming, an absolute knowing that we are already whole and complete. Wisdom must be balanced with compassion, which is the recognition of our oneness with all beings, allowing us to see that we all share a single journey toward unity. When wisdom and compassion unite, we are able to live in the freedom of our true being while embracing all of life wholeheartedly. The integration of wisdom and compassion allows us to celebrate each moment of life as an unfolding journey of freedom and unity.

Kaleshvara is the "Lord of time," and refers to our true being, free from the limitations of time and space that characterize the personality. Kaleshvara mudra directs breath, awareness and energy upward from the heart, our center of love and compassion, to the third eye, our center of clarity and wisdom. The thumbs and index fingers form the shape of a heart, representing compassion. The upward facing triangle formed by the middle fingers represents the wisdom that arises through clear seeing. This gesture reminds us that through the integration of wisdom and compassion, we are able to experience the freedom of our true being while participating fully in creation's infinite beauty.

Systems Balanced:

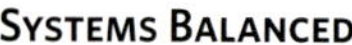

Elements Activated:

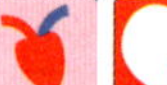

Doshas Balanced:

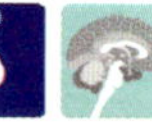
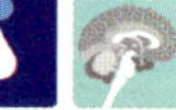

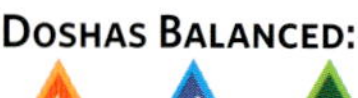

Prana Vayus Nourished:

Chakras Balanced:

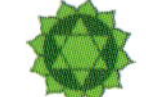
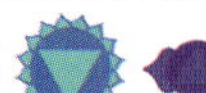

Scale from Calming to Energizing:

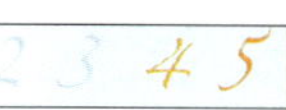
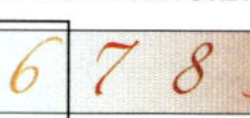

Guided Meditation: Integrating Wisdom and Compassion

- ॐ As you hold Kaleshvara mudra, take several natural breaths to attune to all the feelings and sensations awakened by this gesture.
- ॐ Notice how your breath flows gently upward from your heart to your third eye, naturally uniting your centers of compassion and wisdom.
- ॐ As energy flows more freely between these two centers, you naturally align with your authentic being, releasing your identification with the feelings and beliefs that keep you from experiencing your essential nature as freedom and unity.
- ॐ This integration of wisdom and compassion begins at the level of your material needs.
- ॐ Through the eyes of the heart, you see your desires for material things compassionately as a natural extension of the drive to survive by ensuring your basic needs.
- ॐ Through the eyes of wisdom, you clearly see that nothing that comes from outside can add or subtract to that which is already whole and complete.
- ॐ As compassion and wisdom meet, you are able to release binding desires to possess more than you need while opening to receive all that the universe offers abundantly.
- ॐ Now, sense the integration of wisdom and compassion within your relationships.
- ॐ Through the eyes of the heart, you welcome your feelings compassionately, recognizing that love, affection and trust are a natural part of your journey toward emotional maturity.
- ॐ Through the eyes of wisdom, you clearly see that all of your emotional needs are a reflection of your essential connection and oneness with all beings.
- ॐ As compassion and wisdom meet, you witness your feelings without reacting unconsciously while welcoming love and affection in a natural balance of giving and receiving.
- ॐ Finally, sense the integration of wisdom and compassion at the level of your spiritual journey, including all the teachings and techniques that guide you toward awakening.
- ॐ Through the eyes of the heart, you honor your entire spiritual path, including the practices, teachers and teachings that you have followed with sincerity.
- ॐ Through the eyes of wisdom, you clearly see that, ultimately, there is no spiritual journey, only the experience of pure conscious being, revealed through your process of transformation and awakening.
- ॐ As compassion and wisdom meet, you honor all the great masters and their teachings while resting in the moment to moment presence of your authentic being, beyond all philosophies and beliefs.
- ॐ Aligned with your true being, you live with a sense of freedom and unity while appreciating each moment of life fully and joyfully.
- ॐ Resting in your authentic being, repeat the following three times, aloud or silently: **"As compassion and wisdom unite within my being, I live freely and joyfully."**
- ॐ Slowly release the gesture, taking several breaths to rest in your joyful essence.
- ॐ When you are ready, open your eyes, returning slowly and gently, experiencing the freedom of your essential being.

Annamaya kosha (physical body)

• Directs breath and awareness into the chest, neck and head, creating a massaging effect that improves circulation to the areas of the thymus, thyroid and pituitary glands.
• The uplifting energy may be helpful for depression.
• The mildly energizing effects of this gesture are generally helpful for Kapha imbalance.
• The heart-opening cultivated is generally helpful for Pitta imbalance.
• The enhanced concentration is generally helpful for Vata imbalance.

Pranamaya kosha (energy body)

• Activates Prana and Udana vayus, the upward moving and uppermost currents of energy.
• Opens and balances the fourth, fifth and sixth chakras, centers of unconditional love, spiritual purification and wisdom.

Manomaya kosha (psycho-emotional body)

• Focuses the mind, supporting one-pointed concentration.
• Cultivates an uplifting energy, which may be helpful for depression.

Vijnanamaya kosha (wisdom body)

• The integration of wisdom and compassion naturally opens a doorway to our true being.

Anandamaya kosha (bliss body)

• As the true Self awakens, its innate qualities of wholeness, joy, openness and limitlessness are naturally experienced.

Chapter Sixteen

Cultivating Conscious Presence

MUDRAS FOR MEDITATION

Meditation is a stream of pure Consciousness in which we experience our true being whose nature is freedom and unity. Our true Self is always present, waiting to be recognized, and the various techniques of meditation support the journey of transformation and awakening. We may begin practicing meditation as a way to relax, release stress or find greater inner peace. The positive effects of these initial experiences are usually so satisfying that they encourage us to deepen our practice. In order to progress along the journey of meditation, we need to release the layers of conditioning that keep us from experiencing our true being. As these layers of conditioning are progressively released, the inner and outer conflicts that cause stress and separation are reduced, allowing us to proceed along the journey of meditation more easily. The process of meditation is multifaceted, encompassing five essential steps:

1. Stabilizing Body and Breath

Stabilizing body and breath establishes a firm foundation for meditation. As body and breath are balanced, the mind comes into stillness naturally. The nature of the mind is movement, scanning the environment for opportunities and possible threats. This external orientation is essential for meeting our basic needs, but when our quest is Self-knowledge, this movement of the mind must be gradually decreased. Prajna Prana Kriya mudra calms and stabilizes the body and breath, thereby preparing the mind for meditation.

2. Welcoming Thoughts and Feelings

As body and breath become stable and the mind becomes more serene, thoughts and feelings naturally come to the surface to be seen, integrated and gradually released. Trying to suppress or deny these thoughts and feelings simply empowers them. In this stage of meditation, we learn to welcome thoughts and feelings without resisting. By allowing thoughts and feeling to come and go freely, they gradually lose their power to interfere with the steady stream of consciousness that is meditation. Medha Prana Kriya mudra cultivates openness in which thoughts and feelings can be welcomed easily, allowing our meditation to deepen naturally.

3. Awakening Clear Seeing

The next level of meditation involves developing the ability to witness all that arises in the body and mind. Witnessing goes beyond welcoming, allowing us to distinguish clearly between the conditioned personality and our limitless true being. In witnessing, we explore the limiting beliefs that sustain patterns of thought and feeling, recognizing that they are part of our conditioning and not our essential being. Through this recognition, we gradually release any sense of limitation, inadequacy and subsequent suffering. Jnana mudra enhances one-pointed concentration and clarity that support us in aligning with our true being and releasing conditioning.

4. Effortless Meditation

As identification with thoughts and feelings, as well as the limiting beliefs that sustain them, is released, all facets of our being are integrated naturally. This integration instills a sense of harmony, allowing us to rest in meditation effortlessly. Dhyana mudra supports our ability to rest in the steady stream of meditation.

5. Experiencing Unity

As our meditation journey proceeds, all sense of separation is released, allowing us to merge completely with our true nature as freedom and unity. This sense of unity is initially temporary, but gradually stabilizes, infusing all of our activities. At this level, meditation is no longer a practice, but simply a reflection of our true being. Bhairava mudra supports this experience of unity, cultivating a sense of timeless being in which the movements of the mind naturally come into stillness.

The Steps of Meditation, Related Mudras & Core Qualities

Mudra	Core Quality
Prajna Prana Kriya	Stabilizing Body & Breath
Medha Prana Kriya	Welcoming Thoughts & Feelings
Jnana	Awakening Clear Seeing
Dhyana	Effortless Meditation
Bhairava	Experiencing Unity

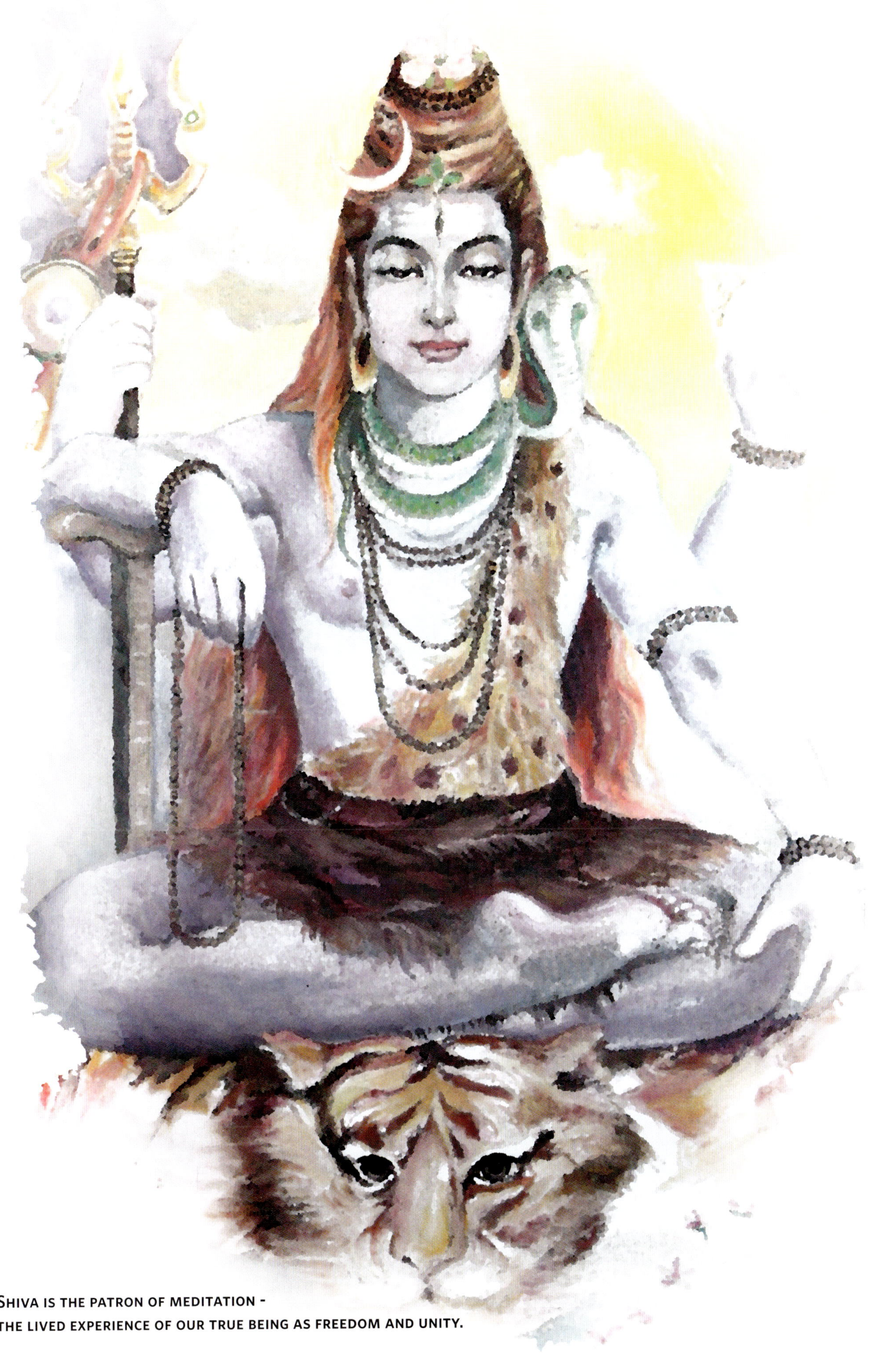

Shiva is the patron of meditation -
the lived experience of our true being as freedom and unity.

100 PRAJNA PRANA KRIYA MUDRA

Gesture of Purifying Wisdom

For Stabilizing Body and Breath

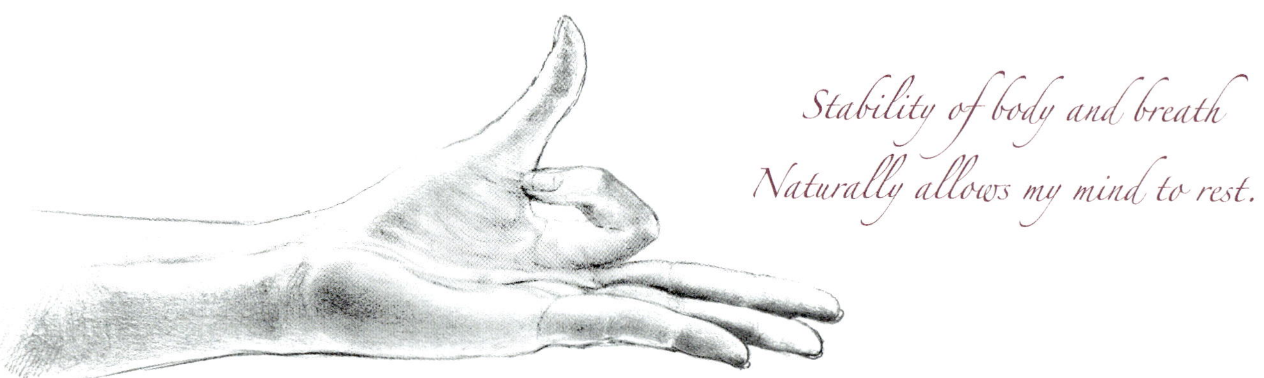

CORE QUALITY

Stabilizing Body and Breath

ESPECIALLY HELPFUL FOR

- Creating a balance of steadiness and comfort within the body and breath as a foundation for entering into meditation.
- Supporting the health of the musculo-skeletal system.
- Relieving stress and anxiety.
- Optimizing the health of the reproductive, eliminatory and urinary systems.
- Supporting slow, rhythmic breathing that calms the nervous system.

MUDRAS WITH SIMILAR EFFECTS

Adhi, Bhu, Chinmaya, Apanayana

CAUTIONS

None

INSTRUCTIONS

1. Press the tips of the index fingers into the lowest joint of the thumbs of each hand, creating an open circular space.
2. Extend the thumbs, little, ring and middle fingers.
3. Rest the backs of the hands onto the thighs or knees.
4. Relax the shoulders back and down, with the spine naturally aligned.

Stabilizing body and breath is a key foundation for meditation, because as they become harmonized, the mind naturally reflects their stability, allowing us to enter into meditation more easily. The body, breath and mind all tend toward movement in order to respond to threats and opportunities to ensure our basic survival needs. Any stimulus draws our attention to the outside world immediately, causing the breath to become more rapid as the body and mind prepare for activity. As we embark on the spiritual journey, our quest for happiness and contentment turns toward our inner being, and stabilizing breath and body forms the foundation of this inward journey.

Prajna means "wisdom," *prana* is "life force energy," and *kriya* is "an action of purification." *Prajna prana kriya* is an action that stabilizes our life force energy, allowing us to enter into meditation more easily. Prajna Prana Kriya mudra directs breath, awareness and energy to the pelvis and base of the body, cultivating a sense of grounding that naturally stabilizes the body and breath. This gesture slows the breath and lengthens the exhalation, calming the lower centers of the brain that regulate heartbeat and breath rate. Prajna Prana Kriya mudra directs breath into the base of the lungs, which has a calming effect, making it excellent for reducing stress and anxiety. This gesture supports the alignment of the spine, which further stabilizes body and breath, forming a firm foundation for meditation.

SYSTEMS BALANCED:

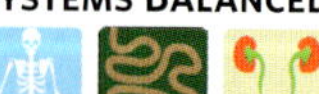
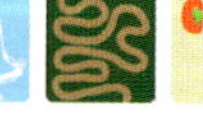
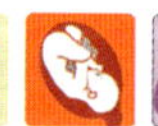
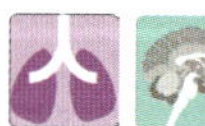
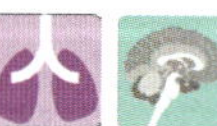
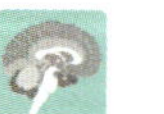

ELEMENTS ACTIVATED:

DOSHAS BALANCED:

PRANA VAYUS NOURISHED:

CHAKRAS BALANCED:

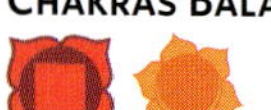

SCALE FROM CALMING TO ENERGIZING:

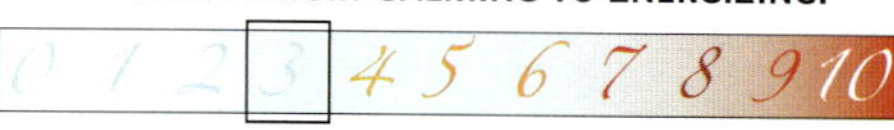

Guided Meditation: Stabilizing Body and Breath

- As you hold Prajna Prana Kriya mudra, take several natural breaths to attune to all the feelings and sensations evoked by this gesture.
- Notice how your breath is naturally directed downward toward the base of your body, instilling a sense of stability and grounding.
- Take several breaths to attune to this growing sense of stability, allowing it to permeate your pelvis, legs and feet, creating a firm foundation for your meditation journey.
- As your lower body becomes more rooted to the earth beneath, take some time to sense how your breath expands at the very base of your lungs, deepening your breathing and enhancing your sense of stability.
- As your body and breath become more stable and serene, your awareness naturally rests at the very base of your brain, the place where the cervical spine meets the cranium.
- Take several breaths to attune to this area of your brain, noticing how your breath becomes even slower and more rhythmic, naturally deepening your sense of stability and serenity.
- Now, sense the base of your body, the base of your lungs and the base of your brain simultaneously, and as stability and serenity permeate your entire being, you rest in absolute stillness and peace, the foundation of your meditation journey.
- Affirm your essential stability, repeating the following three times, aloud or silently: **"With body and breath stabilized completely, I enter into meditation easily."**
- Now, slowly release the gesture, taking several breaths to experience greater stability in your body and breathing.
- When you are ready, open your eyes, returning slowly and gently, sensing a firm foundation for your journey of meditation.

Annamaya kosha (physical body)

• Directs breath and awareness to the pelvis and base of the body, creating a massaging effect that improves circulation to the eliminatory, urinary and reproductive systems.
• Slows the respiration rate, lengthening the exhalation, thereby activating the relaxation response, which is helpful for reducing stress and anxiety.
• Enhances the breath in the lowest portions of the lungs, which may be helpful for those who tend to breathe in the upper chest, which is associated with the stress response.
• The grounding and stabilizing effects of this gesture are generally helpful for Vata imbalance.
• The calming effects are generally helpful for Pitta imbalance.

Pranamaya kosha (energy body)

• Activates Apana vayu, the downward moving current of energy.
• Opens and balances the first and second chakras, centers of safety and self-nourishment.

Manomaya kosha (psycho-emotional body)

• Cultivates a state of deep calm and inner security.

Vijnanamaya kosha (wisdom body)

• Stabilizing body and breath calms our basic survival drives, allowing us to evolve naturally toward the wisdom of our true being.

Anandamaya kosha (bliss body)

• As we experience greater stability, a sense of absolute safety and protection arises naturally.

101 Medha Prana Kriya Mudra

Gesture of Mental Vigor

For Welcoming Thoughts and Feelings

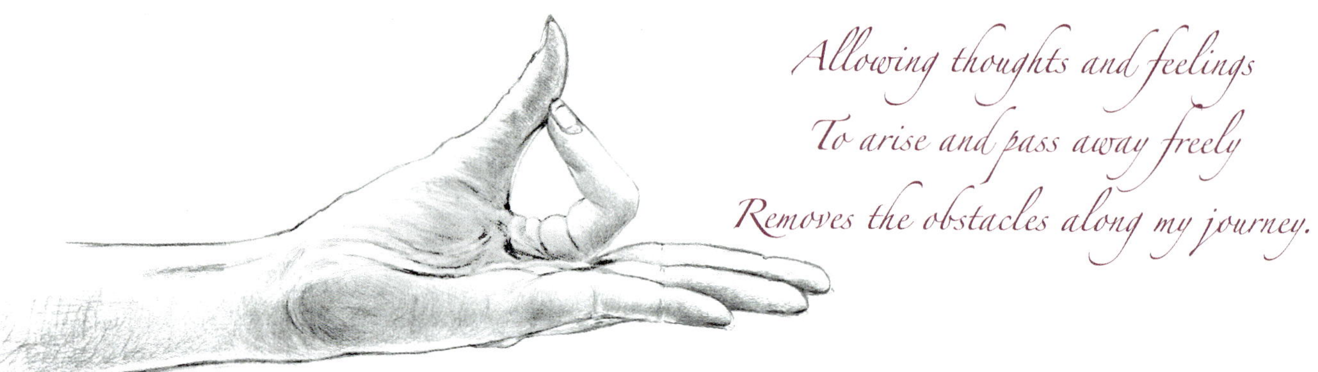

Allowing thoughts and feelings
To arise and pass away freely
Removes the obstacles along my journey.

Core Quality

Welcoming Thoughts and Feelings

Especially helpful for

- Welcoming thoughts and feelings without resisting or reacting to them.
- Vitalizing the respiratory and cardiovascular systems.
- Supporting healthy immunity.

Mudras with similar effects

Urdhvam Merudanda, Vajrapradama, Dirgha Svara

Cautions

None

Instructions

1. Gently press the tips of the index fingers into the middle joint of the thumbs of each hand.
2. Keep the thumbs, little, ring and middle fingers extended straight out.
3. Rest the backs of the hands onto the thighs or knees.
4. Relax the shoulders back and down, with the spine naturally aligned.

After establishing a firm foundation for meditation by stabilizing the body and breath, the next step is cultivating an attitude of non-resistance to all that arises in the mind. During meditation, positive, challenging and neutral thoughts and emotions arise. Our tendency is to embrace the positive and reject, suppress or react to difficult thoughts and feelings. The more we resist, the more thoughts and feelings insist upon gaining our attention. An effective way of dealing with thoughts and feelings, especially those that are challenging, is to welcome them, allowing them to arise and pass away freely in synchrony with our rhythmic breathing, thereby deepening our ability to continue our meditation no matter what is happening in the mind or in our surroundings.

Medha is "mental vigor," *prana* is "life force energy," and *kriya* is "an action of purification." *Medha prana kriya* is an action that purifies our life force energy in order to cultivate mental vigor. Medha Prana Kriya mudra directs breath, awareness and energy to the entire rib cage, enhancing breath capacity, especially in the middle portion of the lungs. This opening supports the health of the entire cardio-respiratory system, providing a massaging effect for the lungs and heart. This gesture also enhances circulation to the area of the thymus gland, supporting the health of the immune system. Medha Prana Kriya mudra calms the emotional processing centers of the brain, allowing us to welcome feelings more easily without repressing or reacting to them.

Systems Balanced:

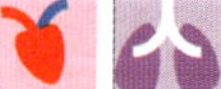
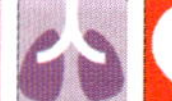
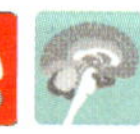
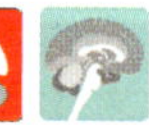

Elements Activated:

Doshas Balanced:

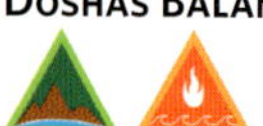

Prana Vayus Nourished:

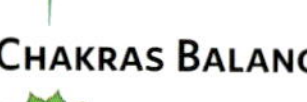

Chakras Balanced:

Scale from Calming to Energizing:

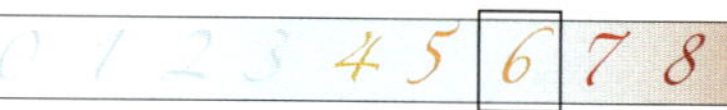

Guided Meditation: Welcoming Thoughts and Feelings

ॐ As you hold Medha Prana Kriya mudra, take several natural breaths to attune to all the feelings and sensations awakened by this gesture.

ॐ Notice how your breath is gently directed into your chest, side ribs and upper back, allowing you to breathe more easily.

ॐ Take some time to attune to the movement of your rib cage, naturally expanding on each inhalation, and softening on each exhalation.

ॐ As you attune more deeply to your middle body breathing, notice how your breath is naturally directed into the middle portion of your lungs, providing the vitality that allows you to rest in meditation more easily.

ॐ As your breath flows freely, allow your awareness to be naturally directed to the middle portion of your brain, your center of emotional processing, cultivating a sense of serenity that supports your meditation journey.

ॐ With greater serenity infusing your psycho-emotional being, you naturally embrace all that arises within your mind more easily, welcoming thoughts and feelings without judging or resisting.

ॐ Take several breaths to embrace openly all positive, challenging and neutral feelings, allowing them to arise and pass away naturally, just like the flow of your rhythmic breathing.

ॐ As you allow all feelings to arise and pass away freely, you experience greater integration and harmony throughout your entire being, allowing you to rest in meditation's steady stream.

ॐ Allowing feelings to simply be, repeat the following three times, aloud or silently: **"By welcoming thoughts and feelings, my meditation naturally deepens."**

ॐ Slowly release the gesture, taking several breaths to rest in meditation.

ॐ When you are ready, open your eyes, returning slowly and gently, with a greater ability to welcome thoughts and feelings in meditation.

Annamaya kosha (physical body)

• Directs breath and awareness to the entire rib cage, creating a massaging effect that enhances circulation to the cardio-respiratory system.
• Enhances circulation to the area of the thymus gland.
• Expands the breath in the middle lungs and also in the mid back, creating a massaging effect in the area of the kidneys and adrenal glands.
• The toning of the muscles of the rib cage enhances breath capacity.
• The expansion of the lungs and the energizing effects of this gesture are generally helpful for Kapha imbalance.
• The opening of the subtle heart is generally helpful for Pitta imbalance.

Pranamaya kosha (energy body)

• Gently activates Prana vayu, the upward moving current of energy.
• Opens and balances the fourth chakra, center of unconditional love.

Manomaya kosha (psycho-emotional body)

• Cultivates emotional balance.
• The mildly energizing effects may be helpful for depression.

Vijnanamaya kosha (wisdom body)

• Welcoming thoughts and feelings without identifying with them so completely, allows us to align with our true inner being more easily.

Anandamaya kosha (bliss body)

• As we welcome thoughts and feelings, we begin to experience them as pure energy, nourishing the seeds for the unfolding of our inherent positive qualities.

102

Jnana Mudra

Gesture of Higher Knowledge

For Awakening Clear Seeing

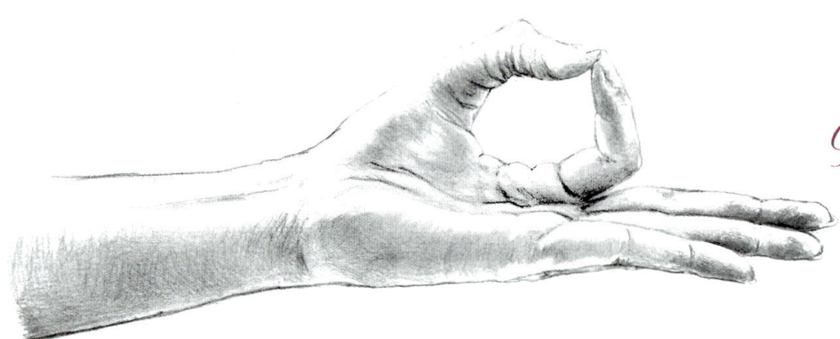

The power of clear seeing
Guides my path toward awakening.

Core Quality

Awakening Clear Seeing

Especially helpful for

- Awakening clear seeing through the power of witnessing.
- Enhancing one-pointed concentration.
- Discerning between the limitless true Self and the limited personality.

Mudras with similar effects

Chin, Citta, Trishula, Sakshi

Cautions

None

Instructions

1. Touch the tips of the index fingers to the tips of the thumbs of each hand.
2. The thumbs and index fingers form a round open circle.
3. Extend the little, ring and middle fingers straight out.
4. Rest the back of the hands onto the thighs or knees.
5. Relax the shoulders back and down, with the spine naturally aligned.

The third stage of meditation is awakening clarity, allowing us to see ourselves, life and other people from the perspective of our true being rather than through the lens of the conditioned personality. Clarity arises through deepening our ability to witness thoughts and feelings as well as the limiting beliefs that sustain them. By witnessing all that arises in the mind without identifying so completely, we are no longer drawn into the mind's "stories." Aligned with our true being, we can explore the beliefs that support patterns of thought and feeling, allowing us to loosen our identification with them in meditation and in all of our interactions and activities.

Jnana means "wisdom," and Jnana mudra supports the clear seeing that allows our authentic being to come to the foreground while our thoughts and feelings are witnessed more objectively. This gesture directs our awareness to the third eye, our center of spiritual clarity and one-pointed concentration, deepening our ability to witness consciously. The placement of the fingers in Jnana mudra serves as a symbol for the meditation process. The index finger, symbolizing the limited personality, curls inward to meet the thumb, representing our limitless true being. The circle formed by the thumb and index finger represents the wholeness and limitlessness of our true being. The little, ring and middle fingers represent the three *gunas*, the qualities of *rajas*, activity; *tamas*, inertia; and *sattva*, purity. In this gesture, these three fingers are released downward, representing the return of the gunas to their primordial state of balance in which they no longer disturb our meditation.

Systems Balanced:

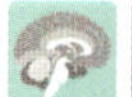  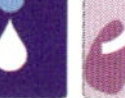 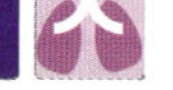

Elements Activated:

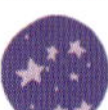

Doshas Balanced:

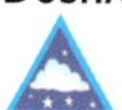 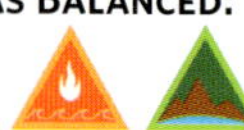

Prana Vayus Nourished:

Chakras Balanced:

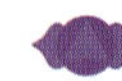

Scale from Calming to Energizing:

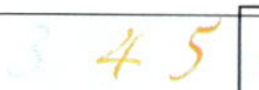

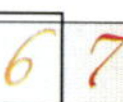

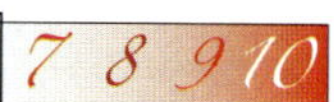

Guided Meditation: Awakening Clear Seeing

- As you hold Jnana mudra, take several natural breaths to attune to all the feelings and sensations awakened by this gesture.
- Notice how your breath is gently directed into your upper chest, neck and head, cultivating a greater sense of clarity.
- Your sense of clarity is enhanced by fuller breathing in the uppermost portion of your lungs, instilling an uplifting feeling that allows you to remain in meditation more comfortably.
- Supported by uplifting energy, your awareness is directed to your frontal brain, your center of higher reasoning, naturally enhancing your sense of clarity.
- Sense the space between your eyebrows, your third eye point, as the center of clarity from which you can witness all that arises in your mind more objectively.
- Within your growing clarity, take several breaths to sense the silent space between your thoughts expanding naturally, allowing you to witness your thoughts and feelings without needing to identify so completely.
- As you rest in this silent space, your mind naturally becomes still and serene, allowing you to align with your authentic being whose very nature is clear seeing.
- Affirm your inherent clarity as you repeat the following three times, aloud or silently: **"Through awakening clear seeing, I experience the silence of my authentic being."**
- Slowly release the gesture, taking several breaths to rest your essential clarity.
- When you are ready, open your eyes, returning slowly and gently, experiencing the clear seeing that allows you to remain in meditation easily.

Annamaya kosha (physical body)

• Directs breath and awareness to the upper lungs, enhancing breath capacity.
• Cultivates a balance of relaxation and alertness.
• Opens both nostrils and supports clearing of the nasal passages.
• Cultivates a sense of balance within both hemispheres of the brain.
• The mildly energizing effects of this gesture are generally helpful for Kapha imbalance.
• The enhanced ability to surrender the personality is generally helpful for Pitta imbalance.
• The enhanced one-pointed concentration is generally helpful for Vata imbalance.

Pranamaya kosha (energy body)

• Gently activates Udana vayu, the uppermost current of energy.
• Opens and balances the sixth chakra, center of wisdom.

Manomaya kosha (psycho-emotional body)

• Cultivates mental clarity and equanimity.
• Creates space between thoughts.

Vijnanamaya kosha (wisdom body)

• With greater clarity, we discern between the limited personality and our limitless true being more easily.

Anandamaya kosha (bliss body)

• Aligned with our true being, effortlessly and continually, an experience of bliss and clarity arises naturally.

103

Dhyana Mudra

Gesture of Meditation

For Experiencing Effortless Meditation

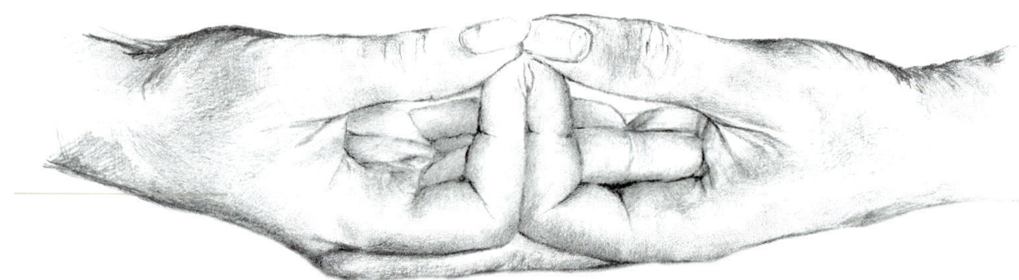

As I rest in the stream of meditation easily,
Body, breath and mind are integrated naturally.

Core Quality
Effortless Meditation

Especially Helpful For
- Supporting effortless meditation.
- Enhancing the health of all body systems.
- Integrating all of the facets of our being.
- Creating space between thoughts to experience inner silence.

Mudras with Similar Effects
Mandala, Hakini, Dharma Chakra

Cautions
None

Instructions
1. Touch the tips of the thumbs to the tips of the index fingers of each hand.
2. Extend the other fingers straight out with no space between them.
3. Rest the right fingers onto the left fingers, bringing the backs of the upper two knuckles of the index fingers together.
4. The tips of the thumbs touch lightly.
5. Rest the hands onto the lap.
6. Relax the shoulders back and down, with the elbows held away from the body and the spine naturally aligned.

As we rest in the steady stream of meditation more easily, all the facets of our being are integrated naturally. These include the lower, middle and upper regions of the body; the three main areas of the lungs; and the three main centers of the brain. Integration at all of these levels naturally leads to an experience of complete harmony. The first three mudras in this family bring awareness to each of the main areas of the body, lungs and brain individually, laying the foundation for the experience of integration cultivated by the fourth gesture, Dhyana mudra. Through this integration, our meditation becomes an effortless stream, allowing us to align more easily with our authentic being. The seamless integration of all facets of being is a powerful support for health and healing within all systems of the body.

Dhyana means "meditation," and Dhyana mudra supports the integration of all aspects of our being, allowing us to remain in meditation for longer periods effortlessly. This gesture facilitates Full Yogic Breathing, supporting the integration of all three main areas of the lungs, body and brain. This gesture creates a steady rhythm in the breath, giving the mind a place to rest, providing a firm support for extended periods of meditation. Dhyana mudra activates the flow of the breath through both nostrils evenly, cultivating equanimity which further supports our meditation. This mudra also lengthens the pauses between breaths, creating space between thoughts, allowing us to glimpse the mind's inherent silence.

Systems Balanced:

Elements Activated:

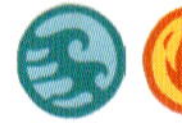
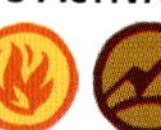
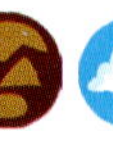

Doshas Balanced:

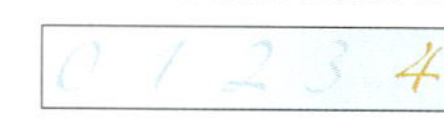

Prana Vayus Nourished:

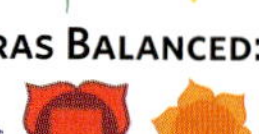

Chakras Balanced:

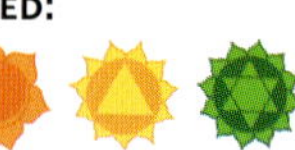

Scale from Calming to Energizing:

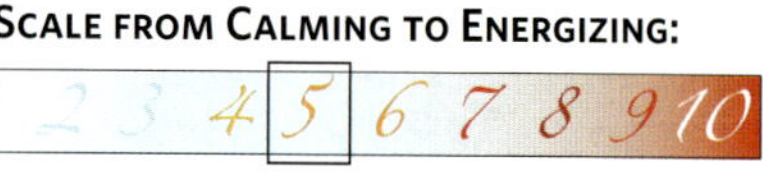

Guided Meditation: Steady Stream of Meditation

- As you hold Dhyana mudra, take several natural breaths to attune to all the feelings and sensations awakened by this gesture.
- Notice how your breath flows smoothly and evenly throughout your entire being, instilling a sense of integration and harmony.
- Begin by experiencing this harmony within your physical being, sensing the lower, middle and upper regions of your body integrated completely.
- Take several breaths to sense how this integration allows you to fully inhabit your body, from the crown of your head to the soles of your feet, enhancing your sense of presence during meditation.
- With a greater sense of integration in your body, your breath naturally becomes more serene, flowing through each of the areas of your lungs - lower, middle and upper - smoothly and evenly.
- Take several breaths to sense your harmonious breathing, as all the areas of your lungs are integrated completely, optimizing lung capacity and vitalizing your entire being, providing abundant energy to sustain your meditation journey.
- With body and breath in perfect harmony, sense all the areas of your brain integrated naturally.
- Take several breaths to sense harmony within your brain's centers of survival, emotional balance and higher reasoning, naturally cultivating the stillness that allows you to remain in meditation's steady stream.
- With your body, breath and brain integrated completely, you rest effortlessly in the steady stream of conscious presence, the essence of your meditation journey.
- Affirm your integration, repeating the following three times, aloud or silently: **"With body, breath and mind integrated completely, I rest in meditation effortlessly."**
- Slowly release the gesture, taking several breaths to rest in meditation's steady stream.
- When you are ready, open your eyes, returning slowly and gently, with an enhanced ability to rest in meditation effortlessly.

Annamaya kosha (physical body)

• Cultivates Full Yogic Breathing, enhancing breath capacity.
• Opens both nostrils evenly, cultivating a balance of rest and alertness that supports optimal health in all body systems.
• The balancing effects of this gesture are generally helpful for Vata, Pitta and Kapha imbalances.

Pranamaya kosha (energy body)

• Balances all prana vayus.
• Balances the first through sixth chakras, with an emphasis on the sixth chakra, center of wisdom.

Manomaya kosha (psycho-emotional body)

• Helps to clear and calm the mind, naturally cultivating equanimity and harmony.
• Creates spaciousness in the mind and slows the train of thoughts.

Vijnanamaya kosha (wisdom body)

• The integration of all the facets of our being serves as a doorway to our true Self, whose essential nature is harmony.

Anandamaya kosha (bliss body)

• As we integrate all aspects of our being, we access deeper states of meditation naturally, along with accompanying experiences of bliss and unity.

104 Bhairava Mudra

Gesture of Shiva's Fearsome Aspect

For Experiencing Unity

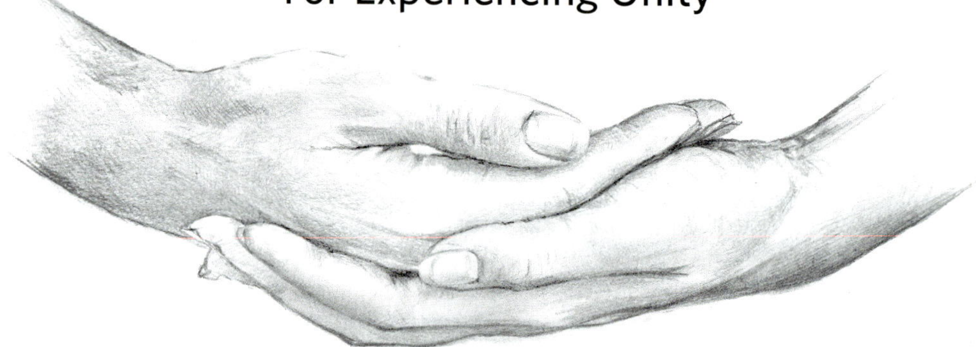

Resting in inner silence and deep peace,
All sense of separation is released.

Core Quality
Experiencing Unity

Especially helpful for
- Supporting the experiencing of our true being as freedom and unity.
- Optimizing the health of all the systems of the body, with a special focus on the nervous, endocrine and immune systems.
- Facilitating an experience of inner silence.

Mudras with similar effects
Ananta, Mandala, Anjali

Cautions
None

Instructions
1. Rest your left hand in your lap, with the palm facing upward.
2. Rest the back of the right hand onto the left hand.
3. The tips of the thumbs may lightly touch.
4. The hands rest naturally on your lap.
5. Relax the shoulders back and down, with the elbows held slightly away from the body and the spine naturally aligned.

The culmination of meditation is the experience of freedom and unity as expressions of our true being. Freedom is characterized by a knowing that we are absolutely whole and complete, independent of anything that is occurring within our personality and in our surroundings. Unity is the recognition that we are one with everything, an integral part of life's ever flowing stream. This experience of freedom and unity may be temporary, occurring during meditation and gradually passing away when our practice is complete. This temporary experience of our true nature is called *Samadhi*. When freedom and unity permeate every moment of our lives as a continual lived experience, it is called *Moksha* or "spiritual liberation."

Bhairava is the "fearsome form of *Shiva*" who destroys the veil of ignorance that obscures our inherent freedom. Bhairava also refers to the bliss of unity that is experienced as limiting conditioning is released. Bhairava mudra, especially when practiced together with the other gestures of this family, offers a glimpse of our essential being as freedom and unity. The simplicity of this mudra, resting one hand in the other, demonstrates clearly that unity is not some distant dream of awakening, but is always present, waiting to be recognized as the very essence of our being. Bhairava mudra supports the experience of *Kevala Kumbhaka*, a natural suspension of the breath that occurs at the end of the exhalation, allowing us to savor the bliss of unity more deeply.

Systems Balanced:

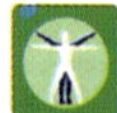

Elements Activated:

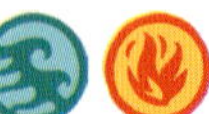

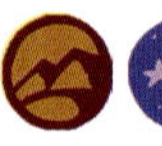
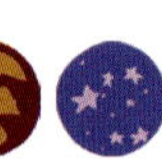

Doshas Balanced:

Prana Vayus Nourished:

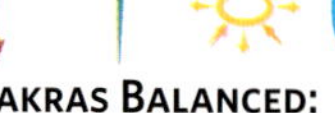
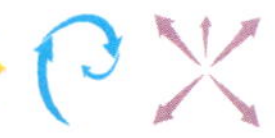

Chakras Balanced:

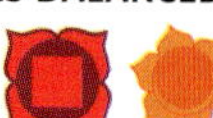

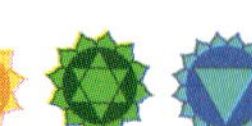

Scale from Calming to Energizing:

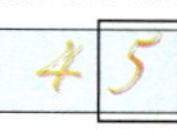

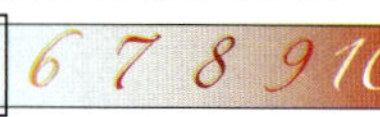

0 1 2 3 4 5 6 7 8 9 10

Guided Meditation: Experiencing Unity

- To integrate all the steps of your meditation journey, you will practice each of the gestures of this family, sensing how they serve as a doorway to the experience of complete unity.
- Begin by bringing your hands into Prajna Prana Kriya mudra. Take several natural breaths to inhabit your lower body completely, allowing you to experience a growing sense of grounding and stability.
- With greater grounding and stability, your breath naturally becomes slow and serene, cultivating a sense of safety as a firm foundation for your meditation journey.
- Now, place your hands in Medha Prana Kriya mudra. Sense your breath expanding your rib cage completely, instilling a feeling of greater opening.
- Take several breaths to sense this opening within your chest, side ribs and upper back, allowing you to welcome thoughts and feelings with greater lightness and ease.
- Next, place your hands in Jnana mudra. Sense energy and breath gently rising into your upper chest, neck and head, allowing your awareness to rest naturally at your third eye point, your center of clear seeing.
- Focused at your center of clarity, you witness all that arises in your mind and body with equanimity while resting in the silence of your authentic being.
- Now, join your hands in Dhyana mudra. Sense how all the regions of your physical body, all areas of your lungs and the main centers of your brain are integrated naturally.
- As you experience this integration of all the dimensions of your being, take several breaths to sense body, breath and mind in perfect harmony.
- Now, allow your hands to rest in Bhairava mudra. Take several breaths to sense the deep inner peace and absolute serenity that naturally permeate your entire being.
- As serenity infuses your entire being, you rest in your essential nature as unity, the culmination of your meditation journey.
- Affirm your meditation journey, repeating the following three times, aloud or silently: **"Resting in absolute serenity, I experience my essential nature as unity."**
- Slowly release the gesture, taking several breaths to rest in your peaceful essence.
- When you are ready, open your eyes, returning slowly and gently, with a greater awareness of your entire meditation journey.

Annamaya kosha (physical body)

• Cultivates Full Yogic Breathing, supporting the health of all the systems of the body.
• Calms the breath, cultivating relaxation.
• The balancing effects of this gesture are generally helpful for Vata, Pitta and Kapha imbalances.

Pranamaya kosha (energy body)

• Gently activates all prana vayus.
• Balances all chakras, with a special focus on the sixth and seventh chakras, centers of wisdom and unity.

Manomaya kosha (psycho-emotional body)

• Cultivates a space of deep inner silence and stillness.

Vijnanamaya kosha (wisdom body)

• As we experience inner silence, we recognize it as the voice of our true inner being from which wisdom arises naturally.

Anandamaya kosha (bliss body)

• As we attune to our essential nature as freedom and unity, feelings of bliss and limitlessness arise naturally.

Chapter Seventeen

Invoking Divine Presence

MUDRAS FOR PRAYER AND DEVOTION

Both prayer and devotion are ways of connecting with the Divine. Prayer invokes Divine support and blessing while devotion communicates our love and longing for the Divine presence. Both prayer and devotion reflect our recognition that we live in a world governed by a higher order beyond our personal control. In prayer, we seek support and guidance through aligning with the Divine source. In devotion, we honor the Divine in a heartfelt way, deepening our level of spiritual connection.

In the *Bhagavad Gita*, the foremost scripture of Indian spirituality, the different levels of prayer and devotion are described beautifully. In chapter 7, verse 16, *Krishna*, as the incarnation of the Divine, describes four kinds of devotees, embodying the four levels of prayer and devotion. Krishna emphasizes that all four types of devotees are beloved to him, but that prayer and devotion reach their culmination when there is no longer any separation between the devotee and the Divine. The four types of devotees are:

Arthi - The Supplicant in Distress
These individuals may not normally invoke a higher power, but when a challenge beyond their control arises, they turn to the Divine for support, solace or a solution.

Artharthi - The Supplicant Making a Request
In this form of prayer, individuals request material abundance, progeny, good health and so on. This request recognizes that all good ultimately comes from the Divine source, and that by attuning to and acknowledging that source, we can enhance our ability to receive its unlimited bounty.

Jijnasu - Seeking Divine Communion through Devotion
This individual is no longer requesting refuge or abundance, but seeking communion with or expressing heartfelt devotion to the Divine. This devotion is often infused with a quality of longing because the spiritual aspirant has experienced a taste of Divine love and now longs for deeper communion. At this level, the Divine often assumes a personal form and the devotee develops a deep personal relationship with his or her chosen deity.

Jnani - Divine Union through Knowledge of the True Self
What is common among the first three types of supplicants is that the Divine is separate from the devotee. Even in profound devotional love, there is still a separation between the lover and the beloved. From the perspective of the *Bhagavad Gita*, the spiritual journey culminates in the recognition of our true Self, which is not separate from the Divine. This recognition of our true being is accompanied by a sense of wholeness, freedom and unity in which all seeking comes to an end. Within this experience of oneness, each moment of life becomes a continual recognition and honoring of all-encompassing unity.

Mudra practice supports all forms of prayer and devotion by focusing and amplifying our intention. Mudras also enhance our energy and vitality, supporting our practice of prayer and devotion. Gestures also facilitate the release of conditioning that keeps us from connecting with the Divine more deeply. Mudras also support the awakening of discernment, allowing us to perceive our true needs and to request them clearly. Ultimately, mudra practice opens us to our true being, inherently whole and complete, wanting and needing nothing, not even to be liberated.

Levels of Prayer and Devotion

Mudra	Level of Devotion
Hridaya	Arthi The Supplicant in Distress
Adhara	Artharthi The Supplicant Making a Request
Tejas	Jijnasu Seeking Divine Union through Devotion
Anjali	Jnani Divine Union through Knowledge of the True Self

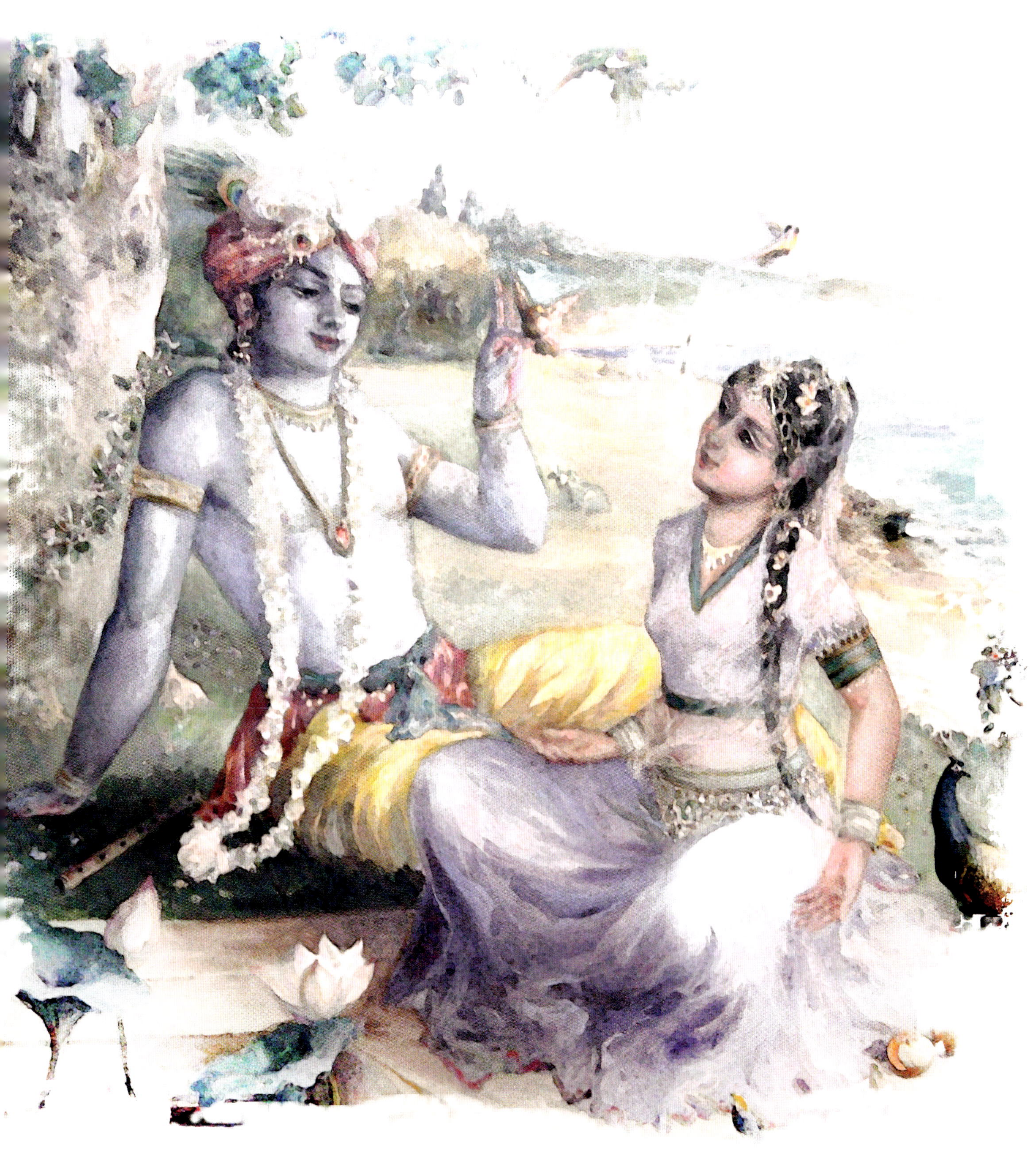

In the Bhagavad Gita, Sri Krishna describes the four types of devotee.

105

Hridaya Mudra

Gesture of the Spiritual Heart
For Seeking Divine Refuge

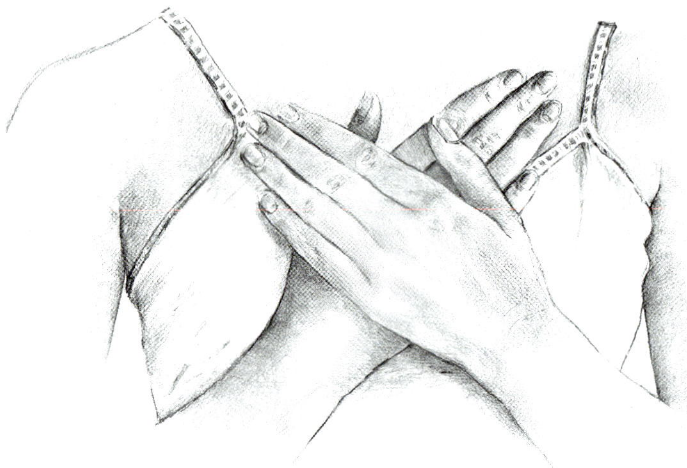

As I open to grace in challenging times, I receive the full support of the Divine.

Core Quality
Seeking Divine Refuge

Especially helpful for
- Seeking the support of the Divine in challenging times.
- Releasing tension from the chest.
- Supporting the health of the immune system.
- Cultivating trust and emotional balance.

Mudras with similar effects
Kapota, Karuna, Purna Hridaya

Cautions
None

Instructions
1. Gently place the right hand over the heart, leaving a slight hollow between the right palm and the heart.
2. Place the left hand over the right hand.
3. Allow the chin to bow slightly forward in a gesture of surrender.
4. Relax the shoulders back and down, with the spine naturally aligned.

When we turn to the Divine in challenging times, we recognize a greater intelligence that can support and guide us through challenging times that seem beyond our control. As we turn to the Divine for support, we open to receive the clarity that allows us to gain a wider perspective of the challenge we are facing, assisting us in finding a solution more easily. Divine guidance can also provide insight and wisdom so that the conditions that created this present challenge are less likely to occur in the future. As we take refuge in the Divine in times of need, our perception of our challenge is gradually transformed and we come to see that every obstacle we encounter serves to guide us along our journey. With this wider perspective, we are able to explore difficult situations, acknowledging their deeper meaning as vehicles for awakening to greater understanding.

Hridaya means "heart," and Hridaya mudra cultivates a space of inner refuge in which we can turn to the Divine for support and solace. This gesture directs breath, awareness and energy into the heart center, cultivating a sense of trust and safety, allowing us to acknowledge our feelings and explore all the dimensions of the challenging situation we are facing. This gesture helps to calm the heart and release stress-related tension from the chest. Hridaya mudra also instills a greater sense of confidence in meeting challenges, which reduces the effects of stress and supports the health of the immune system. The lengthening of the inhaling breath, cultivated by this gesture, provides the energy needed to meet challenges more effectively. The exhalation is also lengthened, instilling a sense of relaxation and release that supports us in dealing with challenges more calmly and objectively.

Systems Balanced:

Elements Activated:

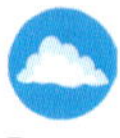

Doshas Balanced:

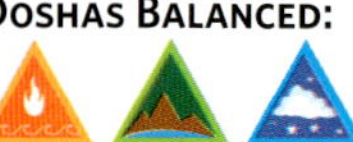

Prana Vayus Nourished:

Chakras Balanced:

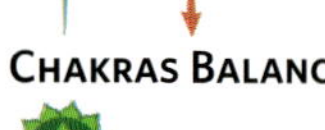

Scale from Calming to Energizing:

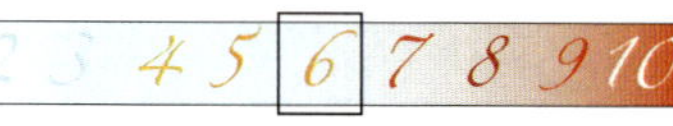

Guided Meditation: **Seeking Refuge in the Divine**

- ॐ As you hold Hridaya mudra, take several natural breaths to attune to all the feelings and sensations evoked by this gesture.
- ॐ Notice how your breath is gently directed into the center of your chest, guiding you inward to your own sacred refuge.
- ॐ As you turn to this refuge in times of need, you receive Divine support and guidance that allows you to move through challenging times more easily.
- ॐ To open to the support of the Divine, bring to mind a challenge that you are facing currently. Take several breaths to receive support and guidance at this moment in your journey.
- ॐ Begin by experiencing the feelings related to this challenge, creating space around them with your breathing, allowing your chest to expand and relax naturally.
- ॐ Take several breaths to attune to the rise and fall of your chest in synchrony with your breathing, embracing all of your feelings more compassionately.
- ॐ As you welcome your feelings, any sense of heaviness gradually begins to release, allowing you to experience greater lightness and ease.
- ॐ With greater lightness, you are able to attune to the Divine refuge within your heart even more deeply, exploring the challenge you are facing with greater clarity in order to come to a place of understanding.
- ॐ Take several breaths to open to see all the dimensions of the challenge you are facing, exploring the factors that may have brought this challenge into being.
- ॐ Now, take some time to reflect on the changes you can make in your perspectives and beliefs that could keep this kind of challenge from reocurring.
- ॐ As you open the doorway to greater understanding, you naturally expand your ability to perceive possible solutions to the challenge you are facing.
- ॐ With this wider perspective, you open to receive guidance and wisdom that allow you to move through this challenging time with greater clarity.
- ॐ Take some time to allow guidance to unfold from within the sacred refuge of your heart.
- ॐ Now, hold an image of the guidance you have received, envisioning the steps that will guide you beyond the challenge you are facing.
- ॐ Now, simply rest within the refuge of your heart, sensing greater peace and serenity, trusting that the Divine is guiding your path at each moment of your life journey.
- ॐ Affirm Divine support as you repeat the following three times, aloud or silently: **"I open to the support and guidance of the Divine at this challenging time."**
- ॐ Slowly release the gesture, taking several breaths to sense Divine protection.
- ॐ When you are ready, open your eyes, returning slowly and gently, sensing the support of the Divine within your sacred refuge.

Annamaya kosha (physical body)

- **Directs breath and awareness to the upper chest and sternum, creating a massaging effect that increases circulation to the area of the thymus gland.**
- **Relaxes the muscles of the chest, releasing tension and constriction.**
- **Instills a sense of trust and confidence in times of challenge that supports immune function.**
- **Supports the expression of emotion, which is generally helpful for Kapha imbalance.**
- **The connection to the heart center cultivated by this gesture is generally helpful for Pitta imbalance.**
- **The sense of support cultivated is generally helpful for Vata imbalance.**

Pranamaya kosha (energy body)

- **Balances Prana and Apana vayus, the upward and downward moving currents of energy.**
- **Opens and balances the fourth chakra, center of unconditional love.**

Manomaya kosha (psycho-emotional body)

- **Cultivates feelings of comfort and emotional balance.**
- **Instills a sense of trust and support.**

Vijnanamaya kosha (wisdom body)

- **As we seek refuge in the Divine in difficult times, we gradually begin to see that the Divine is present at each moment of our journey.**

Anandamaya kosha (bliss body)

- **As we sense greater support, feelings of trust and release begin to unfold from the heart center naturally.**

106 Adhara Mudra

Gesture of Support

For Receiving Abundantly

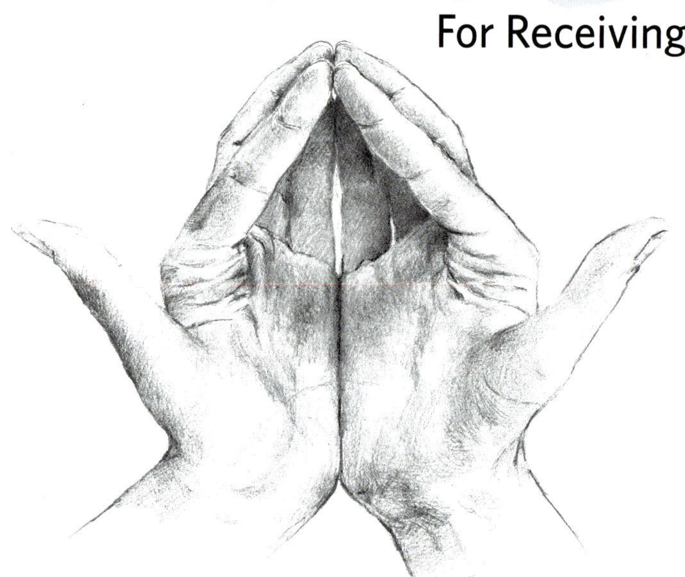

With greater openness to receive,
The Divine provides for all my needs.

Core Quality

Opening to Receive Abundantly

Especially helpful for

- Creating a natural sense of openness to receive abundantly.
- Supporting digestion.
- Releasing tension from the mid back.
- Supporting the health of the kidneys and adrenal glands.
- Cultivating self-esteem, which helps to remove beliefs of unworthiness and inadequacy.

Mudras with similar effects

Avahana, Hastaphula, Kubera

Cautions

None

Instructions

1. Bring the palms together in prayer position in front of the abdomen, with the fingertips facing forward.
2. Keeping the fingertips and the wrists together while spreading the thumbs out to the sides like open wings, creating space between the palms.
3. Relax the shoulders back and down, with the forearms resting against the abdomen and the spine naturally aligned.

Prayer can be used to support the fulfillment of our personal requests. In this type of prayer, we submit our intentions to the Divine source, seeking support. To enhance the effectiveness of this type of prayer, we must clarify what we need, which involves looking beyond our surface-level desires. For example, a perceived material need, when examined closely, may reveal deeper emotional or spiritual needs, such as love, security or a desire for connection to our true being. Satisfying the material need may provide some relief, but will never be a substitute for clarifying and meeting the deeper need. With a clearer sense of our true needs, the next step is to release any beliefs that we are unworthy of receiving. Finally, we surrender our request to the Divine who always knows what we need, both to support us materially and to provide for our deeper needs.

Adhara means "foundation," and refers to the Divine as the source of all abundance. Adhara mudra directs breath, awareness and energy into the solar plexus, cultivating a sense of enthusiasm and self-esteem that supports us in recognizing that we are worthy to receive abundantly. The open hands reflect our willingness to receive, as well as our intention to release the limiting beliefs that keep us from receiving. This gesture also enhances our ability to focus one-pointedly, allowing us to clarify our needs and make our request more objectively. Adhara mudra instills a sense of trust that we always receive everything we need at the right moment along our journey.

Systems Balanced:

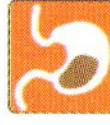

Prana Vayus Nourished:

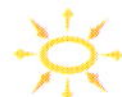

Elements Activated:

Chakras Balanced:

Doshas Balanced:

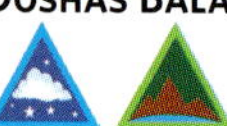

Scale from Calming to Energizing:

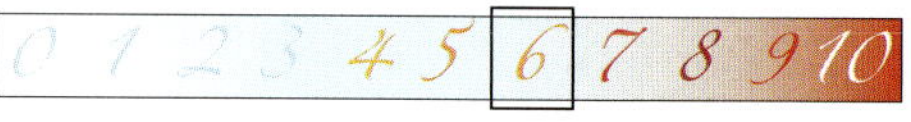

Guided Meditation: Opening to Receive Abundantly

- As you hold Adhara mudra, take several natural breaths to attune to all the feelings and sensations evoked by this gesture.
- Notice how your breath is gently directed into your solar plexus, creating a space of receptivity in which you naturally open to receive more abundantly.
- Take several breaths to attune to the space within your hands as a symbol of your openness to receive all of life's bounty.
- Your open hands also affirm that you are ready to release any beliefs of unworthiness or inadequacy that could keep you from receiving.
- Take some time to reflect on that which you are asking to receive, noticing both your surface-level need as well as your deeper intention for love, self-worth or inner peace.
- Now, make your request to the Divine source, choosing words that reflect your intention clearly from the deepest part of your being, repeating your request three times silently.
- Next, visualize that which you have requested within your hands as a manifest reality, envisioning all the ways that it will support your life journey.
- Finally, surrender your request to the Divine source, recognizing that the universe always provides exactly what you need, allowing you to continue your journey with openness and receptivity.
- Affirm your openness to receive, repeating the following three times, aloud or silently: **"I open to receive abundantly by aligning my needs with the one source energy."**
- Now, slowly release the gesture, taking several breaths to sense your complete receptivity.
- When you are ready, open your eyes, returning slowly and gently, with a willingness to receive abundantly.

Annamaya kosha (physical body)

- **Directs breath and awareness to the solar plexus, creating a massaging effect that increases circulation to the digestive system.**
- **Enhances the horizontal movement of the diaphragm, strengthening the main muscle of respiration.**
- **The enhanced movement of the diaphragm in the back body massages the area of the kidneys and adrenal glands while releasing tension from the mid back.**
- **The energizing effects of this gesture are generally helpful for Kapha imbalance.**
- **The one-pointed concentration cultivated is generally helpful for Vata imbalance.**

Pranamaya kosha (energy body)

- **Gently activates Samana vayu, the horizontal current of energy.**
- **Opens and balances the third chakra, center of personal power.**

Manomaya kosha (psycho-emotional body)

- **Enhances self-esteem.**
- **Focuses the mind, cultivating the ideal environment for manifesting intentions.**

Vijnanamaya kosha (Wisdom body)

- **As we open to receive, we also recognize that the Divine is the source of everything.**

Anandamaya kosha (bliss body)

- **With enhanced self-esteem, feelings of inner wealth and radiance arise naturally.**

107

Tejas Mudra

Gesture of Light

For Cultivating Devotional Love

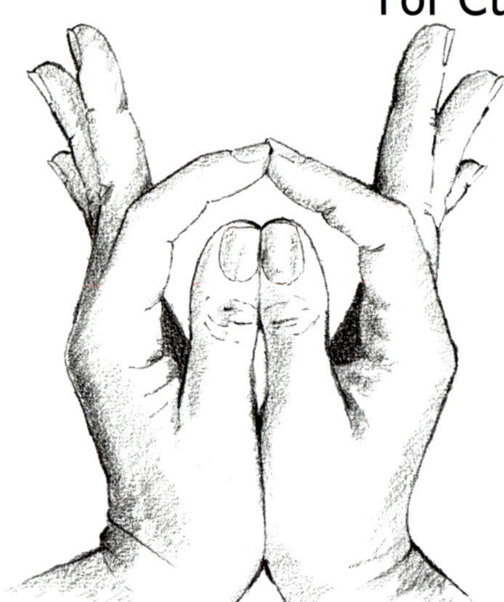

Through heartfelt devotion to the Divine,
Radiant light encompasses my heart and mind.

Core Quality

Cultivating Devotional Love

Especially helpful For

- Cultivating devotional love.
- Strengthening the immune system.
- Instilling a sense of optimism, enthusiasm and uplifting energy.

Mudras with similar effects

Padma, Karuna, Purna Hridaya

Cautions

Those with hypertension or heart conditions should carefully monitor the effects. Purna Hridaya, which is less energizing, can be used as a substitute.

Instructions

1. Hold the hands in prayer position in front of the heart.
2. Bend the index fingers, forming a halo around the thumbs without touching them.
3. Keep the thumbs joined along their length while spreading the other fingers wide apart.
4. Relax the shoulders back and down, with the elbows held slightly away from the body and the spine naturally aligned.

Bhakti, "spiritual devotion," is a profound love and longing for the Divine presence. This seeking is often so intense and all-encompassing that it is compared with the longing of the lover for the beloved. This heartfelt devotion is often directed toward a particular deity using a *mantra*, a "sacred word" or "phrase," repeated continuously in order to connect more deeply. Within the Indian culture, there is a wide variety of deities that embody specific qualities. For example, *Ganesha* represents loving protection and the removal of obstacles. *Shiva* embodies spiritual purification leading to liberation. *Sarasvati* is the essence of knowledge and creativity. *Krishna* is the embodiment of both wisdom and loving compassion. As we deepen our connection to and devotional love toward our chosen deities, we gradually embody their essential qualities, naturally supporting us along our spiritual journey.

Tejas means "light" or "brilliance," and Tejas mudra awakens the light of devotional love that unites the seeker with his or her chosen deity and related qualities. This gesture directs breath, awareness and energy to the heart center, creating a sense of a Divine sanctuary in which we welcome and communicate more easily with our chosen deity. Tejas mudra cultivates optimism and a feeling of well-being that helps us to deepen our love and affection naturally. This gesture gently stimulates heart rate and blood pressure, cultivating energy and vitality that allow us to remain focused upon our chosen deity for longer periods. The shape of the hands represents the radiant flame of spirit that infuses our entire being as we connect with the Divine deeply and sincerely, guiding our path and allowing us to embody all of the qualities of our chosen deity.

Systems Balanced:

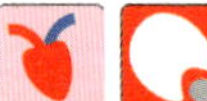
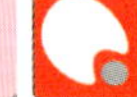

Elements Activated:

Doshas Balanced:

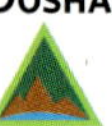

Prana Vayus Nourished:

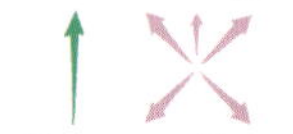

Chakras Balanced:

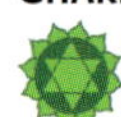

Scale from Calming to Energizing:

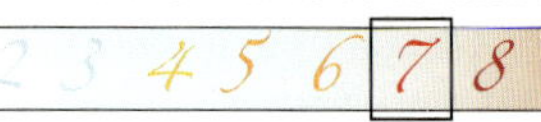

Guided Meditation: Light of Devotion

- As you hold Tejas mudra, take several natural breaths to attune to all the feelings and sensations awakened by this gesture.
- Notice how your breath is gently directed into your heart center, instilling a feeling that you are entering a sacred sanctuary where you can attune to the Divine more deeply.
- At the center of your sanctuary, visualize a candle flame as an expression of Divinity, taking several breaths to rest your attention upon it, lightly and lovingly.
- Take some time to allow the luminosity of your candle flame to radiate throughout your being, infusing you with the light of Divinity.
- As radiant light bathes your entire being, you embody the qualities that allow you to enter into Divine communion more deeply.
- Begin by opening to receive the quality of tranquility, a knowing that you are absolutely safe at each step of your journey, embraced in the loving arms of Divinity.
- With greater tranquility, you receive the clarity that allows you to see the Divine in all of creation, deepening your sense of unity, experiencing everything as a reflection of Divinity.
- Seeing the Divine in everything, your appreciation for life expands naturally, taking several breaths to sense your growing ability to receive each moment as a learning and a blessing.
- With greater appreciation for each moment of living, you embrace your entire life journey wholeheartedly, releasing any sense of unworthiness by understanding that everything has its own purpose and meaning, guiding you toward the light of Divinity.
- As you embrace your life more completely, you recognize that the Divine has always been present, guiding you at each step of your journey.
- Blessed by the Divine presence, a sense of surrender arises naturally, allowing you to let go completely into the arms of Divinity, as the light of love infuses your entire being.
- Take some time to rest in Divine embrace, as your heart is filled with silence and grace.
- Affirm the light of Divinity as you repeat the following three times, aloud or silently: **"As Divine light fills my heart, I experience deep devotional love."**
- Slowly release the gesture, taking several breaths to rest in the Divine presence.
- When you are ready, open your eyes, returning slowly and gently, infused with the light of Divinity.

Annamaya kosha (Physical body)

• Directs breath and awareness to the heart area, creating a massaging effect that enhances circulation to the upper chest, including the thymus gland.
• The cultivation of positive emotions, such as love and compassion, supports the health of the immune system.
• The vitalizing effects of this gesture are generally helpful for Kapha imbalance.

Pranamaya kosha (Energy body)

• Activates Prana vayu, the upward moving current of energy, as well as Vyana vayu, the all-pervading current, moving from center to extremities.
• Opens the fourth chakra, center of unconditional love.

Manomaya kosha (Psycho-emotional body)

• Cultivates inner light and energy that can be directed toward a devotional deity.
• Instills a sense of focus and centering.

Vijnanamaya kosha (Wisdom body)

• Bhakti, heartfelt devotion, serves as a doorway to our true Self, whose essence is love.

Anandamaya kosha (Bliss body)

• As devotional love flows throughout our being, we experience its essential qualities, including wholeness, serenity, reverence, trust and peace.

108

Anjali Mudra

Gesture of Reverence
For Invoking Divine Union

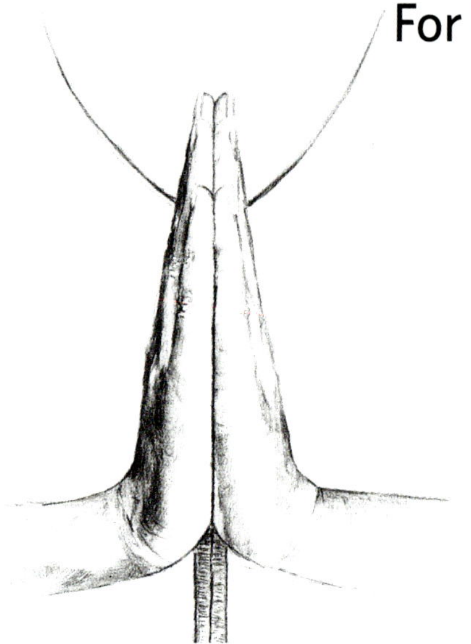

With a gesture of reverence to each one I meet, I affirm our essential unity.

Core Quality
Invoking Divine Union

Especially Helpful for
- Invoking a sense of Divine union.
- Drawing the senses inward, which calms the mind, reducing stress and blood pressure.
- Releasing tension from between the shoulder blades.
- Supporting the health of the immune system.
- Cultivating inner silence.

Mudras with similar effects
Kapota, Karuna, Citta

Cautions
None

Instructions
1. Join the hands in front of the heart, with the fingers together, facing upward.
2. Allow a slight space of openness at the center of the palms.
3. The outer borders of the thumbs may rest against the sternum, or be held slightly away from the body.
4. Relax the shoulders back and down, with the elbows held slightly away from the body and the spine naturally aligned.

In the previous types of prayer and devotion, there is a separation between the one who is praying and the one to whom the prayer is addressed, between the devotee and the Divine. Along the journey of spiritual awakening, this separation is gradually released, allowing the devotee and the Divine to merge as a seamless unity. From the perspective of the *Bhagavad Gita*, all forms of prayer and devotion support us along our journey, but in the ultimate sense, they are all reflections of our quest for unity. The seeker in times of need finds support by embracing a greater unity beyond the limited perspective of the personality. The person who wishes to receive abundantly aligns with the Divine as the source of all bounty. Devotional love is a taste of the unity that is the essence of our true being. As we reach the culmination of the spiritual journey, all sense of separation is released, and we recognize that all we seek is already present as the essence of our own being.

Anjali means "reverence," and refers to an honoring of the Divinity within ourselves and all beings. Anjali mudra invokes this unity by bringing the hands together, symbolizing the integration of all of the polarities within our being. This gesture directs breath, awareness and energy into the center of the chest, supporting us in turning inward toward our authentic being, allowing our sense of oneness with the Divine to deepen naturally. By recognizing creation's all-encompassing unity, life's doubts, questions and problems are resolved completely. This gesture is also used as a greeting and it is a way of communicating to each person that we meet that we recognize our essential unity.

Systems Balanced:

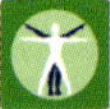

Elements Activated:

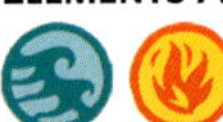

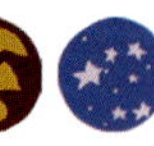
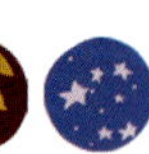

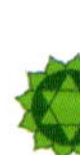

Doshas Balanced:

Prana Vayus Nourished:

Chakras Balanced:

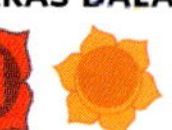

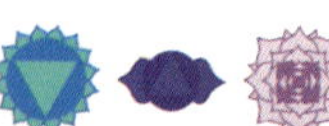

Scale from Calming to Energizing:

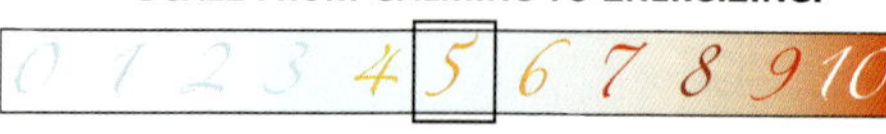

Guided Meditation: Invoking Unity

- As you hold Anjali mudra, take several natural breaths to attune to all the feelings and sensations awakened by this gesture.
- Notice how your breath is gently directed into your heart center, inviting your senses to rest naturally inward.
- As you rest more deeply at the center of your being, take several breaths to experience a sense of integration and unity that arises naturally.
- You will deepen your experience of integration by exploring some of the complementary polarities within your being, sensing them merging as a seamless unity.
- Begin by bringing your awareness to the right side of your body, naturally focusing your breath within your right nostril.
- Take some time to sense greater warmth and vitality throughout the entire right side of your body, awakening your active polarity, related to doing and achieving.
- Next, bring your awareness to the left side of your body, naturally focusing your breath within your left nostril.
- Take some time to sense greater refreshment and ease throughout the entire left side of your body, reflecting your receptive polarity, related to a sense of surrender and release.
- For your next few breaths, sense the plane of contact where your palms meet, allowing your awareness to encompass both sides of your body evenly, instilling a sense of complete integration and harmony.
- Next, bring awareness to your right hand as a symbol of wisdom, the sum total of understanding and clarity that you have gained along your spiritual journey.
- Now, bring awareness to your left hand as a symbol of compassion, your ability to see that we all share a common journey toward awakening.
- For your next few breaths, sense the plane of contact where your palms meet, experiencing the integration of wisdom and compassion, knowing that only through their unity can you experience complete awakening.
- With wisdom and compassion united, take some time to focus on your right hand as a symbol of yourself as a devotee, having a personal relationship with the Divine from whom you seek blessing.
- Now, take some time to focus on your left hand as a symbol of the Divine itself, the destination of your spiritual journey, the Divine source who receives your prayers, devotional love and offerings.
- For your next few breaths, sense the plane of contact where your palms meet, experiencing the devotee and the Divine as a seamless unity.
- Take several breaths to rest in complete oneness with the all-encompassing Divinity whose light is the source and essence of all things.
- Affirm unity at all levels of being, repeating the following three times, aloud or silently: **"Through the integration of all polarities, I experience my very essence as unity."**
- Slowly release the gesture, taking several breaths to rest in your Divine essence.
- When you are ready, open your eyes, returning slowly and gently, allowing your sense of oneness to guide your journey.

Annamaya kosha (physical body)

• Directs breath and awareness to the front of the chest, creating a massaging effect that increases circulation to the thymus gland.
• Expands the breath between the shoulder blades, releasing tension from this area.
• The integrating effects of this gesture are generally helpful for Vata, Pitta and Kapha imbalances.

Pranamaya kosha (energy body)

• Balances Prana and Apana vayus, the upward and downward moving currents of energy.
• Opens and integrates the entire chakra system, with a special focus on the fourth chakra, center of unconditional love.

Manomaya kosha (psycho-emotional body)

• Cultivates equanimity.
• Directs the senses inward.
• Instills a sense of reverence.

Vijnanamaya kosha (wisdom body)

• As we become calm and centered, we experience unity as a reflection of our true being.

Anandamaya kosha (bliss body)

• As we experience greater integration, feelings of wholeness and unity arise naturally.

APPENDIX A - Mudras for Supporting the Main Yoga Postures

Asana	Name in Sanskrit	Supporting Mudra	Benefits Enhanced by the Mudra
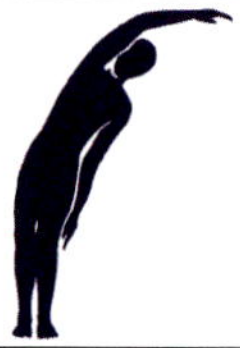	**Ardha Chandrasana** *Standing Half Moon*	Medha Prana Kriya mudra with the raised hand 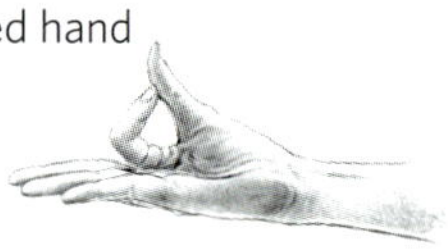	Opens and expands the sides of the rib cage, cultivating fuller breathing while facilitating longer holding.
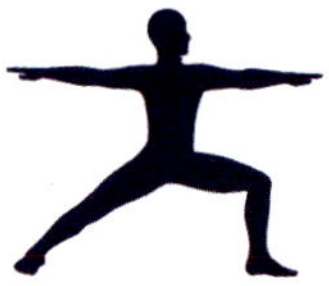	**Virabhadrasana II** *Hero II*	Merudanda mudra 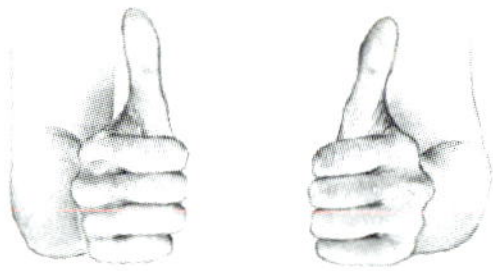	Directs the breath into the solar plexus, cultivating strength, energy and stability. Enhances focus and supports the alignment of the spine, perpendicular to the earth.
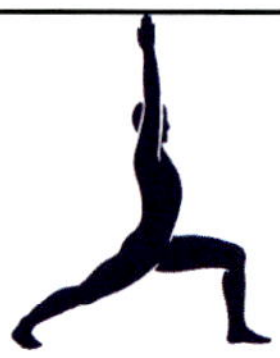	**Virabhadrasana I** *Hero I*	Vajrapradama mudra 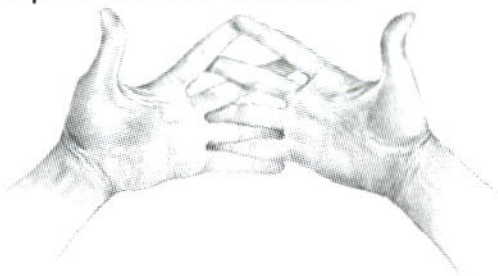	This gesture is held in front of the chest. Expands all four sides of the rib cage, cultivating the qualities of courage and fortitude, and the ability to face life with an open heart.
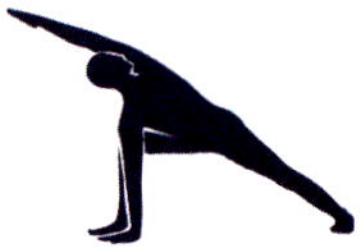	**Parsvakonasana** *Lateral Angle*	Vayu mudra 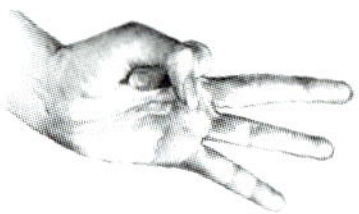	This gesture is held with the raised hand. Activates the air element, expanding the sides of the rib cage, facilitating its opening and rotation. Instills a sense of lightness and ease that supports in aligning the spine diagonally.
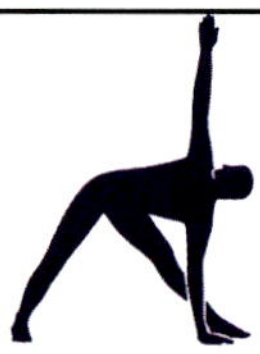	**Trikonasana** *Triangle*	Prana mudra with the raised hand Apana mudra with the lower hand 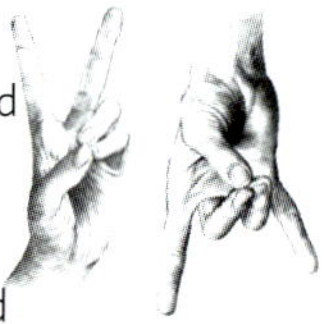	The combination of these gestures harmonizes Prana and Apana vayus, the upward and downward moving currents of energy, supporting the alignment of the spine.
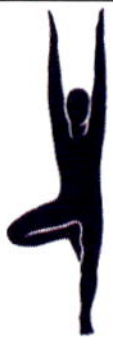	**Vrikshasana** *Tree*	Vyana Vayu mudra 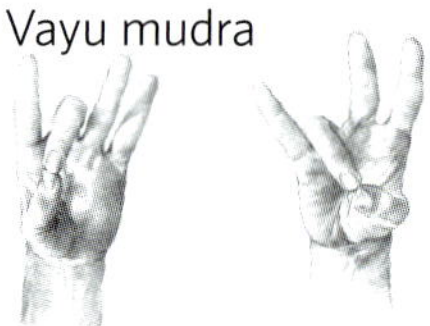	Enhances body awareness, supporting balance while lengthening and tractioning the entire spine.
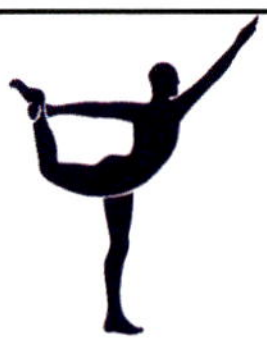	**Natarajasana** *Dancer*	Hansi mudra with the forward hand, palm facing upward 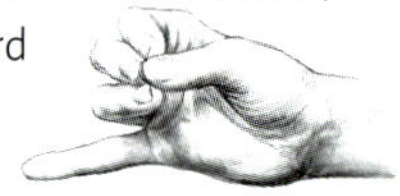	Cultivates stability in the pose, supporting balance. Releases tension from the face, cultivating joy and gracefulness, allowing for a deeper chest opening and facilitating longer holding.
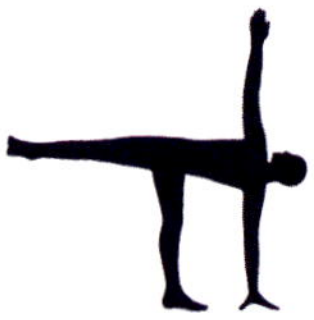	**Ardha Chandrasana** *Balancing Half Moon*	Anushasana mudra with the raised hand 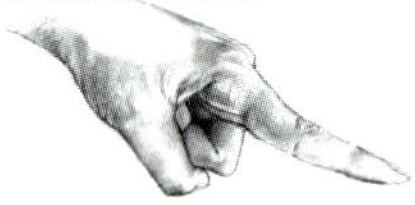	Enhances focus and body awareness while supporting the radiation of energy from center to periphery.
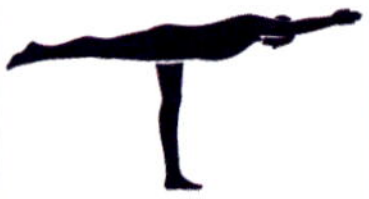	**Virabhadrasana III** *Hero III*	Surya mudra 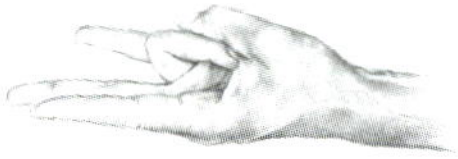	Directs the breath to the solar plexus, cultivating vitality, facilitating longer holding while conserving energy.
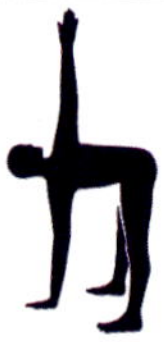	**Parivritta Prasarita Padottanasana** *Rotated Separate Leg Forward Fold*	Vayu mudra with the raised hand 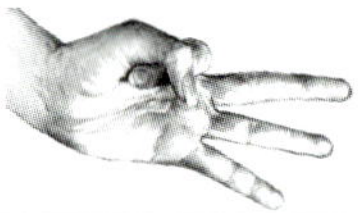	Expands the sides of the rib cage, facilitating its opening and rotation.

APPENDIX A - MUDRAS FOR SUPPORTING THE MAIN YOGA POSTURES

Asana	Name in Sanskrit	Supporting Mudra	Benefits Enhanced by the Mudra
	Adhara Utkatasana *Firm Foundation*	Adhi mudra	Enhances grounding and facilitates the flow of subtle energy through the body. The increased energy facilitates longer holding.
	Malasana Variation *Squat Balance*	Shivalingam mudra	Enhances balance and centering as well and supports the lengthening of the spine. Increased energy facilitates longer holding.
	Malasana *Squat*	Murti mudra	Activates Apana vayu, the downward moving current of energy, enhancing grounding and stability, and supporting the purification of the body.
	Dandasana *Staff Pose*	Anushasana mudra	Activates Vyana vayu, the all-pervading current of energy, supporting the lengthening of the spine and the activation of the extremities.
	Paripurna Navasana *Seated Boat*	Vyana Vayu mudra	Activates Vyana Vayu mudra, enhancing body awareness, cultivating strength and energy at the center of the body while radiating energy outward to the extremities.
	Baddha Konasana *Bound Angle Butterfly*	Mira mudra	Directs breath and energy to the pelvis, supporting the opening of the hip joints, assisting in forward bending with the spine in alignment.
	Upavista Konasana *Separate Leg Forward Fold*	Pranidhana mudra	Lengthens the exhalation, cultivating relaxation and the release of muscular tension, especially from the thighs. Brings breath to the spine, supporting its alignment.
	Virasana *Seated Hero*	Prithivi mudra	Enhances grounding and a sense of support, allowing the base of the body to release onto the earth more easily.
	Vajrasana *Thunder Bolt*	Adhi mudra	Cultivates embodiment and a sense of deep grounding and stability, as well as a firm foundation for the natural lengthening of the spine.
	Mandukasana *Frog*	Jalashaya mudra	Directs breath and energy into the pelvis and base of the body, supporting the opening of the hips as well as an enhanced sense of grounding and stability.

APPENDIX A - Mudras for Supporting the Main Yoga Postures

Asana	Name in Sanskrit	Supporting Mudra	Benefits Enhanced by the Mudra
	Deviasana *Goddess*	Vajrapradama mudra	This gesture is held in front of the chest, deepening the expansion of the rib cage. Supports the natural lengthening of the spine and a sense of lightness that allows for longer holding.
	Chakravakasana *Sunbird*	Surya mudra with the raised hand	Activates the solar plexus, cultivating strength and energy that facilitates longer holding while conserving energy.
	Ardha Matsyendrasana *Seated Twist*	Palli mudra with the raised hand	Supports deeper rotation while maintaining the natural alignment of the spine.
	Ardha Mandalasana *Half Circle*	Vayu mudra with the raised hand	Expands all four sides of the rib cage. Also provides lightness for longer holding.
	Vashistasana *Side Arm Balance*	Prana mudra with the raised hand	Cultivates lightness, energy and vitality, facilitating longer holding.
	Supta Navasana *Lying Boat*	Anushasana mudra	Directs breath and energy from the center of the body to the extremities, facilitating longer holding and tractioning of the spine.
	Supta Virasana *Reclining Hero*	Pushan mudra	Enhances the massaging effects of the pose on the digestive and eliminatory systems. Increases grounding and facilities longer holding.
	Jathara Parivartanasana *Knee Down Twist*	Medha Prana Kriya mudra with the hand of the extended arm	Expands the breath in the chest and sides of the rib cage, deepening rotation, while supporting the natural alignment of the spine.
	Apanasana *Knee to Chest*	Murti mudra	Activates Apana vayu, the downward moving current of energy, lengthening the exhalation and deepening the massage of the abdomen. Supports the alignment of the spine.
	Padmasana *Lotus*	Jnana mudra	Stabilizes the pose and increases the level of comfort in the legs. Also directs energy upward toward the sixth chakra, facilitating concentration and meditation.

APPENDIX B - Mudras for Supporting the Main Pranayamas

Name and Description	Supporting Mudra	Benefits Enhanced by the Mudra
Kaki Pranayama *Crow's Beak Breath* Inhale through the nostrils; lengthened exhalation through the mouth with the shape of a beak.	Bhu mudra	Facilitates the lengthening of the exhalation while cultivating grounding and stability. Enhances embodiment, integrating the purifying effects of this pranayama throughout the entire body.
Sedanta Pranayama *Refreshing Breath* Inhale through the joined teeth and exhale slowly through the nostrils with the mouth closed.	Svadhisthana mudra	Lengthens both the inhalation and the exhalation, enhancing the cooling effects of this breath.
Dirgha Pranayama *Full Yogic Breath (front of the body)*	Purna Svara mudra	Enhances Full Yogic Breathing up and down the front of the body.
Dirgha Pranayama *Full Yogic Breath (back of the body)*	Anudandi mudra	Enhances Full Yogic Breathing up and down the back of the body.
Dirgha Pranayama *Full Yogic Breath (entire body)*	Hakini mudra	Enhances Full Yogic Breathing throughout the entire body.
Viloma Krama *Exhalation in Three Steps* Inhale through the nostrils, followed by an active, short exhalation in three steps.	Shivalingam mudra	Expands the total volume of air exhaled.
Anuloma Krama *Inhalation in Three Steps* Gently inhaling in three steps, followed by a natural exhalation.	Madhyama Sharira mudra	Expands the total volume of air inhaled.
Kapalabhati Pranayama *Skull Shining Breath* A passive inhalation in which the abdomen expands fully, followed by a short, active exhalation.	Merudanda mudra	Facilitates the complete inhalation as well as the active exhalation.
Suryanuloma Pranayama *Right Nostril Breathing* **Chandranuloma Pranayama** *Left Nostril Breathing*	Pingala mudra Ida mudra	Directs the breath into the right nostril, right lung & right side of the body; the solar aspect of our being. Directs the breath in the left nostril, left lung & left side of the body; the lunar aspect of our being.
Nadi Shodhana Pranayama *Alternate Nostril Breathing* Inhale left nostril, pause, exhale right, pause; inhale right nostril, pause, exhale left, pause. Repeat.	Ida mudra - left nostril Pingala mudra - right nostril	Facilitates the alternation of the breath from one nostril to the other and also cultivates the lengthening of the natural pause at the end of the inhalation and at the end of the exhalation.

Brahmarpanam Mantra with Mudras

This prayer is a verse from the Bhagavad Gita, chapter 4, verse 24. It is commonly used before meals to remind us that all we receive is a gift from the Divine.

Pushpanjali
brahmarpanam
Brahman is the instrument of offering

Avahana
brahma havir
Brahman is the ghee that is offered

Tejas
brahmagnau
into the fire that is also Brahman

Hastaphula
brahmana hutam
offered by Brahman,

Achala Agni
brahmaivatena
Brahman is only

Hakini
gantavyam
reached

Shivalingam
brahma karma samadhina
by the one who sees Brahman in all actions

Gayatri Mantra with Mudras

The Gayatri Mantra is one of the best known and loved mantras within the Vedic tradition. It is an invocation to the sun god, Savitri, as the embodiment of the one source Consciousness. The following sequence was developed by Joseph and Lilian Le Page.

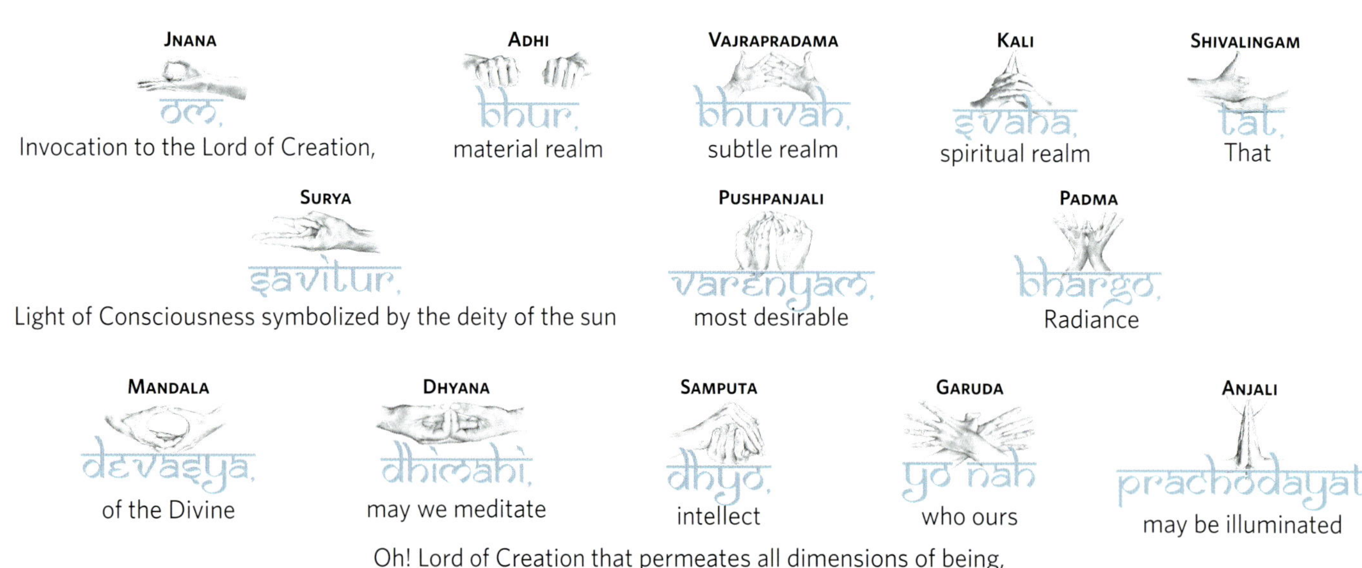

Oh! Lord of Creation that permeates all dimensions of being,
May we meditate upon that radiant Divine Light that inspires and guides us.

Loka Samasta Sukhino Bhavantu

Loka Samasta is a Vedic mantra that invokes happiness and comfort for all beings.

Hakini
loka
All realms, worlds, universes

Dharma Pravartana
samasta
All beings

Hansi
sukhino
Transcendental (all-pervading) Happiness

Hridaya
bhavantu
May be

May All Beings Be Happy

Sahanavavatu Mantra

The Sahanavavatu mantra is one of the shanti (peace) mantras which has its origins in the Taittiriya Upanishad. This mantra is often used as a "universal" prayer of peace and prosperity. The mantra is especially used to invoke God's blessings for harmony amongst teachers and students.

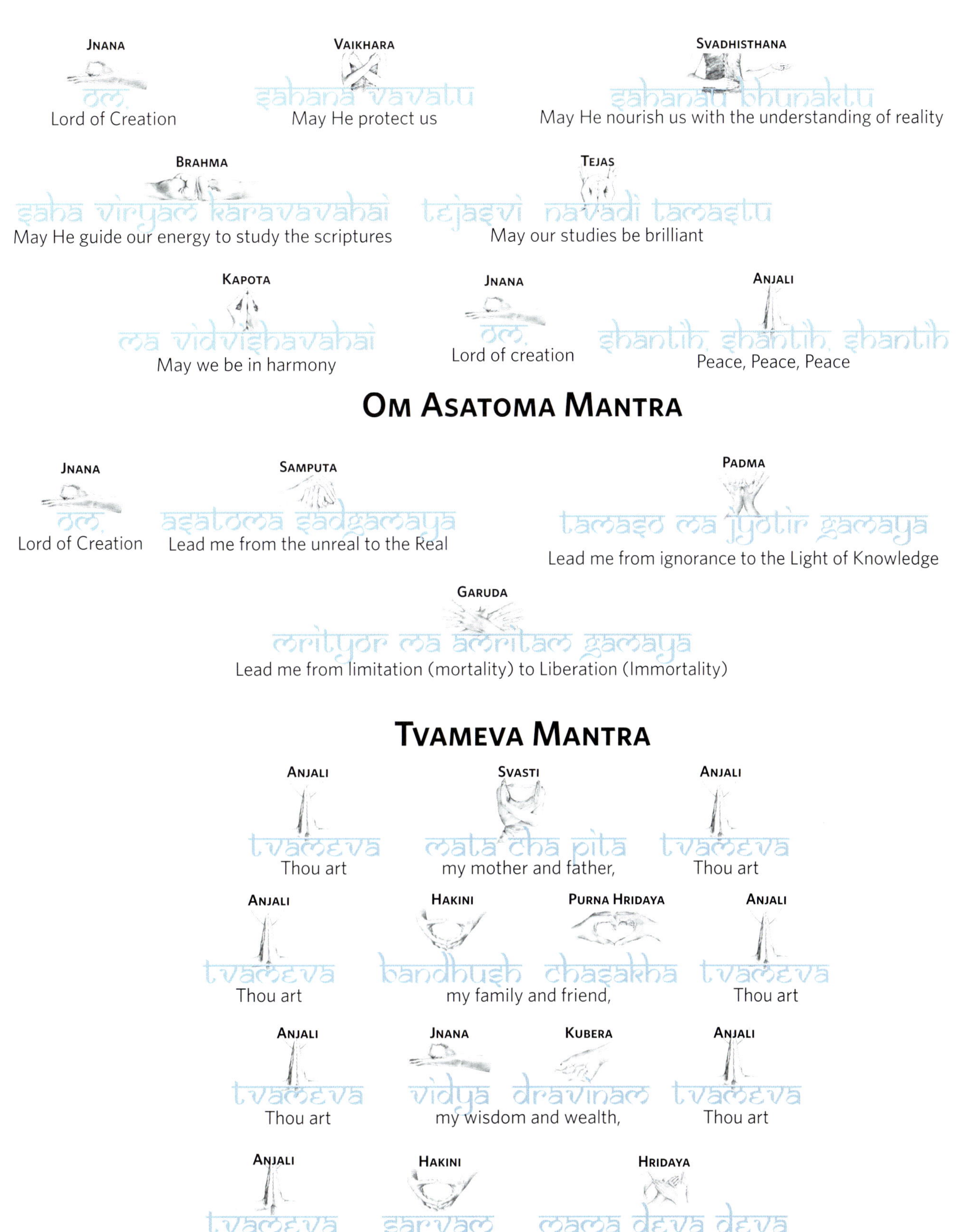

Mudras in Yoga Therapy

Yoga Therapy is the specific application of the philosophy, psychology and techniques of Yoga for healing the whole person. Yoga Therapy is applied to the specific needs of individuals or special focus groups, such as those with hypertension, cancer or back pain. ***Integrative Yoga Therapy***, a pioneer in the field, has developed a unique Yoga Therapy methodology based on a ten-week therapeutic program in which each class has a special theme designed to promote optimal healing.

Each of the classes within the ten-week program is organized within the ***Integrative Yoga Therapy*** ten-step process. The Yoga postures, breathing exercises and other techniques each play an essential role in the healing process. Mudras together with accompanying affirmations are especially important because they are interspersed throughout all parts of the program, weaving all the segments of the class together into an integrated whole.

THE INTEGRATIVE YOGA THERAPY TEN-STEP PROCESS

Each class in the ten-week program is composed of ten steps:

1. **Check-in** - the mudra and theme from the previous week is reviewed, together with the homework.
2. **Educational Theme** - the Yoga therapist introduces a theme in order to awaken a specific Core Quality or facet of healing.
3. **Awareness Exercise** - a guided awareness exercise allows the students to explore a particular Core Quality.
4. **Sharing** - students share their experience with the group.
5. **Mudra & Affirmation** - a specific mudra, along with an affirmation, is presented in order to support the Core Quality for that class.
6. **Breathing Exercises** - specific breathing techniques support the theme.
7. **Warm-ups & Yoga Postures** - Yoga sequences are given that are appropriate for the specific group or condition. Mudras and affirmations are woven throughout the practice, helping to integrate the theme.
8. **Yoga Nidra (guided relaxation)** - a specific Yoga Nidra is presented each week to integrate the Core Qualities more deeply.
9. **Meditation** - the mudra and affirmation for the week form the foundation of the meditation practice.
10. **Closing** - each participant offers a word that encapsulates their experience, integrating the class. Homework is given in which practicing the mudra and affirmation are a key component.

THE INTEGRATIVE YOGA THERAPY TEN-WEEK PROGRAM

The ***IYT Healthy Heart Program*** is an example of the Integrative Yoga Therapy approach in which mudras play a key role.

Week 1: Visualizing Optimal Health "I visualize a new dawn of perfect health." **Core Quality:** New Possibilities	Ushas mudra
Week 2: Stress Reduction "I am completely relaxed and at ease." **Core Quality:** Relaxation	Dvimukham mudra
Week 3: Body Awareness "I trust and honor my body." **Core Quality:** Healthy Embodiment	Prithivi mudra
Week 4: Correct Postural Alignment "My body and spine are naturally aligned." **Core Quality:** Optimal Alignment	Merudanda mudra
Week 5: Optimal Breathing "My breath flows freely and easily." **Core Quality:** Breathing Completely	Vajrapradama mudra
Week 6: Self-nourishment "I awaken to my own spring of inner healing." **Core Quality:** Self-nourishment	Svadhisthana mudra
Week 7: Awakening the Senses "I awaken my senses to live each day more vibrantly." **Core Quality:** Living More Fully	Hakini mudra
Week 8: Gratitude "I treasure each moment of life as a precious gift." **Core Quality:** Gratitude	Samputa mudra
Week 9: Opening the Heart "My heart beats in synchrony with the heart of all beings." **Core Quality:** Compassion	Padma mudra
Week 10: Life's Deeper Meaning "I align with my life's deeper meaning." **Core Quality:** Purpose and Meaning	Anjali mudra

The Science of Mudra

By Matthew J. Taylor, PT, PhD, ERYT-500

The publication of this book is an advancement in the science of mudra, because it allows for the observation and experimentation of the effects of mudra on health and well-being in a more comprehensive way than has been presented previously. The knowledge produced by such investigation will invite further scrutiny through the lens of the scientific method in order to develop a theoretical explanation of how mudras "work." This appendix is intended to invite further explorations of this subject.

What is Published About Mudras?

A review of the literature in April 2013 found no published peer-reviewed studies that looked specifically at mudra as a phenomenon or a treatment variable. There are a few Kundalini studies that utilized movements, mantra and mudra in combination, but the practice was not isolated to mudra and no specific discussion of the theoretical explanation of mudra was published. A review of the few available books on mudra found that beyond the relaxation response and elemental model descriptions of possible explanations, there was no discussion reflecting emerging neuroscience and the complexities of human movement and behavior.

How Might Mudras Work?

The latest science findings reveal a level of complexity and integration of function and form that leaves behind the parts models of right/left brain, brain as mind, and isolated anatomical function and location. The revelations of epigenetics, neuroplasticity and interpersonal mind that were mere speculation at the turn of the century are now accepted facts. The reductionist process has revealed an integrative reality suggesting many possible explanations for the role of mudra. This appendix offers a short list of ideas intended to spur further investigation.

Considerations for Future Inquiry:

• Both the motor and sensory cortices (exteroceptive system) allot nearly one third of their surface to the hands vs. less than a third to the trunk and extremities. Additionally, the discovery of an interoceptive system in the right anterior insula proximate to a more primitive exteroceptive representation suggests that the introspective practice of attention through mudra to subtle experience (pain, temperature, itch, buzz, visceral sensation, vasomotor activity and more) will influence the subjective image of the material self as emotional awareness.

• Touching fingers and hands together promotes cross-lateralization and sensorimotor integration in human development. Correlated with objective movement, function and quality of life scales investigations might include inexpensive scale reporting through high-tech movement analysis and imaging studies.

• Rhythmic movement and sound inhibit a sense of separation and isolation. Differentiation from traditional mudra and sham movements or other control activities might illuminate whether any such activity yields benefit or if these classic patterns generate specific responses.

• Cognitive reframing and new narrative generation create both intra and interpersonal behavioral changes. The meaning of accompanied mantras and symbolism of the mudras alters narratives that affect prefrontal and limbic activity. Altering novice orientation groups from traditional explanation, neuroscience explanation, mixed explanations and sham explanations could be examined to isolate the effect of subjective narrative and its role in mudra response generation.

• Altered position and function of the upper extremities affect postural control, respiration patterns and subsequently autonomic nervous system biasing. Simple measures of respiratory recruitment, surface muscle activity, chest and abdominal volumetric changes within and between mudras might suggest interregional relationships between observable biomechanical measurements and subjective experiences of mudras such as the chakra series where regional variation is often reported.

• Visual and guided imagery accompanying mudras are known to change motor performance and exteroceptive and interoceptive body images. Constructing imageries focused on anatomical attention, qualitative attention, and variation of neutral/detached observation vs. healing outcome stories presents a possible research direction.

• Regular motor practices generate synaptogenesis in the brain, increasing integration and establishing new associative relationships not limited to particular regional activity. Attention to emotional responses without reaction leads to enhanced resilience and increased empathy. Mapping these changes of "hard-wiring" has been done with meditation with well-documented changes in anatomy, recruitment patterns to stimuli and subjective behavioral changes.

• Distraction eases the experience of pain and isolation. Case reports to diagnostically related groups (e.g., headache, back pain, GERD, etc.) with controls are possibilities for observation and reporting.

• Attention to breathing and somatic and emotional experience alters genetic expression and produces the relaxation response. Mudra practice may generate similar epigenetic responses in isolation or combination with known practices.

• Introspective capacity enhances creativity and generates increased inclusiveness, compassion, patience and empathy. Matching these responses with classic mudra is a field of possible study.

The Potential at Our Fingertips

This is just a small list of possibilities to invite deeper consideration of "How mudras work." When matched with advancing technologies of measurement (fMRI, PET scans, body image scaling, surface EMG's, etc.), more robust research methodologies (quantitative, qualitative and mixed methods), data management and statistics through software, transcription and thematic extraction, there are tremendous possibilities.

For more information or discussion on this subject, contact research@matthewjtaylor.com.

APPENDIX F - MUDRA CORE QUALITIES

MUDRA NAME	CORE QUALITY
1. Kanishtha	Connection to the Earth
2. Anamika	Self-healing
3. Madhyama	Balanced Energy
4. Tarjani	Opening the Heart
5. Angushtha	Inner Listening
6. Hakini	Integration
7. Kanishtha Sharira	Lower Body Breathing
8. Madhyama Sharira	Middle Body Breathing
9. Jyeshtha Sharira	Upper Body Breathing
10. Purna Svara	Complete Breathing
11. Adhi	Stillness
12. Adho Merudanda	Centering
13. Merudanda	Alignment
14. Urdhvam Merudanda	Expansiveness
15. Prithivi	Embodiment
16. Vittam	Free Flow of Vital Energy
17. Purna Hridaya	Honoring Thoughts & Feelings
18. Citta	Awakening the Inner Witness
19. Hansi	Unfolding Positive Qualities
20. Rupa	Healthy Skeletal System
21. Anudandi	Back Pain Relief
22. Matsya	Healthy Joints
23. Apanayana	Balanced Elimination
24. Varuna	Healthy Urinary System
25. Yoni	Female Reproductive Health
26. Shankha	Male Reproductive Health
27. Trimurti	Harmonious Life Transitions
28. Pushan	Balanced Digestion
29. Brahma	Awakening Energy & Vitality
30. Mira	Easeful Breathing
31. Vayan	Optimal Circulation
32. Apana Vayu	Healthy Heart
33. Mahashirsha	Headache Relief
34. Garuda	Balanced Metabolism
35. Vajrapradama	Enthusiasm for Living
36. Pala	Anxiety Relief
37. Vyana Vayu	Healthy Nervous System
38. Bhramara	Healthy Immunity
39. Mani Ratna	Global Healing
40. Bhu	Stability of the Earth
41. Jala	Fluidity of Water
42. Surya	Radiant Energy of Fire
43. Vayu	Lightness of Air
44. Akasha	Vastness of Space
45. Dharma Pravartana	Balancing All Five Elements
46. Achala Agni	Optimal Digestion
47. Abhaya Varada	Fearlessness
48. Jalashaya	Serenity
49. Ratna Prabha	Vitality
50. Apana	Purifying Current of Energy
51. Prana	Uplifting Current of Energy
52. Matangi	Radiating Current of Energy
53. Linga	Clarifying Current of Energy
54. Anushasana	All-Pervading Current of Energy

MUDRA NAME	CORE QUALITY
55. Chinmaya	Security
56. Svadhisthana	Self-nourishment
57. Vajra	Self-empowerment
58. Padma	Unconditional Love
59. Kali	Spiritual Purification
60. Trishula	Non-duality
61. Ananta	Unity Consciousness
62. Dharma Chakra	Integrating All the Chakras
63. Ida	Receptivity
64. Pingala	Dynamism
65. Shakata	Spiritual Unity
66. Vaikhara	Protection from the Forces of Nature
67. Svasti	Protection from Negative Energy
68. Gupta	Protection from Our Limiting Beliefs
69. Ganesha	Protection for New Beginnings
70. Dvimukham	Deep Relaxation
71. Kurma	Reducing Sensory Overload
72. Pranidhana	Letting Go
73. Ushas	Opening to New Possibilities
74. Kapota	Non-violence
75. Samputa	Truthfulness
76. Hastaphula	Non-stealing
77. Kubera	Conservation of Energy
78. Pushpanjali	Non-grasping
79. Vishuddha	Purity
80. Chaturmukham	Contentment
81. Mushtikam	Spiritual Discipline
82. Sakshi	Self-study
83. Chin	Surrender to the Divine
84. Murti	Steady and Comfortable Posture
85. Dirgha Svara	Expansion of Life Force Energy
86. Ishvara	Withdrawal of the Senses
87. Abhisheka	One-pointed Concentration
88. Dharmadhatu	Meditation
89. Mandala	Spiritual Union
90. Shivalingam	Spiritual Commitment
91. Shunya	Opening to Transformation
92. Palli	Trusting Inner Guidance
93. Avahana	Heartfelt Acceptance
94. Karuna	Compassion
95. Purna Jnanam	Spiritual Discernment
96. Varahkam	Equanimity
97. Shakti	Awakening Spiritual Energy
98. Uttarabodhi	Self-mastery
99. Kaleshvara	Spiritual Freedom
100. Prajna Prana Kriya	Stabilizing Body & Breath
101. Medha Prana Kriya	Welcoming Thoughts & Feelings
102. Jnana	Awakening Clear Seeing
103. Dhyana	Effortless Meditation
104. Bhairava	Experiencing Unity
105. Hridaya	Seeking Divine Refuge
106. Adhara	Opening to Receive Abundantly
107. Tejas	Cultivating Devotional Love
108. Anjali	Invoking Divine Union

APPENDIX G - MUDRAS AND HEALTH CONDITIONS

HEALTH CONDITION	PRIMARY MUDRA	SECONDARY MUDRAS
Addiction	Svadhisthana	Anamika, Dvimukham, Shankha, Matsya
ADHD	Chinmaya	Bhu, Murti, Prithivi, Abhisheka
Allergies	Bhramara	Anjali, Purna Svara, Hakini, Dharma Chakra
Anemia	Merudanda	Vajra, Kubera, Surya, Pushan
Anger Management	Padma	Kapota, Purna Hridaya, Jalashaya, Svadhisthana
Anxiety	Pala	Bhu, Chinmaya, Dvimukham, Pranidhana
Asthma	Mira	Vittam, Medha Prana Kriya, Dirgha Svara
Back Pain	Anudandi	Dirgha Svara (upper), Vajra (middle), Yoni (low)
Cancer	Kapota	Dvimukham, Avahana, Hakini, Svadhisthana
Chronic Stress	Pranidhana	Bhu, Dvimukham, Chinmaya, Jalashaya
Cold Hands & Feet	Vyana Vayu	Anushasana, Dharma Chakra
Colds & Flu	Prana	Bhramara, Madhyama Sharira, Dirgha Svara
Constipation	Apana	Apanayana, Pranidhana, Jala, Prajna Prana Kriya
Cystitis & Urinary System	Varuna	Jala, Dvimukham, Matsya, Mira
Dementia & Alzheimer's	Dhyana	Trishula, Jnana, Ushas, Ishvara, Dvimukham
Depression	Vajrapradama	Padma, Purna Hridaya, Dirgha Svara, Kaleshvara
Diabetes (Type 2)	Madhyama	Pushan, Dharma Chakra, Hakini, Vajra
Digestive Conditions	Pushan	Achala Agni, Vajra, Kubera, Svadhisthana
Eating Disorders	Hakini	Karuna, Svadhisthana, Pushan, Chinmaya
Fibromyalgia	Matsya	Jalashaya, Jala, Svadhisthana, Vyana Vayu
Chronic Fatigue	Vajra	Hakini, Mandala, Dharma Pravartana
Headaches & Migraine	Mahashirsha	Pranidhana, Dvimukham, Apana, Chinmaya
Hearing Conditions	Shunya	Mandala, Kaleshvara, Garuda, Akasha
Heart Conditions	Apana Vayu	Vayan, Padma, Purna Hridaya, Hansi
Hypertension	Vayan	Chinmaya, Dvimukam, Apana, Jalashaya
Irritable Bowel Syndrome	Apanayana	Apana, Pranidhana, Jalashaya, Hakini
Immune Conditions	Purna Hridaya	Bhramara, Dharma Chakra, Hakini, Kaleshvara
Insomnia	Dvimukham	Apana, Pranidhana, Chinmaya, Svadhisthana
Menopause	Trimurti	Yoni, Mira, Dharma Chakra, Mandala
MS & Nervous System Conditions	Vyana Vayu	Anushasana, Hakini, Mandala, Dharma Chakra
Osteoarthritis & Joint Conditions	Matsya	Jala, Vyana Vayu, Mira, Svadhisthana
Osteoporosis & Skeletal Conditions	Rupa	Jalashaya, Bhu, Adhi, Palli, Anudandi
Phobias	Pala	Adhi, Shankha, Svadhisthana, Abhaya Varada
PMS & Female Reproductive Conditions	Yoni	Mira, Matsya, Trimurti, Jalashaya
PTSD	Svadhisthana	Dvimukham, Pala, Ushas, Ishvara, Abhaya Varada
Respiratory Problems	Dirgha Svara	Mira, Shakti, Medha Prana Kriya, Vayu
Prostate & Male Reproductive Conditions	Shankha	Prajna Prana Kriya, Adho Merudanda, Apana
Scoliosis	Merudanda	Anudandi, Bhu, Prithivi, Palli, Linga
Self-Esteem	Vajra	Kubera, Matangi, Brahma, Surya, Merudanda
Sinusitis	Bhramara	Matsya, Vittam, Svadhisthana
Stroke	Ida/Pingala	Dharma Chakra, Hakini, Mandala
Thyroid & Endocrine Conditions	Garuda	Kaleshvara, Vishuddha, Angushtha
TMJ Dysfunction	Chinmaya	Dvimukham, Mahashirsha, Matsya
Weight Management	Brahma	Matangi, Mushtikam, Ganesha, Surya

APPENDIX H – Sanskrit Pronunciation Guide

The names of the mudras are in Sanskrit, an ancient Indian language, especially used for spiritual texts. The Sanskrit alphabet has 50 letters as compared to 26 in English; therefore, a series of diacritical marks, comprised of dots above and below letters as well as lines above letters, are used with our alphabet to show the additional letters. Below is a guide to pronouncing the letters of the Sanskrit alphabet.

VOWELS:

A long vowel (e.g. ā) is held twice as long as its corresponding short vowel (e.g. a).

a – short a as in drama; example: yoga
ā – long form of a, like the a in water; example: āsana; mudrā
i – as in sift; example: maṇipūra
ī – long form of i, like the ee in seen; example: īśvara
u – as in bull; example: guru
ū – long form of u, like the oo in boo; example: pūrṇa
ṛ – rolled r followed by a very short i, like fiber; example: Kṛṣṇa
ṝ – rolled r followed by a long i, like starring; example: pitṝṇām
ḷ – short l followed by a rolled r, like cavalry; example: kḷp
ḹ – long l followed by a rolled r, like cavalry (held longer);
no example is found in Sanskrit
e – as in say; example: Vedānta
ai – as in high; example: chaitanya
o – as in open; example: Gopāla
au – as in bow; example: śauca
ṅ or ṃ – a nasal n or m; example: śāṅkha, oṃ
ḥ – a final unvoiced aspirated h sound; example: namaḥ

CONSONANTS:

k – regular k as in kite; example: karma
kh – like the kh in bunkhouse; example: duḥkha
g – regular g as in good; example: Gāṇeśa
gh – like the gh in ghee; example: ghat
ṅ – as in sing; example: piṅgalā
c – regular ch as in church Example: cakra
ch – like the chh in coach house Example: chāyā
j – regular j as in jam; example: jīva
jh – like the geh in hedgehog Example: jhalā
ñ – as in banyan; example: Patañjali
ṭ – like the letter t in taste; example: muṣṭi
ṭh – like the th in anthill; example: svādhiṣṭhāna
ḍ – like the d in god; example: daṇḍa
ḍh – like the dh in adhesive; example dṛḍha
ṇ – like the letter n in not; example: prāṇa
t – like the letter t in tongue; example: tantra
th – like the th in lighthouse; example: atha
d –like the d in dorm; example: doṣā
dh – like the dh in buddha; example: buddha
n – like the n in now; example: nāḍī
p – regular p as in pop; example: Pārvatī
ph – like the ph in uphill; example: phala
b – regular b as in boy; example: bāla
bh – like the bh in clubhouse; example: bhakti
m – regular m as in man Example: mālā

SEMI-VOWELS:

y – as in yes; example: yoga
r – as in run; example: rajas
l – as in long; example: Lakṣmī
v – as in victory; example: vāyu

SIBILANTS:

ś – similar to the sh sound in sugar; example: Śiva
ṣ – as in sharp; example: upaniṣad
s – as in safe; example: sādhana

ASPIRATE:

h – aspirated h as in hello; example: hari

COMPOUNDS:

kṣ – like the ksh in backshift; example: mokṣa
jñ – like the gy in Guyana; example: jñāna

APPENDIX I - Alphabetical Listing of Mudras & Sanskrit Pronunciation

MUDRA	TRANSLITERATION	PAGE
Abhaya Varada (47)	abhaya varada	120
Abhisheka (87)	abhiṣeka	212
Achala Agni (46)	acala agni	118
Adhara (106)	adhāra	256
Adhi (11)	adhi	40
Adho Merudanda (12)	adho merudaṇḍa	42
Akasha (44)	akāśa	112
Anamika (2)	anāmikā	118
Ananta (61)	ananta	152
Angushtha (5)	aṅguṣṭha	24
Anjali (108)	añjali	260
Anudandi (21)	anudaṇḍi	64
Anushasana (54)	anuśāsana	136
Apana (50)	apāna	128
Apana Vayu (32)	apāṇa vāyu	86
Apanayana (23)	apanayana	68
Avahana (93)	āvāhana	226
Bhairava (104)	bhairava	250
Bhramara (38)	bhrāmara	98
Bhu (40)	bhū	104
Brahma (29)	brahma	80
Chaturmukham (80)	caturmukham	198
Chin (83)	cin	204
Chinmaya (55)	cinmaya	55
Citta (18)	citta	56
Dharma Chakra (62)	dharmacakra	154
Dharma Pravartana (45)	dharmapravartana	114
Dharmadhatu (88)	dharmadhātu	214
Dhyana (103)	dhyāna	248
Dirgha Svara (85)	dīrghasvara	208
Dvimukham (70)	dvimukham	176
Ganesha (69)	gaṇeśa	172
Garuda (34)	garuḍa	90
Gupta (68)	gupta	170
Hakini (6)	hākinī	26
Hansi (19)	haṅsī	58
Hastaphula (76)	hastaphulla	190
Hridaya (105)	hṛdaya	254
Ida (63)	iḍā	158
Jala (41)	jala	106

BIBLIOGRAPHY

1. Barks, Coleman. The Essential Rumi. New York: Harper Collins, 1995.
2. Berry, Thomas & Swimme, Brian. The Universe Story. New York: Harper Collins, 1992.
3. Borysenko, Joan. Minding the Body, Mending the Mind. Canada: Bantam, 1988.
4. Bunce, Frederick W. Mudras in Buddhist and Hindu Practices: An Iconographical Consideration. New Delhi, India: DK Printworld, 2009
5. Daty, K.K. Yoga and Your Heart. Mumbai: Jaico Publishing House, 2003.
6. Dev, Keshav Acharya. Mudras for Healing. New Delhi: Aacharya Shri Enterprises
7. Dienstfrey, Harris. Where the Mind Meets the Body. New York: Harper Perennial, 1991.
8. Dychtwald, Ken. Bodymind. New York: Tarcher Penguin, 1950.
9. Eliade, Mircea. Yoga Imortalidade e Liberdade. Sao Paulo: Editora Palas Athenas, 1996.
10. Eraly, Abraham. Gem in the Lotus. New Delhi: Penguin Books, 2000.
11. Feuerstein, Georg. The Yoga Tradition. Arizona: Hohm Press, 1998.
12. Feuerstein, Georg. Wholeness or Transcendence?, New York: Larson Publications, 1992.
13. Feuerstein, Georg. Yoga The Technology of Ecstasy. Los Angeles: Jeremy P. Tarcher, Inc., 1989.
14. Fried, Robert. The Breath Connection. New York: Insight Books, 1935.
15. Hermogenes, Jose. Saude Plena com Yogaterapia. Rio de Janeiro: Nova Era, 2005.
16. Hirschi, Gertrud. Yoga in Your Hands. Maine: Samuel Weiser In.,2000.
17. Johari, Harish. Chakras the Energy Centers of Transformation. Vermont: Destiny Books, 2000.
18. Judith, Anodea. Eastern Body Western Mind. Berkeley, CA: Celestial Arts Publishing, 1996.
19. Kabat-Zinn, Jon. Full Catastrophe Living. New York: Dell Publishing, 1990.
20. Kupfer, Pedro. Mudra Gestos de Poder. Florianopolis, 1999.
21. Lefevre, Clemence. Manuel Pratique des Mudras. France: Editions Exclusif, 2006
22. Levine, Stephen. Healing into Life and Death. New York: Doubleday, 1987.
23. Morrison, Judith H. The Book of Ayurveda. New York: Fireside, 1995.
24. Ornish, Dean. Love and Survival. New York: Harpers Collins Publishers, 1997
25. Radha, Sivananda Swami. Hatha Yoga the Hidden Language. Boston: Shambala Publications, 1987.
26. Ramm-Bonwitt, Ingrid. Mudras, as Maos como Simbolo do Cosmos. Sao Paulo: Editora Pensamento Ltda., 1987.
27. Sapolsky, Robert M. Why Zebras Don't Get Ulcers. New York: W. H. Freeman and Company, 1998.
28. Saraswati, Karmananda Swami. Yogic Management of Common Diseases. India: Bhargava Bhushan Press, 1983.
29. Saraswati, Niranjanananda Swami. Prana Pranayama Prana Vidya. India: Bihar School of Yoga, 1994.
30. Saraswati, Satyananda Swami. Asana Pranayama Mudra Bandha. Bihar, India: Bihar Yoga Bharati, 1996
31. Saraswati, Swami Satananda. A Systematic Course in the Ancient Tantric Techniques of Yoga and Kriya. Bihar, India: Bihar School of India, 1981.
32. Sargeant, Winthrop. The Bhagavad Gita. New York: State University of New York Press, 2009
33. Saunders, E. Dale. Mudra a Study of Symbolic Gestures in Japanese Buddist Sculpture. New Jersey: Princeton University Press, 1960.
34. Singleton, Mark. Yoga Body. New York: Oxford University Press,2010.
35. Tirtha, Sada Shiva Swami. The Ayurveda Encyclopedia. New York: Ayurveda Holistic Center Press, 1998.
36. Tulku, Tarthang. Conhecimento da Liberdade. Sao Paulo: Dharma Publishing, 1984.
37. Upadhaya, PT. Rajnikant. Mudra Vigyan. New Delhi: Diamond Books
38. Upadhyay, R.P. Mudras, Postures and Mantras for Health, Fitness and Happiness. Delhi: Health and Harmony, 1999.
39. G.P. Bhatt & Pancham Sinh. The Forceful Yoga. Delhi: Motilal Banarsidass Publishers, 2004.
40. Venkatesananda, Swami. Enlightened Living. Canada: Anahata Press, 1999
41. Worthington, Vivian. A History of Yoga. London: Arkana, 1989.
42. Zambito, Salvatore. The Unadorned Thread of Yoga. Washington: The Yoga Sutras Institute Press, 1992.

REFERENCES Notes

1 - G.P. Bhatt & Pancham Sinh. The Forceful Yoga. Delhi: Motilal Banarsidass Publishers, 2004

2- Online Etymology Dictionary: www.etymonline.com

3. Grana, W. (2011). Osteoporosis. *Orthopedic Knowledge Online, from the American Academy of Orthopedic Surgeons.* Retrieved November 30, 2011, from http://www5.aaos.org/

4. Low back pain fact sheet. (Reviewed June 15, 2011). In *National Institute of Neurological Disorders and Stroke*. Retrieved January 2, 2012 from http://www.ninds.nih.gov/disorders/backpain/detail_backpain.htm

5.Osteoarthritis. (Reviewed November 26, 2011). *In A.D.A.M. Medical Encyclopedia.* Retrieved December 29, 2011, from http://www.ncbi.nlm.nih.gov/pubmedhealth/PMH0001460/

6. U.S. Department of Health and Human Services, National Digestive Diseases Information Clearinghouse (NDDIC). (September 2007). *Irritable Bowel Syndrome.* NIH Publication No. 07-693. Retrieved December 8, 2011, from http://digestive.niddk.nih.gov/ddiseases/pubs/ibs/

7. Our main resource for the effects of stress on health is *Why Zebras Don't Get Ulcers. Sapolsky, Robert M.* New York: W. H. Freeman and Company, 1998.

8. U.S. Department of Health and Human Services, Women's Health. (April 14, 2010). *Interstitial cystitis/bladder pain syndrome fact sheet.* Retrieved December 13, 2011, from http://www.womenshealth.gov/publications/our-publications/fact-sheet/interstitial-cystitis.cfm

9. Potter, J., Bouyer, J., Trussell, J., & Moreau, C. (2009). Premenstrual syndrome prevalence and fluctuation over time: results from a French population-based survey. *Journal of Women's Health, 18*(1), 31-39. doi: 10.1089/jwh.2008.0932

10. http://www.eocinstitute.org/Meditation_boosts_Serotonin_levels_s/435.htm

11. Enlarged Prostate. (Reviewed December 14, 2011). In *A.D.A.M. Medical Encyclopedia*. Retrieved December 31, 2011, from http://www.nlm.nih.gov/medlineplus/ency/article/000381.htm

12. Lummus, W., & Thompson, I. (2001). Prostatitis.(3), 691-707. doi: 10.1016/S0733-8627(05)70210-8

13. Mayo Clinic. (July 23, 2011). *Menopause.* Retrieved December 15, 2011, from http://www.mayoclinic.com/health/menopause/DS00119

14. Lad, V. (2002). *Textbook of Ayurveda: Fundamental Principles of Ayurveda, Volume 1.* Albuquerque, New Mexico: The Ayurvedic Press.

15. U.S. Department of Health and Human Services, National Institute of Diabetes and Digestive and Kidney Diseases (NIDDK). (April 2008). *Your digestive system and how it works. NIH Publication No. 08-2681.* Retrieved January 9, 2011, from http://digestive.niddk.nih.gov/ddiseases/pubs/yrdd/

16. Obesity. (Reviewed July 11, 2011). In *A.D.A.M. Medical Encyclopedia.* Retrieved December 30, 2011, from http://www.ncbi.nlm.nih.gov/pubmedhealth/PMH0004552/

17. Mayo Clinic. (May 27, 2010). *Asthma.* Retrieved December 7, 2011, from http://www.mayoclinic.com/health/asthma/DS00021

18. National Headache Foundation. (2011). *Resources from the National Headache Foundation.* Retrieved December 2, 2011, from https://www.headaches.org

19. Nussey, S., & Whitehead, S. (2001). *Endocrinology: An integrated approach.* Oxford: BIOS Scientific Publishers.

20. U.S. Department of Health and Human Services, National Institute of Mental Health (NIMH). (2011). *Depression.* NIH Publication No. 11-3561. Retrieved December 9, 2011, from http://www.nimh.nih.gov/health/publications/depression/complete-index.shtml

21. U.S. Department of Health and Human Services, National Institute of Mental Health (NIMH). (2011). *Anxiety Disorders.* NIH Publication No. 09-3879. Retrieved December 11, 2011, from http://www.nimh.nih.gov/health/publications/anxiety-disorders/nimhanxiety.pdf

22. Multiple Sclerosis. (Reviewed December 3, 2011). In *A.D.A.M. Medical Encyclopedia.* Retrieved December 26, 2011, from http://www.ncbi.nlm.nih.gov/pubmedhealth/PMH0001747/

23. U.S. Department of Health and Human Services, National Institute of Allergy and Infectious Diseases. (December 6, 2011). *Immune System.* Retrieved December 13, 2011, from http://www.niaid.nih.gov/topics/immuneSystem/Pages/default.aspx